Case Studies In Health Policy and Management

CALUM PATON
AND
STEPHEN BACH
Centre for Health Planning and Management
University of Keele

Nuffield Provincial Hospitals Trust

Published by the
Nuffield Provincial Hospitals Trust
3 Prince Albert Road, London NW1 7SP

ISBN 0 900574 75 5

Designed by Bernard Crossland
PRINTED IN GREAT BRITAIN BY
BURGESS & SON (ABINGDON) LTD
THAMES VIEW, ABINGDON
OXFORDSHIRE

THE AUTHORS

Dr Calum Paton

is Senior Lecturer, Centre for Health Planning and Management, University of Keele. He is Director of the Case Study research and writing programme, funded by the Nuffield Provincial Hospitals Trust, of which this book is the product. He has published on British and US health policy, political theory and political economy; is co-Director of the MBA (Health Executive) programme and has worked as consultant to the Overseas Development Administration in Asia, Africa and the Caribbean. He is also co-Editor of the *International Journal of Health Planning and Management*. Previously he was Assistant Secretary, Nuffield Provincial Hospitals Trust.

Mr Stephen Bach

is Research Fellow, Centre for Health Planning and Management, University of Keele. He joined the Centre to work full-time on the Case Study programme and now teaches and researches in health policy and industrial relations and management of human resources. He has published in particular on competitive tendering in the NHS and contracting after the implementation of the NHS White Paper, *Working for Patients*. Previously he worked in North East Thames Regional Health Authority where he entered the NHS as a National Management Trainee.

CONTENTS

PART II. POLICY PRIORITIES

LIST OF TABLES

Introduction

THE RATIONALE

This book contains six case studies which address a wide range of topics in health policy and management. They have been selected with a view to broad coverage of salient policy issues which pose important challenges for health service managers. The aim is that they be used by managers, practitioners, and students of health policy and management for a number of purposes: to understand policy-making, the implementation of policy and the links between these two processes; to predict likely consequences of actions and the effect of institutional structures and cultures upon them; to reinterpret events in order to understand 'how' and 'why' things happened; to trace the influences upon and even causes of successes and failures (taking care to set out criteria for these value judgements); to examine particular chronologies of events and configurations of power to aid overall analysis; to understand how power is distributed within organisations and within society; and to use insights gained to become better managers, advisers or analysts.

In short: the book is intended to improve both the understanding and practice of management. It will be used, we hope, in the NHS, in the policy community as a whole and particularly in academic settings where health service managers and policy-makers undertake courses and degrees.

THE APPROACH

The Director of the Case Study Writing Programme studied at the John F Kennedy School of Government, Harvard University, and encountered the lengthy narrative case study in a US environment. The book is a contribution to the task of filling a dearth of such material in Britain, where the 'case study' often means merely a few pages-long simulated exercise or alternatively a conventional narrative. A case study ought to be structured to highlight key events, individuals, and centres of power, initiative and resistance to policies and their implementation.

The case study, however, ought not to sacrifice theory on the altar of chronology and empiricism. Events are influenced by individuals, but often constrained, or directed by, circumstances, social factors or environmental features (in the broadest sense of that term). It is hoped that the issues chosen are analysed with an awareness of this. To this end the often huge quantities of detail and (deliberate) eschewal of theory in a US context is not replicated here.

This book is a joint product by the two authors, who have enjoyed enough similarity of perspective and approach to make the tasks of both researching and writing rewarding and cooperative. Dr Paton, as Director of the programme, has been responsible for its overall ambitions, shape and direction and Mr Bach, the full-time Research Fellow, has carried out much of the empirical work. Both are responsible for the theoretical perspectives adopted, and for the writing.

THE ISSUES

The issues are: the transition to community care for people with a mental handicap; the outcome of a district plan for future services in a provincial NHS district; the outcome of a radical strategy to reorient and rationalise services in a large London district (which serves as an interesting comparison with the former study); the approaches of regions to resource allocation as, post-White Paper, competition replaces 'bureaucratic' determination of priorities as the new NHS watchword; an attempt by an NHS unit to tackle waiting lists; and the continuing saga of competitive tendering.

The geographical range is wide, as is the list of topics and the range of NHS settings explored.

USING THE STUDIES

The studies cover a range of issues in a range of geographical and social settings. The aim is that health managers and students analyse decision-making processes at a detailed level in a 'classroom' situation, while readers of the book generally will find rigorous analysis of policy as well as explanation of the implementation process.

Case studies face a 'problem of empiricism': one cannot generalise from specific circumstances. One can however seek, without dogmatic interpretation, to understand how contexts constrain and enable; how managers can mobilise support or opposition; how short-term decisions affect the long-term and how preferences can be 'traded off' by bargaining actors; how bureaucratic decision-making can rely on established procedures; and how 'rational actors' can seek to implement their chosen mix of policies (Allison, 1971). Personalities and styles of behaviour are important but not determinant in themselves (Steinbruner, 1974). Structures and social factors may be central in some cases, less so in others.

THEORETICAL PERSPECTIVES

This leads naturally to methodology. No one theoretical perspective is assumed. For example, some social analysts are pluralists (Paton, 1990), some point to 'elitism' in policy-making and others take perspectives grounded in political economy which interpret social policies as derivative of economic policy.

Our aim has been deliberately to avoid abstract choice from among such different perspectives, but to suggest that the reader is aware of these options in analysing policy. Who holds central power in the NHS? How pluralistic, diffuse, or centrifugal is policy-making? How pluralistic, fragmented, or coherent is policy implementation within Districts? What concepts and methodologies can one supply to illuminate such debates?

UNDERSTANDING THE PAST AND PREDICTING THE FUTURE

It is a major role of the case study to stimulate discussion of *how* the past shapes the future, albeit liberally and loosely. Thus a case study may often be segmented so that the teacher can 'take stock', in a classroom, as to what *so far* has happened; who has been influential and why; which decision-making machinery has been significant and why; and so on. Then, a simple exercise in prediction can be followed by an unfolding of what actually happened. It is anticipated that some of the studies can be used in this way. This book meanwhile represents the 'literary' and academic output, while of course organised fully on the case study principle, and thereby usable for workshop-style classroom study in itself, by health service managers, postgraduate students of health policy and management, and a variety of other students.

INTERPRETING OR INTERVENING

It is important to identify managerial scope for influencing as well as understanding—cerebral work is a prelude, for the manager, to informed actions. Another central purpose of the case study is to allow groups to analyse when and why managerial actions were effective or ineffective, and thereby—again with restraint and awareness of pitfalls—to build up expertise for the future. Again the present studies are constructed with a view to enabling this form of study.

POLICY AND IMPLEMENTATION

The book takes as its backdrop the ideologies, political structures and political forces which define the policy debate and influence policy.

Then it explores the forces affecting the implementation of policy—structures, individuals, social forces and economic constraints to name but a few. It ranges from the centre, to regions, to districts and down to units and departments within the NHS with—broadly—the district as core focus. It considers successes and failures; incentives open to managers; constraints facing managers; and how policies evolve, affecting chances of local influence. In short, it highlights key determinants of outcome rigorously without being artificial or naive—in other words, it adopts the case study approach.

THE CHANGING HEALTH SERVICE

It has become a commonplace to observe that the NHS is experiencing a period of rapid change. The Conservative administration of the 1980s embarked on a major restructuring of the public sector, and the NHS was gradually incorporated into this process. (Three White Papers in as many years in the late 1980s testify to this.) However, the Government has not always been prescriptive about the manner in which policy should be implemented. Instead the onus has been placed on management to fashion policy in the most appropriate way to meet central objectives.

A much greater role has therefore been assigned to management in bringing about change in the organisation. The magnitude of change has also increased the emphasis on managers' ability to understand change and to develop the skills needed to bring about change. However, although there is a considerable literature on the management of change, this tends to be orientated to the private sector. One current orthodoxy is to emphasise the universality of the management function across the private and public sector. The appropriateness of the private sector models for the NHS however has recently been questioned, albeit after some years of searching for parallels. In particular the central role of government in a tax-funded service, the plethora of interest groups in and around the NHS and the absence of a narrow commercial dynamic to NHS activities have been the features most frequently cited in arguing that differences in approach must be set firmly against any similarities in comparing private with public.

The striking feature of this type of debate is the thin empirical evidence on which claims and counter claims are based. For example, the debate on the impact of the Griffiths Inquiry Report's implementation is marked by the cautiousness of the conclusions drawn (see for example, Harrison *et al*, 1989). This reflects the difficulty in gauging the impact of management on the degree of change in the NHS.

Consequently, there is a need to document the process of policy-making in the NHS in an evolving context and to assess the factors that contributed to that change. The case studies in this volume are a part of that process.

THE EMERGENCE OF GENERAL MANAGEMENT

During the 1980s there has been a surge of interest in the nature of management. The leaders of industry have seen their books become best sellers. This interest has encompassed the public sector, where improved management has become a central plank of government policy to improve organisational effectiveness.

This trend has diverse origins. Concern with the performance of the British economy is not a new phenomenon but the solutions espoused in the 1980s have moved away from earlier 1970s 'corporatist' type solutions and have focused analysis on the internal dynamics of organisations at local level. Management as well as trade unions attracted blame (from a variety of political perspectives) for economic performance. This pattern was not confined to the UK as influential management thinkers in the USA notably Tom Peters (Peters and Waterman 1982; Peters 1987) were calling for nothing less than a management revolution to revitalise the competitive position of US industry.

The election of the Conservative Government in 1979 provided a political focus for this nascent management thinking. Criticism of management in the 1960s had often been from a 'pro trade union' stance. Now, the Government was critical of the public sector (including public sector management), viewing it as immune from the discipline of the market place and competition, which created large insensitive bureaucracies. A corollary of this analysis was that management in the public sector was lacklustre due to the absence of incentives for better performance. 'Management' behaviour was essentially administrative, passively concerned with channelling inputs to professional groups rather than having a leading role in making decisions about priorities and resource allocation and subsequently monitoring performance against established objectives. For a government committed to the reduction of public expenditure there was a need to improve the effectiveness of resource use in the face of continued demands upon government expenditure.

This approach was significant for the NHS where the management role had traditionally been ill-defined and geared to serving the needs of professional staff. After the 1974 reorganisation this had admittedly begun to alter as a more professional tier of management began to emerge. Later, the appropriateness of consensus management was increasingly challenged, in a harsher financial climate.

servative Government therefore was committed to improv-
ciency of the NHS, and looked towards the private sector for
models. A series of measures was introduced in the early
group of initiatives was intended to increase the account-
he NHS to the centre (the Department of Health) in order to allow the implementation of government policy to be monitored at local level. Regional reviews were introduced and carried out annually to enable Ministers to alert regions to current ministerial aims and review progress in the previous year. Similarly, the development of performance indicators—which measured clinical manpower and financial activity in health authorities—implied a desire for tighter monitoring of performance and for the first time raised the possibility of comparing health authorities' performance.

A second series of initiatives injected both market and management disciplines into the NHS. This took a variety of forms. Prominent individuals from private industry were invited to review the NHS in order to carry out scrutinies of activity using (hitherto) private sector bench marks as measures of effectiveness. Lord Rayner of Marks and Spencers undertook a diverse range of 'value for money' studies, varying from the examination of the collection of traffic accident fees to the organisation of catering services. Concerning management techniques, practices adopted in the NHS since 1982 have included the subjection of capital investment to option appraisal process which incorporates a form of cost benefit analysis.

A policy of mandatory competitive tendering was introduced in 1983 for ancillary services. Health authorities were asked to test the cost effectiveness of their domestic, catering and laundry services. Acceptance of the lowest tender was required unless 'compelling reasons' dictated otherwise. This led to some services being contracted out and major changes in working practices even where services were retained in-house.

Finally the Government recognised that the success of its strategy required a cadre of managers to implement their agenda of changes. This reflected an increased understanding in government that the achievement of policy goals had often been foiled by the diffuse decision-making process in the NHS. Consequently, following the recommendations of the 1983 NHS Management Inquiry (The Griffiths Report) which identified the need for a chief executive role in the NHS, general managers were appointed at health authority and unit level.

General management aimed to increase the authority of management in the NHS and sharpen decision-making by vesting responsibility for decisions in one individual. In addition to short-term contracts, since 1987, general managers' pay has included a performance related element based on the achievement of objectives. General managers have therefore been given powerful incentives to achieve change.

The emphasis on improved managerial effectiveness has been reiterated in the NHS White Paper *Working For Patients* (Department of Health, 1989a). This has assigned a central role to management in fashioning the NHS reform package at local level. Management influence has been enhanced by an increased role in deciding on the nature of services to be purchased and provided through contracting systems. The White Paper's reforms are therefore set to usher in an accelerating pace of change as the provider market is established, following the timetable set out in the Health Services Bill presented to Parliament in November 1989.

In sharp relief to this picture of rapid organisational change and acceptance of the need for strategic management to bring about change, the applied literature, on the manner in which both policy-making and implementation occurs in the NHS, remains limited.

EDUCATION AND TRAINING

Education and training in the NHS prior to Griffiths was orientated to professional needs with the acquisition of professional skills as the central concern. This led to criticism from managers that professionals had little understanding of the management process. Efforts to remedy this situation included demands that clinical training should include the rudiments of management. Management training itself was under-developed in the NHS although the foundation of the National Health Service Training Authority separately from but around the time of the Griffiths Report was intended to address this.

There has been a greater recognition of management training needs post-Griffiths. The balance between professional needs and management needs, however, remains contested.

Attempts to develop management in the NHS have therefore been limited and professional training has continued to be dominant. However, there are signs that this situation is altering. A series of reports (Constable, 1987) have highlighted the paucity of management training in the UK and the Handy Report recommended an increase in the number of managers undertaking MBA programmes. There has generally been recognition of the need for higher level 'strategic' management education for current and future 'top management' programmes. To achieve these ends, programmes have drawn heavily on case study material. This teaching method has been adopted by the leading British business schools, but health care management centres, while flirting with the case study method, have been deterred by the limited amount of case study material available. Furthermore, detailed narrative case studies on the 'Harvard model' have often been wholly absent in a British context.

LEARNING THROUGH CASE STUDIES

The changing definition of case studies reflects their evolution from simple statements of problems through to complex educational tools grounded in intensive field research. Case studies of the latter sort are intrinsically connected with Harvard University in the USA where they were developed. Early cases, under the aegis of the Harvard Business School, were confined to private sector experience and portrayed (for example) a company's situation at a particular historical point in time. As they have developed studies have become richer, drawing on a greater range of internal and external documentation and present an evolving situation over time. This allows the nature of decision-making in the organisation to unfold before the reader. The Director of the research reported in this book experienced public sector case studies at Harvard's Graduate School of Government.

A case is a structured record of events faced by management in an organisation, requiring analysis to promote planning and decisions as to the appropriate course of action. The information on which decisions were made, be it quantitative or qualitative in nature, and details of the *process* of decision-making, are provided. Case studies are intentionally selective, in that the removal of extraneous detail leads to a clearer picture of the key actors, key events, and key institutions involved in the decision-making process.

Case studies, by drawing on current policy-making and management, can inform managers about the nature of decision-making and allow them to reflect on existing practice. Case studies therefore are a departure from wholly traditional knowledge-based systems of education. Instead the emphasis is on training managers to enhance their decision-making skills. By peeling away the layers of the management process to expose the core decisions managers face, this enables management to think explicitly about the choices they face.

THE GROWING RELEVANCE OF CASE STUDIES TO THE NHS

It has become commonplace to observe that the NHS has, prior to the White Paper of 1989, rationed health care through implicit rather than explicit criteria. Waiting lists have been the visible outcome of this system. The instigation of a 'provider market' will, it is believed, make rationing more explicit as managers will need to draw up contracts for the services they require. This trend may be reinforced by government emphasis on the devolution of decision-making to managers who—albeit within a centrally defined framework of key objectives—will have increased autonomy to fulfil those objectives in the manner they see fit. This will result in managers more starkly facing the consequences of their actions and being held responsible for them.

Case studies, by illuminating the decision-making process, parallel the manager's situation. Cases make explicit the relevant considerations for policy-making, enabling managers to draw their own conclusions about the appropriate trade-offs among factors such as political considerations, economic necessity, the importance of safeguarding access, improving the quality of clinical care, staff needs, and the needs of patients.

POWER AND THE MANAGER

An additional feature of case studies is their ability to highlight where power lies in organisations. The management literature is predominantly silent on this issue, yet 'solutions' advocated in evangelical management texts will be vacuous unless they can be successfully implemented. Success clearly depends on galvanising support externally and within the organisation for change and having the power to proceed with desired solutions. Management literature however tends to assume that managers have this authority rather than acknowledging that their power may be contested, constrained by structures, or biased by social forces.

In the NHS the locus of power has been the source of intense debate particularly since the adoption of general management. Proponents have argued that general management has eroded the power of clinicians while sceptics point to the continuing dominant position of the medical profession.

The case studies in this volume illustrate such issues. For example, it might have been anticipated that the closure of a long-stay hospital would have created opposition primarily from the workforce, concerned about its future. In practice the views of the local community had a greater impact when concerns were raised about the policy for care in the community. How can this be explained? Was it due to particular managerial practices; the inevitable outcome of a government policy widely distrusted by the local community; or the consequence of divisions between the trade unions involved? What more *universal* lessons can be drawn from the *particular* outcomes described in this book? This is the challenge of the case-study method—to draw lessons without illegitimate or hasty generalisation.

CHOICE OF TOPICS

The selection and development of case studies was based on the following principles:

1. The need to select issues which would have a continuing importance; were relevant for management practice over time; and which were not simply issues currently in vogue.

2. Linked to the above, a commitment to examine within each study the unfolding nature of decision making over time in order to diminish the risk of focusing on atypical events and using these occurrences to draw faulty conclusions.

3. A commitment to selecting research sites where significant outcomes (be they positive or negative) had resulted. This enabled a small number of key variables to be identified in order to trace how these factors could explain the eventual policy outcome.

4. The need to select cases which illustrated the diversity of policy making in the NHS. Consequently, case studies were drawn from the unit level (Coventry/'Greenbelt'/Macclesfield) reflecting the importance of decision making at this level; the district level (Northville, Riverside) and the Regional level (Resource Allocation) with actors from other levels (e.g. national) also considered. Similarly, a national geographical spread was necessary in order to capture the impact of government policy in different parts of the country.

5. The desirability of using different types of case study:

(a) *Organisational and behavioural case studies*

This type of study traces the fate of a policy or initiative over time. This may be the implementation of a national policy (e.g. competitive tendering) at local level or a policy that has evolved locally in response to local needs but which is sensitive to national or regional policy guidelines, e.g. the Northville case study of planning new acute service provision.

These studies identify the main actors in the decision-making process, the main interests affected, the political, social and economic environment and the various outcomes over time through an examination of the decision-making process. This is the predominant model of case studies adopted.

(b) *Analytical case studies*

This type of study complements the behavioural case study. It explores particularly problematic areas of health services management—in this volume waiting lists and resource allocation—analysing the policy arena and examining particular management initiatives to overcome these difficulties. The focus is therefore more results orientated than the organisational and behavioural case studies and has a 'macro' rather than a predominantly 'micro' orientation.

RESEARCH APPROACH

The field work for these studies was undertaken between July 1988 and August 1989. The choice of studies reflected the guiding principles outlined above. Prior to field research a thorough review was carried out of existing research. These reviews formed the basis for the overviews of the current debates which precede each case study. This places each study in its policy context in order to help draw out the dilemmas faced by management in the studies.

The field work used a number of parallel research techniques. Interviews with key actors in the decision-making process was the bed-rock. Interviews did not follow a rigid format. Nonetheless particular questions were asked of all participants and a number of similar issues were addressed. Interviews not only included the traditional key actors as defined by organisational structures—district and unit general managers, regional and district officers, chairman of health authorities, community health council and trade union representatives—but also included important actors who fell outside these orthodox hierarchies. For example, in the Riverside case study the Health Authority's plans spawned a number of opposition groups which exerted an influence on the management process. Similarly, the impact of the media can be significant in altering managerial conduct. In the contracting arena, bad publicity about private contractors has deterred certain health authorities and private contractors themselves from tendering for contracts.

Interviews were complemented by documentary evidence. This included not only formal documentation such as minutes and reports of the district/regional health authority and other management fora, including regional reviews, but in addition less formal letters, memoranda and papers between officers. Documentation gave an indication of the importance of the issue to management and the process of decision-making. Diligence is needed to prevent a bias towards decisions and a neglect of non-decisions as well as the exclusion of issues that never reached the forum decision fora. This can be partially overcome by being sensitive to differences highlighted by individuals in interviews which do not accord with the formal documentation. These differences needed to be explored at interview until a satisfactory explanation emerged.

CONFIDENTIALITY

It will be noted that some of the studies use 'fictitious' health authority names. This is to protect those who preferred confidentiality. Others use actual names; again, this reflects the preferences of those involved.

SPECIAL THANKS

Many people have helped us, some of whom have had to remain anonymous. Without them and those named below, the studies would have been impossible.

Mr David Knowles: District General Manager, Riverside District Health Authority.

Mr Hugh Ross: Unit General Manager, City Unit, Coventry and Warwickshire Hospital, Coventry Health Authority.

Dr Fleur Fisher: Unit General Manager, Community and Mental Handicap Unit, Macclesfield Health Authority.

We would also like to thank Professor Kenneth Lee, Mr Geoffrey Hoare and Mr Michael Rigby of the Centre for Health Planning and Management, University of Keele, both for advising on and reading a number of these studies. Naturally the usual disclaimer applies. We also thank Rose Plimbley for preparing the manuscript.

PART I

PLANNING

CHAPTER 1

Planning: A theoretical approach

INTRODUCTION

The 1980s have witnessed the slide from favour of the concept of planning. The Conservative government's approach has been characterised by its commitment to the market as the best means to regulate economic activity. In the Health Service the encouragement of market forces has been through the introduction of competitive tendering for ancillary services and encouraging the private sector, thereby generating greater competition. The recent White Paper *Working for Patients* (Department of Health, 1989a) which advocates the establishment of a provider market in the NHS and greater use of market discipline (for example in the establishment of pay levels) is set to extend this trend. The development of a provider market will have a major impact on the ability of districts and regions to fulfil their planning responsibilities.

The paradox is that the need for effective planning remains paramount. In a period of increased expectations about what health services can provide, increased possibilities from advanced technology as well as an ageing population coupled with a period of resource restraint, there is a clear need to decide on priorities and plan accordingly. However, in such an era planning may be especially contentious not only because change is inherently distasteful to those adversely affected but because the losers may outweigh those who gain. Consequently, planners need to recognise the political nature of the planning process and accommodate potential opposition.

WHY PLAN?

Planning involves making choices about how the future will differ from the past thereby making subject to calculation that which was previously left to chance. By exploring future changes in the environment in which the organisation operates the aim is to adapt as necessary to ensure the organisation can continue to fufil its objectives. Planning also facilitates the integration of all parts of the organisation to ensure that work is focused on common goals.

The rationale for planning in the NHS embodies similar logic to the arguments for allocating resources in an economy by planning rather than market mechanisms. British economic policy, while predominantly market orientated, has adopted planning as a response to market failure either when externalities have existed or where consumer sovereignty has been absent. In health care it has traditionally been argued that consumers were unable to make informed choices about their needs for health care and this has under-pinned the existence of the NHS. Consequently, as the state has taken over the provision of health care, planning linked to the establishment of priorities has been used to allocate resources.

At the district health authority level the benefits of planning are four-fold. First, an organisation to achieve its objectives needs to make rational decisions about the future. In the absence of market signals and the clear objective of profit, other means have to be established to decide on priorities and translate this into action, and planning is a means of achieving this. Second, plans will only be achieved if resources are available to fund them and in a period of financial stringency some priorities will have to be discarded. Consequently, planning provides a link between setting objectives and funding schemes to fulfil those plans. Third, schemes which are agreed need to be phased as some elements of a plan will take longer to come to fruition than other aspects, if each part of a scheme is not planned the final outcome will not be adequately integrated. Finally planning is a means to try and reduce the uncertainty of the future by making predictions about the future and drawing up contingency plans for differing eventualities.

THEORIES OF PLANNING

Planning theory and practice has demonstrated the difficulty of translating these potential benefits into tangible results. For example, the orthodox view of planning neglects the impact that the planning process will have on those affected and the possibility that interest groups will act to modify the plans to achieve their objectives. Instead the comprehensive rational planning model views the planner as a technician who remains neutral and seeks out objective solutions to particular problems. The planning process is rational and comprehensive in that all the opportunities for intervention are listed and the consequences of each action are considered. The course of action selected is chosen to fulfil the objectives of the plan and to maximise output. This type of model, moving from goals to strategies and then seeking resources to match those strategies, is familiar. The underlying assumption is that the application of the scientific method to policy-making ensures a rational outcome.

This approach has increasingly been criticised. The most influential critique was launched by Lindblom (1959–79). He argued that the notion of rational decision making was flawed. It was usually not possible to establish clear objectives in organisations which faced competing claims on resources. Furthermore the rational planning model assumes that planners have all the necessary information to evaluate competing options. Yet if the information is not available or is too expensive to gather and analyse, then the basis of decision-making is vulnerable to distortion.

The boundaries of the rational planning model are also not specified. In the arena of health care it has frequently been argued that an individual's state of health is influenced by social class (Townsend, Davidson, 1982) and other related variables, for example housing, which are beyond the boundaries of health planning. Consequently, the scope of the rational planning model is not delineated. However, it can scarcely be viewed as comprehensive if the approach does not include factors central to health status yet which may be beyond the influence of health planners.

The rational planning approach is insufficiently flexible to accommodate the inherent uncertainty of the future. A pertinent example of this has been the emergence over a short period of time of AIDS which has required an adjustment to the strategic plans of health authorities. The rational planning approach is unable to accommodate uncertainty, in that it specifies long-term objectives and a pathway to those objectives which are not readily changed.

Lindblom's response to his rejection of the rational planning model was advocacy of a strategy of disjointed incrementalism. This was premised on his view that rational decision-making was not possible and consequently it was better to confine policy-making to tinkering with current policies. Lindblom was therefore arguing for adoption of an approach which marginally altered the status quo and by implication accepted that the choices open to planners were in practice severely limited. In this model the planner's role was less central than in the rational planning approach, where the planners orchestrated all the other actors. In Lindblom's approach the planner becomes a referee who seeks to involve all the parties and presides over an institutionalised bargaining system but does not direct the parties to a particular favoured outcome as in the rational planning model.

Although Lindblom's approach has merit in its recognition of power relations in the planning process and its attempt to establish limits to the planning process, it posits an essentially pessimistic view of the possibilities of change in organisations. Decisions made at the margin tend only to consider marginal areas of the organisation's activity. The weakness of the incremental approach can be illustrated by the manner in which budgets have traditionally been established in the NHS. The starting point for the coming year's budget is the previous year's budget and adjustments may be made at the margin. This leaves the bulk of activity unchanged and not scrutinised. A response to these difficulties has been attempts to develop zero based budgeting.

Attempts to find a middle way between the rational planning approach and the incrementalist approach have inevitably tried to blend the best elements from each model. Etzioni (1967) argued that it was possible to achieve this by providing two sets of mechanisms, one for making fundamental decisions and the other for incremental decisions. Etzioni refers to the approach as mixed scanning because of his emphasis on a rapid investigation of all the options from which are selected a small number of options for detailed analysis. The selection procedure revolves around which issues are viewed as of fundamental importance and justify detailed planning work and a prior step to selection is a review process of the current situation in the particular authority.

This approach by being consciously selective is more systematic and rational than the over ambitious rational planning approach which will fail to meet its objective of evaluating all options (Lee and Mills, 1982). Nonetheless, the mixed scanning approach leaves a number of questions unanswered. First, there is little guidance on how to select issues of fundamental importance for further consideration. If clear criteria are not established for this selection then an *ad hoc* selection of issues will result, threatening the rationality of the approach. Second, it suffers from the deficiency of the rational planning approach in not being able to incorporate political constraints or the uncertainty of the planning process.

The challenge of successful planning is to inject rational criteria into the decision-making process but still accommodate diverse interest groups. Planning will inevitably be contentious because plans will promote particular constituencies interest and erode others. Furthermore, there is likely to be resistance (even amongst gainers!) to having decisions removed from their sphere of influence and technical analysis introduced into a process which previously relied predominantly on personal judgements and political influence. This might be expected particularly from professional groups who have enjoyed a large degree of autonomy in the past and who would be reluctant to relinquish this power.

The production of technical information enables planners to assess the performance of professionals against objectives and reduces planners dependence on professionals for technical information. However, it is advantageous to obtain the cooperation of those affected. Although the participation of those affected may enable them to galvanise support against particular proposals at an early stage if potential opposition elements are not incorporated this may simply lead to the postponement of controversy. Furthermore participation will commit individuals to the plan and prevent them from disowning the plan as easily.

It is through recognition of the political nature of the planning process and the uncertainty of planning future services, while trying to harness support for clear objectives that some of the difficulties in planning, during a period of rising demand and limited resources, can be overcome. This type of approach is different from the planning systems that were instigated in the NHS during the 1970s which met with limited success.

THE EVOLUTION OF PLANNING IN THE NHS

Prior to 1976 there was no formal system of planning in the NHS. The Guillebaud Report on the cost of the NHS published in 1956 argued that no convincing case had been made out on the transfer of hospital services to local authority control but acknowledged the need for a more systematic method of planning services through strong regional organisation. Nonetheless, planning remained the province of the Department of Health which periodically announced national plans most notably the Hospital Plan of 1962. At the periphery planning was incorporated into routine administrative work and was of an incrementalist nature.

Ham's (1981) study of Leeds Regional Hospital Board illuminates the planning process in the early years of the NHS. Officers were cautious about the redistribution of beds due to fear of antagonising the medical staff. The Board was reluctant to accept bed norms which were a corollary to the 1962 Hospital Plan for similar reasons, even though norms represented the first attempt to formulate national standards of provision since 1948. The Hospital Plan ushered in the break with the previous *laisser-faire* attitude of the Department but was dominated by capital planning with emphasis firmly on bed norms.

The emphasis on capital planning was to be superseded by the shift to service planning which was embodied in the 1976 planning system. The origins of the system lay in development in the NHS which was making increasing demands on the country's resources and faced a proliferation of high technology medicine. This required a more rational use of resources if priorities were to be established. The year of 1976 also witnessed the first attempt to establish systematic priorities throughout the health and personal social services services by care group which linked to the service planning approach adopted in the new planning system.

Developments in central government also favoured the adoption of a national planing system which would link to the central government expenditure planning system (PESC) and the programme budget approach at the Department of Health. Finally the 1970s was a period of development for corporate planning and this influenced the direction of the NHS particularly through the advice of the management consultants McKinseys who helped to formulate the 1974 reorganisation (Hambleton, 1986).

The 1976 planning system attempted to introduce a comprehensive planning system into the NHS. The system compelled regional health authorities to compile strategic plans every decade, which were meant to focus on broad service developments over the decade and establish clear priorities. Operational plans were to be detailed programmes of action for the following two to three years. The rational planning system was subject to a barrage of criticism, as difficulties emerged.

The process was extremely laborious. Planning teams were established with large memberships which were unable to agree on priorities leading to the deferment of decisions. The time consuming nature of the planning process discouraged clinicians from becoming involved. Clinicians who did participate were reluctant to portray their colleagues' views for fear of abrogating their clinical freedom. There was ambiguity about the new care groups which were outlined in the priorities document which prevented logical service planning. Finally the use of a bidding system was also flawed as not all departments lodged bids, leading to incoherent plans which owed as much to departmental aspirations as to an assessment of need based on common criteria.

The operational difficulties faced by planning teams were accentuated by the hierarchical nature of the planning system where plans were meant to be guided by central directives on bed norms and standards of provision. The guidelines were of limited value as they failed to disaggregate sufficiently between specialisms and the whole approach of norms was being criticised. Norms failed to distinguish between different levels of social deprivation prevailing in different areas nor did they provide any information on quality of outputs, focusing as they did on inputs. Consequently, regional health authorities did not follow the guidelines and this made comparisons of plans difficult as they were not consistent.

The regional plans that were produced were weak on how they proposed to meet the objectives outlined. Regions lacked adequate information on which to make these decisions and this was further exhibited in the lack of manpower planning in the regional plans. There was also a failure to assess the capital costs of the proposed plans leading to many regions being over committed on their capital programme which subsequently served to undermine revenue plans.

PLANNING UNDER THE CONSERVATIVE GOVERNMENT

The shortcomings of the 1976 planning system were recognised and with the advent of a new Conservative Government in 1979 the emphasis shifted away from comprehensive planning to a stronger devolved management function with the district as the central focus for planning acticity. This tried to overcome the problem that planning had been viewed as a bureaucratic activity with no clear benefit for districts, leading to the production of plans which were seen as an end in themselves, rather than the pathway to future service provision. By establishing the district as the main focus for planning activity it was hoped to avoid planning becoming an annual event divorced from the other management functions of the district.

Consequently the 1982 reorganisation which abolished the area tier in the NHS focused on a strengthened management function at unit level also modified the planning machinery. The system was simplified and although strategic plans were retained the emphasis shifted to district level planning. Operational planning was divided between the operational programme which was the district's action plan for the forthcoming year and the forward programme for the following year which contained provisional proposals. The time-scales on updating strategic plans were also modified. To prevent the vague objectives embodied in the first round of regional plans the responsibility was placed on the Department of Health to issue national guidance to regions, prior to the preparation of strategic plans. The emphasis on comprehensiveness was reduced and instead specific areas of activity were to be targeted.

Although the changes modified the over ambitious expectations of what the planning system could deliver and introduced helpful simplifications, for example the use of annual programmes, a number of difficulties were not addressed. In essence the nature of the system had not altered. The system remained hierarchical with the centre instructing the periphery on the composition of the plan. Instead expectations about the outcomes from the planning system were lowered. This made it difficult to convince districts that planning was a useful exercise which would further their own management needs rather than a task which was imposed to strengthen the role of the centre. This perception that planning was irrelevant was strengthened by the lack of any attempt to link resource allocation to planning. Finally the use of a norm based approach was seen as increasingly inappropriate in a service which in the 1980s has tried to orientate itself towards examining the appositeness and quality of its outputs, not simply the quantity.

Planning is no longer favoured in the manner it was during the 1970s. However, a number of recent developments may paradoxically have strengthened the role of planning in the NHS. The implementation of the Griffiths report and the appointment of general managers at authority and unit level has sharpened managerial decision-making in the NHS and this has led to the compilation of planning documents which no longer merely state good intentions but are scheme-specific action plans with clear deadlines.

General managers on short-term contracts with a performance related element available on achievement of specific objectives have a clear incentive to ensure that planning timetables are realistic and achievable. Furthermore in an era of resource retraint the incrementalist drift of earlier methods in the NHS is not feasible and managers are forced to establish clear priorities. Planning is an essential tool in disentangling competing claims for resources.

The 1980s have seen a stream of initiatives which have contributed to an improvement in planning even though they were not introduced primarily for that purpose. A severe weakness that planners faced in the NHS was the lack of timely, accurate and relevant information available on which to plan future service provision. The Steering Group on Health Services Information (Körner Group) reviewed the future development of health services information systems and made a series of recommendations including the establishment of district minimum data sets intended to increase the information available for planning purposes. The Resource Management Initiative (RMI) and its predecessors have provided a further stimulus to the development of information systems which will prove useful for operational purposes. After the 1989 White Paper, resource management will be extended considerably.

The Government has also pressed for better management of the NHS estate by emphasising that the NHS should not regard the estate as a free good. By compelling health authorities to have estate operational plans in place by December 1989 the planning brief for authorities has been widened and further helped to strengthen the planning function. Demographic changes have led to fears that the NHS faces acute manpower shortages and this has acted as a catalyst to bolster the neglected area of manpower planning.

The resilience of planning under a government firmly committed to the market place, may seem surprising. However, although the government has emphasised its commitment to devolution of responsibility to management at local level to enhance effectiveness and reduce central interference there are limits to the independence that central government will tolerate. The danger for government is the spectre of local management using their autonomy to deviate from central government objectives. This paradox was expressed by Len Peach in the following manner:

> As Chief Executive of the NHS I like wild ducks, but I like them to fly in formation.

Formal planning procedures help the government to resolve this dilemma by retaining control over the direction of district management actions and this is reinforced by the annual review process. For planning can also be a useful device as a means to limit professional autonomy by reducing dependence on professional channels of information and by reference to national priorities in establishing objectives.

The prospects for a more robust future for planning contrasts with the incrementalist drift of earlier planning in the NHS. Detailed studies have lamented the lack of progress to emerge from the planning process. Ham (1981) concluded that planning was an intensely political process with the outcomes decided by the distribution of power. This was weighted heavily towards the clinicians who effectively vetoed the planners intentions through their immediate control over resources and their appeals to clinical knowledge (which proved difficult to challenge) and the influence they exerted through membership of regional and district health authorities. However, he suggests that this was being challenged in the 1970s by trade union action and the increasing authority of management. The White Paper *Working for Patients* is a further step in strengthening the management role.

Rathwell's (1985) examination of strategic planning in the NHS concurs with Ham's pessimistic conclusions. He argues that planning teams failed to live up to expectations due to planners not being given clear objectives and the emphasis on the imposition of the plan rather than the end product. He also found that power tended to be used in a negative way to block change. Consequently, it might seem that past experience does not augur well for the future.

THE FUTURE OF PLANNING

The 1989 White Paper made a case for 'managed' competition to replace bureaucratic versions of planning. However, the main challenge then facing the NHS was the reconciliation of competitive forces with planning. After all, regions—although 'slimmed down'—were still responsible for the strategic mix of resources within their boundaries. Indeed, given the need to ensure the practicality of 'competing' strategies for provision within and between districts, this strategic role may unintentionally have been strengthened.

Already, by the end of 1989, some regions are seeking to redraw district boundaries, geared to ensuring more global district 'purchasers' of care and more control of 'providing' hospitals and units within larger authorities. 'Directly managed' units, for which districts are responsible, mean that the district health authority is in a somewhat schizophrenic position—on the one hand, purchaser; on the other hand, provider. As a result, a regional planning role is needed to prevent *either* a 'market' oriented policy becoming its opposite as districts merely finance their own units *or* radical uncertainty as units expand and contract unpredictably.

Furthermore if districts are to be put on their resource allocation targets quickly, there will be losers and gainers on a significant scale. Inner-city districts, for example, may have to lose money to reach their target, as populations decline, *even* if the new formulae would help *some* areas of London relative to the old RAWP formulae. (There is no hard and fast rule—different measures combining social deprivation and mortality benefit different areas of the country and different districts.) Even beyond this, such districts may lose more money still from their target as 'cross-boundary' inflows are no longer rewarded through the formula.

As a result, some regions—by the end of 1989—were amending the pure assumptions of the 'internal market' model by continuing to *fund* cross-boundary flow payments through their district allocations, thereby in effect mandating certain inter-district flows (or at least forcing districts to 'pay twice' if they wanted to refer elsewhere, since they had already 'paid' given the region's allocation policy).

In practice, the regions were experimenting with a market/planning mix after the White Paper had set the scene for a new NHS. The Department of Health was at this stage open to such 'pragmatic' behaviour, as it also recognised that wholesale 'market' uncertainty could lead to hospitals and units unfunded, doctors and managers uncertain as to where to refer, and a chaotic service. The Department was in fact divided into those who saw competition as a radical force and those who saw it as rhetoric to be 'managed' along with other flavours of the month.

Indeed 'competition' may be viewed as a means of achieving unmet planning goals of past decades. For example, the movement of services out of London, and the rationalisation of London's provision, ran aground on the rocks of the medical profession's hostility in the 1960s and 1970s. Now, as health authorities contract for services on the basis of price and other factors, expensive London services may prove unattractive in some cases. While self-governing trusts in London may prosper with government help and private sector business, other services may decline. *Money* may partially 'return' to London as the RAWP formula's amendments work out, but *services* may move out. Ironically this is the opposite scenario to Alain Enthoven's 'internal market', which he saw as a means of continuing to redistribute money out of London yet protecting London's services—by allowing extra-London purchasers to contract for London's services. (The 'grinding down' of the great teaching hospitals such as Guy's, St Thomas's and St Bartholomew's was the initial observation which led Enthoven to reflect on a new model of purchasing.) Overall then if planning is dead, as Mr Duncan Nichol, Chief Executive of the NHS, is alleged to have declared, 'long live planning'. Regions continue to plan services on the basis of formulae and methodologies which gauge the need of local populations and model access to services. Planning may be less mechanistic than before, and 'flexibility' may be the watchword. But simplistic conclusions should be avoided.

The criticism of planning in the NHS found in the academic literature rarely places the NHS experience in an international context where a more favourable interpretation of events is possible. The United Kingdom, by adopting planning mechanisms albeit rather mechanistically, has avoided the duplication and incoherence of health services in market led systems as exemplified by the USA. The NHS is universally acknowledged to be good value for money and this derives in part from the planning of comprehensive services to avoid waste.

The adoption of planning in the UK dates from the mid-1970s which coincides with a period of increasing organisational turbulence in the NHS. Planning which entails the translation of national priorities into local action has been muddied by this rapidly changing national picture. For example, in the early 1980s the Government proclaimed community care as its central priority. However, in the mid-1980s as cuts in expenditure led to ward closures in the acute sector and ferocious criticism of govenment policy, as a short-term political expedient government re-routed resources into the acute sector. Clearly planning is made extremely difficult in this type of environment.

Furthermore although corporate planning has always entailed making choices between competing options due to limited resources, in the 1980s the corporate planning process has faced starker choices and been asked to decide where service reductions should be imposed. This has clearly tarnished the image of the planning process. Nonetheless there are other more hopeful signs. Planning is becoming more integrated with management, with a shift to district and increasingly unit planning.

The improvements in information available to the NHS and movement away from an obsession with structural solutions to improve planning and an increasing focus on the process of change should contribute to more robust planning. However, uncertainties remain over the future direction of planning in the NHS particularly in the light of the White Paper *Working for Patients* which will dramatically alter the role of planning in the NHS. Finally the central problem of reconciling local needs and national priorities may have been recast with the implementation of general management, but the difficulty of resolving these tensions between the centre and the periphery still places a heavy burden on the planning process.

CHAPTER 2

Case study: Riverside

HEALTH SERVICES IN LONDON

The existence of a National Health Service has sometimes disguised the degree of variation that exists in health services across the UK. London, as the capital city, has provided to an unparalleled extent teaching and research facilities for the remainder of the country, and has been home to a cluster of famous and historic hospitals. A unique feature of London, significant for planning purposes, has been that it is covered by more than one regional health authority. This has created difficulties in planning in a coordinated way across London, and spawned attempts at the beginning of the 1980s to plan seriously across regional boundaries.

The difficulties London Hospitals have faced during the 1980s has stemmed from the implementation of the 1976 Resource Allocation Working Party (RAWP) recommendations which produced ways of securing through resource allocation the means to ensure that there would eventually be equal opportunity to access to health care for people at equal risk. The RAWP formula was used to calculate target shares of national resources. This exercise revealed that the four London Thames Regions were significantly over-target with, in particular, North-West, North-East and South-East Thames Regions recognising that they would face an unfavourable resource allocation context for the 1980s.

This situation was further complicated by the overall financial stringency and search for efficiency savings that the Government instigated. Consequently, the process of RAWP adjustment became more painful, as health authorities which had been prepared for a process of differential growth, began to receive no growth monies, creating a need to make radical changes in service configuration. The Thames Regions were also internally diverse, stretching from inner-city Districts with declining populations but historically satisfactory provision, to shire counties with an expanding population but a legacy of sparse provision. However, as with other population migrations this tended to leave a disproportionate amount of dependent groups remaining with special needs exacerbated as the Acheson Report highlighted by the maldistribution of GPs in London.

The final piece of the jigsaw has been the changing context of medical education in London. The historical evolution of medical education was unusual in that teaching was focused around teaching hospitals rather than universities which led to a disparate system of twelve fiercely independent medical schools. In 1968 Lord Todd's Royal Commission on medical education recommended that the (undergraduate) medical schools should be brought together in six groups to take advantage of economies of scale and to cover the expanding medical syllabus adequately. The schools rejected Todd but the continuing squeeze on London University finances led to a further working party under Lord Flowers.

This was established by Lord Annan, Vice Chancellor of London University which reported in 1980 and argued that financial viability made it imperative that larger schools were formed. Meanwhile a flurry of interest in pan London planning resulted in the establishment of the Department of Health's London Advisory Group under Sir John Habakkuk and the influential London Health Planning Consortium.

The Consortium believed it was wrong to let the historical legacy decide the future number and position of hospitals in London. They recognised that with population decline in central London and the need to develop priority services a thorough re-evaluation of acute services in London was needed. They were blunt in their diagnosis:

> The problem in London is in essence, that the level of clinical facilities needed to support the medical schools concentrated in the centre can no longer be justified on service grounds.

The evidence was clear in the number of medical schools who were increasingly sending students further out of London to complementary hospitals to work with general medical 'firms'. The consequences were increasingly fragmented medical schools straddling many sites.

The Consortium identified the required level of acute hospital services in London to the end of the 1980s and tried to link the needs of the medical schools to this revised acute bed configuration. The estimated 20–25 per cent reduction of acute beds in London, from 44,495 beds to 39,560 required that teaching facilities needed to be shared by coupling inner and outer London hospitals in a coherent manner. This was essentially a pragmatic approach which recognised existing links but which did not preclude pairings between existing inner and outer London health authorities. An obstacle to this strategy was the need for separate authorities to come together and rationalise services inevitably raising the spectre of gainers and losers.

The emergence of new super-districts, first Bloomsbury, then Riverside, and more recently Parkside with more in the offing, has enabled rationalisation to take place and the pattern envisaged by the consortium gradually to emerge. For example, the Middlesex and University College Hospitals are now both in Bloomsbury and are served by a single medical school. There are plans to build a single hospital to replace them both. The formation of Parkside in 1988 led to the pairing of the Central Middlesex and St Mary's, Paddington and in October 1989 the North-West Thames Regional Health Authority approved a plan to concentrate acute services on these two sites.

Mergers of districts however, still leaves unresolved coordination of planning between regions. The lack of progress in this area was brought home by a critical report from the King's Fund (1987) which examined the pressures on London's health services during 1987 and concluded that:

> Despite their best endeavours Regions have not been able to coordinate their approach to planning on a London-wide basis. The tendency for planning horizons to be effectively restrained by the Regional boundaries is the basis for our title *Back to Back Planning*.

The difficulties highlighted included variations in planning data and differences in methodology between the four Thames Regions. The lack of progress demonstrated that few incentives existed to encourage coordinated planning between regions due to the lack of a reimbursement system. Consequently, although within a region it was recognised that mergers of districts would enable resources to be liberated (due to the rationalisation of services) freeing up resources for other districts, between regions no such financial incentives existed. This created anxieties between regions about the impact of unplanned closures in another region on their workload. In the Riverside case study, described further on, there was concern at St Thomas' Hospital in South-East Thames Regional Health Authority about the flow of patients after the temporary closure of St Stephen's Hospital. As no formal cross charging systems existed any compensation involved protracted negotiation. This is one of the difficulties recent government proposals are designed to resolve.

The provider market outlined in the White Paper had its origins in the work of Alain Enthoven who recognised the perverse incentives of the NHS. His original outline of an internal market was an attempt to ensure that the London teaching hospitals were compensated for the cross-boundary flows that were drawn to them, by allowing funding to follow patients. The degree to which this will occur and enable the London teaching hospitals to remain financially viable has been thrown into doubt by the revised funding system outlined in the White Paper.

By moving to a system of funding based on resident population this will result in large reductions for some London health authorities with declining populations but historically high levels of provision. The future of these hospitals could also be jeopardised by their unfavourable competitive position due to higher labour costs and capital charges. The irony is that Enthoven's vision of compensating London hospitals for inflows of patients may be reversed with London Districts exporting patients out of London in search of cheaper treatment.

THE ORIGIN OF RIVERSIDE

Riverside Health Authority (HA) was created in April 1985 by the merger of the former Victoria and Hammersmith and Fulham Health Districts. The merger followed from the creation in 1984 of the combined Charing Cross and Westminster Medical School.

The academic and financial problems besetting London's teaching hospitals had led Lord Annan, Vice Chancellor of London University to set up a working party under Lord Flowers. The Westminster Medical School managed to partially stave off the Flowers axe on its medical school but could not prevent merger with the Charing Cross Hospital. The fusion was intended to safeguard both schools, and the whole rationale of Flowers was to create bigger more viable units. However, the linkage of the schools revived the debate about the future role of the Westminster Hospital.

The merger of the Medical School was a catalyst for the establishment of Riverside Health Authority. The Districts had to examine the delivery of services across the area covered by the new medical school, where previously there had been no natural link between the Charing Cross Hospital and the Westminster Hospital. There was a perception that the two Districts were too small to remain viable particularly as the resident population was in decline. It was also a period when the impact of the RAWP formula was beginning to bite into the resource situation of the Thames Regions. This raised the spectre of reductions in service for the Victoria District and they would be easier to achieve in a larger district, where more opportunities for rationalisation would exist. The opposition from CHCs and Victoria to the merger signalled their anxieties that the amalgamation was to be a precursor to a reduced level of acute services.

DESCRIPTION OF THE DISTRICT

Riverside Health Authority was situated in the North-West Thames Regional Health Authority and covered an area of West London bounded to the south by the River Thames. To the east lies Bloomsbury Health Authority (North-East Thames RHA); to the north, the new Parkside Health Authority and to the west and north-west, Hounslow and Spelthorne Health Authority and Ealing Health Authority.

The District included Hammersmith, Fulham, Chelsea, South Kensington, and South Westminster with a population of 287,000 and a revenue budget in 1987/88 of £140m. It crossed the boundaries of three London Boroughs: the City of Westminster; the Royal Borough of Kensington and Chelsea; and the London Borough of Hammersmith and Fulham. It had three District General Hospitals (DGH): Charing Cross Hospital; St Stephen's Hospital and Westminster Hospital.

The provision of acute hospital and related services managed by Riverside Health Authority are concentrated on six main sites:

1 Charing Cross Hospital. Fulham Palace Road, SW6
(*7 hectares*)

The hospital was completed in 1972 and includes the majority of the Charing Cross and Westminster medical school. Academic departments are also located at Westminster, St Stephen's and West London Hospitals as well as using facilties in other health authorities. Charing Cross provides accident and emergency services and a full range of acute specialties. A number of regional specialties—neurosciences, plastic surgery and cancer services are either located on the site or were due to be located there in the future. The size of the investment in Charing Cross and the accretion of regional specialties at the site ensured its long-term future in any reconfiguration of acute services. In 1986 there was an average of 719 available beds.

2 Westminster Hospital, Dean Ryle Street, SW1
(*0·75 hectares*)

The hospital in its current location dated from the 1930s. It provided an accident and emergency service and a comprehensive range of acute specialties. There is also a maternity and special care baby unit. The facilities for cancer services provided at the hospital were to be moved into the single unit based on the Charing Cross site. The hospital had faced threats of closure due to its comparatively small size, small local catchment area, and high costs but had strong political support from the Palace of Westminster, who locked to the hospital for their medical care. In 1986 there was an average of 340 available beds.

3 St Stephen's Hospital, Fulham Road, SW10
(*3·08 hectares*)

The hospital was established in 1878 as the infirmary to a workhouse. The buildings are in the main from two eras—the West Wing being Victorian, the East Wing a later 1960s development consisting of some low rise developments and a multi-storey block containing ward accommodation. Although the West Wing had been subject to upgrading to include beds for the elderly, the age and disparate lay out of the buildings across the site made an increase in the activities on this wing improbable. The East Wing although of comparatively recent construction also required refurbishment.

The hospital provided an accident and emergency service and a range of acute specialties. There was also a large genito-urinary medicine clinic. Approximately 25 per cent of the national caseload for HIV related disease used Riverside services which were concentrated on the St Stephen's site. The hospital had the character of a district general hospital with a case mix that was distinct from the more medical school orientated hospitals of Charing Cross and Westminster. Consequently, it had less lobbying strength than either of the teaching hospitals and was therefore potentially vulnerable if an acute hospital had to close. In 1986 there was an aveage of 343 beds available.

4 West London Hospital, Hammersmith Road, W6
(*1·09 hectares*)

The main hospital was built in the 1880s and included maternity services, a special care baby unit and beds for elderly long-stay and acute elderly mentally ill people. In July 1986 the Authority consulted on the closure of the hospital but withdrew the proposal at the beginning of 1987. In 1986 there was an average of 116 available beds.

5 St Mary Abbot's Hospital, Marloes Road, W8
(*3·95 hectares*)

The majority of the buildings dated from the early 1900s. The site included beds for the continuing care of elderly and mentally ill people and an acute adult mental health unit. In 1986 there was an average of 161 available beds.

6 Westminster Children's Hospital, Vincent Square, SW1
(*0·16 hectares*)

The hospital was purpose built at the turn of the century, but was subsequently extended. The hospital provided an accident and emergency service and a full range of facilities for acutely ill children which included a bone marrow transplant unit. In 1987 the Authority proposed that the hospital close and its services be moved to Westminster hospital. However, the cost of reprovision at £4·5 million was not made available by the Regional Health Authority and the scheme was shelved. In 1986 there was an average of 67 available beds.

A bed profile of these hospitals summarising the average number of available beds in 1986 by clinical specialty, is shown in Table 1. The location of services in Riverside and the local authority boundaries are illustrated in Tables 2 and 3.

TABLE 1. *Riverside Health Authority: Bed Profile of Acute Services and Related Services*

SPECIALTY	CXH	MH	SSH	WLH	SAM	WCH	TOTAL
General Medicine	100	73	85			25	258
General Surgery	85	70	53			25	233
Paediatrics	25	1	15			26	67
Dermatolgy	5		10				15
Trauma & Orthopaedics	69	37	50			7	163
Rheumatology	24	3	8				35
Rehabilitation	8						8
Gynaecology	22	12	20				54
Urology	31	12	9				52
Cardiology	24	21	5				50
ENT	27					2	29
Opthalmology	27						27
Neurosciences	60	15				6	81
Plastic surgery	3						3
Cancer services	52	42	9				103
Thoracic services	14						14
Oral surgey	4	4	1			1	10
Other acute	11	4	3				18
Sub-total	591	294	268			67	1,220
Maternity		37		42			79
Special Care Baby Unit		9		12			21
Elderly	89		75	46	116		326
Mental Illness	39						39
Elderly mentally ill				16	45		61
Total	719	340	343	116	161	67	1,746

SOURCE: SH3–Average Available Beds 1986 (all numbers rounded)

KEY TO HOSPITALS

CXH: Charing Cross
WH: Westminster
SSH: St Stephen's
WLH: West London
SMA: St Mary Abbot's
WCH: Westminster Children's

The management structure of the Authority had to alter dramatically to accommodate the merger of the two Districts, and the establishment of general management. Initially the merger was not complete with the management of community services remaining divided between two

TABLE 2. *Riverside DHA with Local Authority Boundaries*

KEY TO MAP

Hospitals □

1 Hammersmith Hospital
2 Queen Charlotte's Maternity Hospital
3 West London Hospital
4 Charing Cross Hospital
5 St. Mary Abbots Hospital
6 St. Stephen's Hospital
7 Brompton Hospital
8 Royal Marsden Hospital
9 Chelsea Hospital for Women
10 The Gordon Hospital
11 Westminster Children's Hospital
12 Westminster Hospital

Health Centres and Clinics ○

13 The Health Centre, White City
14 The Grove Health Centre
15 Glenthorne Road Health Clinic
16 St. Dunstan's Health Centre
17 Milson Road Health Clinic
18 Fulham Road Chiropody Clinic
19 Parsons Green Health Clinic
20 Wandsworth Bridge Road Health Clinic
21 Earls Court Child Guidance Clinic
22 Holland Street Clinic
23 South Kensington Clinic
24 World's End Health Centre
25 Cheyne Centre for Spastic Children
26 Violet Melchell Clinic
27 Ebury Bridge Clinic
28 Alderney Street Clinic
29 Bessborough Street Clinic

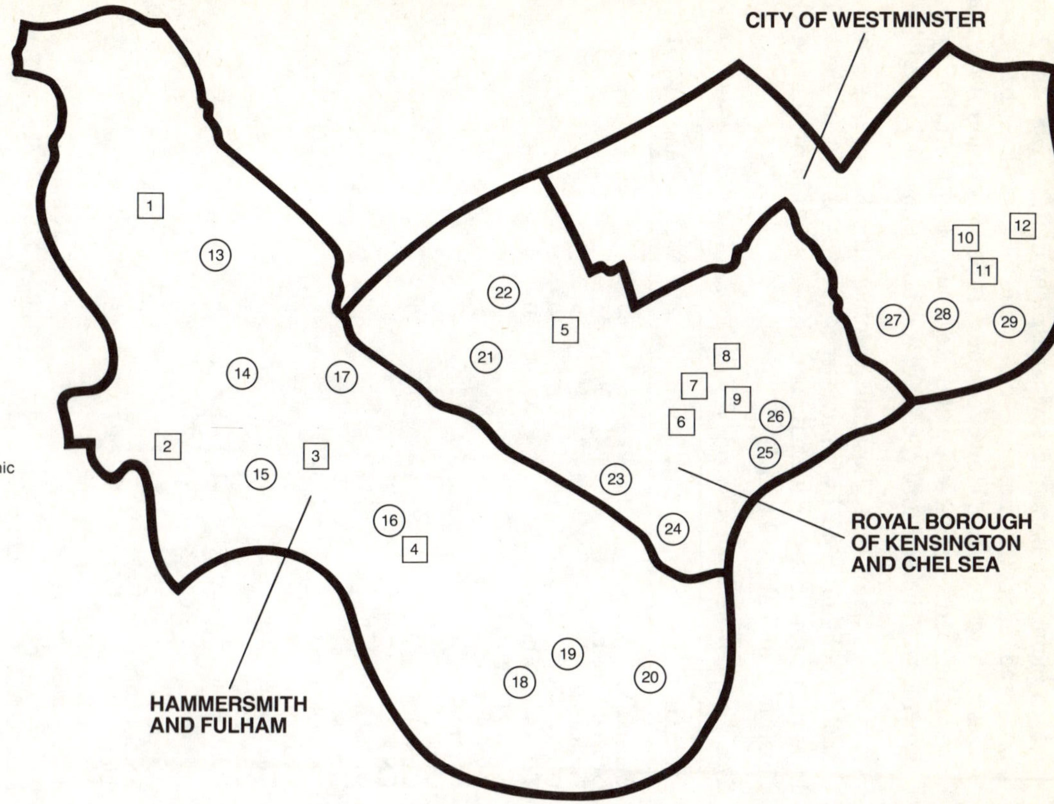

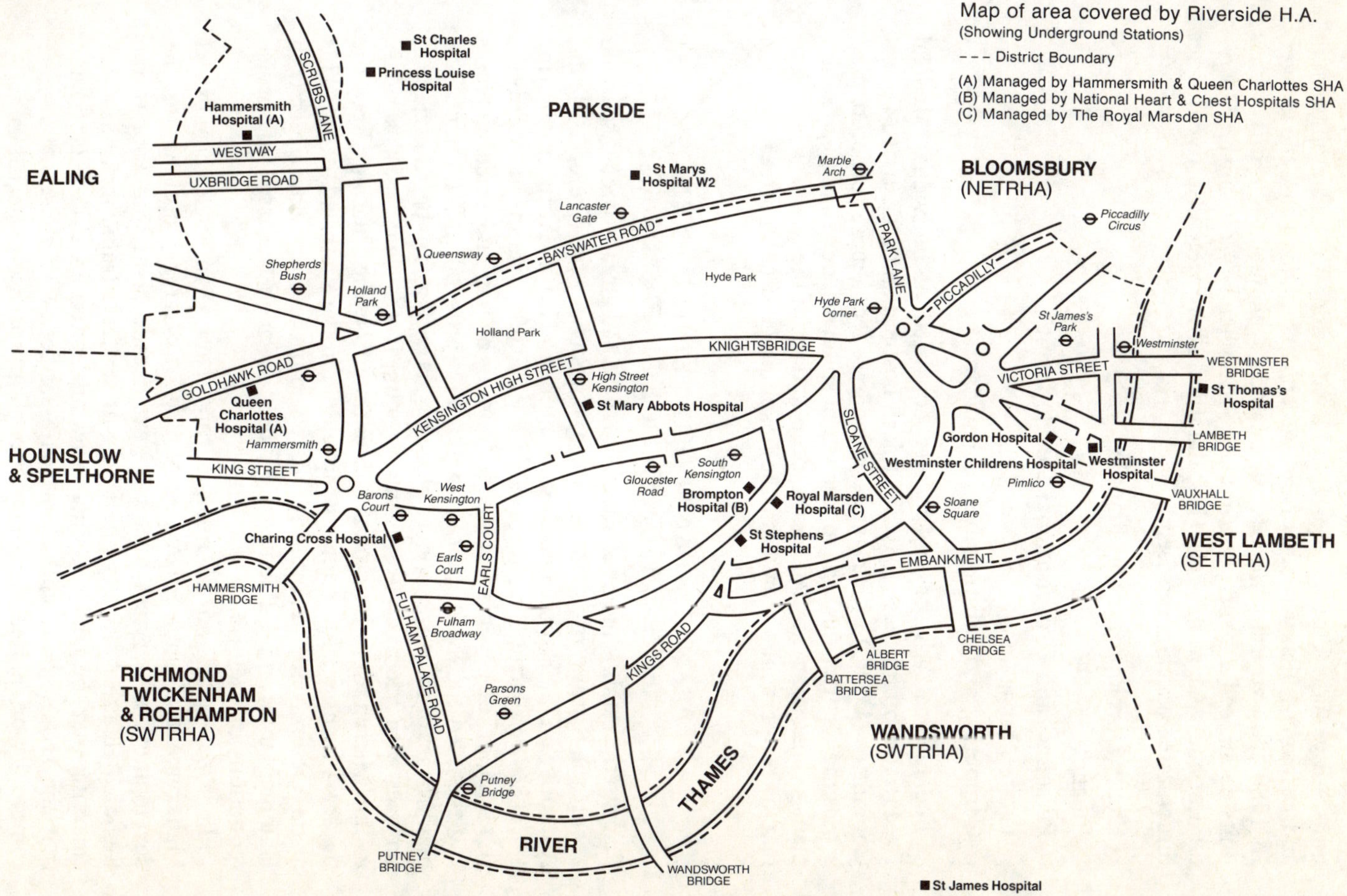

TABLE 3. *Map of area covered by Riverside Health Authority*

units—Riverside East (Victoria) and Riverside West (Hammersmith and Fulham) which was one of the agreements made to ease the merger. In 1988 the two units were amalgamated as planned. The three other units comprised a mental health unit, St Stephen's/Westminster Hospital unit and a Charing Cross Hospital unit. There were also five district directorates which comprised:

Policy Development and Planning
Finance
Personnel and Organisational Development
Estate Management
Computing and Information Technology

The medical advisory machinery consisted of individual Medical Executive Committees (MECs) at each hospital and a District Medical Committee (DMC) which was designed to reflect a more corporate view across the District than the individual hospital orientated MECs. Senior management concentrated on the deliberations of the DMC as it tried to take a less parochial view than the hospital based committees.

PLANNING ACTIVITY PRIOR TO THE ESTABLISHMENT OF RIVERSIDE

Prior to the establishment of Riverside there had already been discussion about the future of acute services particularly in Victoria Health Authority. The Hammersmith and Fulham Health Authority during 1983/84 were struggling to prevent a £600,000 overspend due to the combination of government under-funding of pay and price increases and the need for the Authority to move towards its RAWP target. The main thrust of its acute services planning activity was to begin reviewing services with Victoria Health Authority but it was clear that as services in the District were becoming concentrated on the Charing Cross site the main focus for future change would lie in the Victoria District. This made Victoria Health Authority wary about the proposed merger with Hammersmith and Fulham as it would re-open the issue of service reductions in Victoria.

This was not a novel situation for Victoria. In 1982 the District Management Team initiated a review of strategic options for the development of services over the next decade. This was prior to the Regional Health Authority publishing its strategic framework but it was emerging that the resource situation would deteriorate for Victoria and that the focus would shift from acute services to a concern for more community orientated, non-institutional approaches to health care.

In 1983, the Victoria Health Authority published *Evaluation of Health Services in Victoria: A Strategic Framework for the Future;* Volume 1. This had three elements:

1. a comprehensive review of existing health services;
2. a detailed analysis of the constraints and opportunities relevant to identification of optimal strategies for the future;
3. it identified the criteria to be employed for the evaluation of strategic proposals. The criteria included the need for flexibility, realistic resource assumptions, accessibility and acceptability both internally to the Authority and externally to the wider community.

The document was the first stage of a phased process. Options were not identified in this first document in order to focus debate on the existing situation and the evaluative criteria to be used in evaluating future options. A further volume of the strategy was produced which examined options for reductions in hospital services as a consequence of the reduction in Victoria's revenue allocation by between £7-10m per annum. It assumed:

i. a substantial reduction in the number of beds in the District;
ii. the relocation of the Westminster Children's Hospital;
iii. the closure of at least one of the three major hospital sites.

The last assumption was stated in the strongest terms:

> 'Given the scale of the revenue savings that have to be achieved in Victoria, it is impossible to define any strategies for the totality of health care which do not involve hospital closure.'

Five options were selected for review which are summarised in Table 4 with the evaluative criteria used. The document did not specifiy which option it viewed as the preferred option as this would not have been in keeping with the approach which Victoria was beginning to adopt. This explored alternative planning methods moving away from fixed point planning, to more flexible approaches which left a range of options available to the Authority. This did not mean senior management had no preferences, rather options were indicated which needed more detailed assessment, consultation and negotiation.

The most favoured option in consultation was Option A which retained DGHs at the Westminster and St Stephen's site and closed St Mary Abbott's. This option had a number of advantages:

(a) it retained the commitment to the two sectors of Victoria and, therefore, ensured services would remain accessible;
(b) it could be implemented quickly and phased as appropriate;

TABLE 4. *Options for reductions in hospital services:* Victoria Health Authority

Option	*Flexibility*	*Resources*	*Needs*	*Accessibility*	*Acceptability*	*Context*	*Timetable*
A	high	low	medium	high	medium	medium	high
Bi	low	high	low	low	low	low	medium
Bii	low	high	medium	low	low	low	medium
C	medium	medium	medium	medium	low	medium	low
D	low	high	medium	medium	medium	high	medium

KEY TO OPTIONS

OPTION A:
Westminster: DGH
St Stephens: DGH
St Mary Abbotts: closed

OPTION Bi:
Westminster: DGH
St Stephens: closed
St Mary Abbotts: priority services

OPTION Bii:
Westminster: closed
St Stephens: DGH
St Mary Abbotts: priority services

OPTION C:
Westminster: specialist acute with no A&E
St Stephens: DGH
St Mary Abbotts: closed

OPTION D:
Westminster: closed
St Stephens: closed
St Mary Abbotts: DGH

Flexibility and robustness: the need for the strategic framework to be capable of being adjusted to meet changes in the social, economic, medical and technological environment, within which is determined both the range and the level of services provided.

Resources: will the cost of proposals match the best judgement of any future resource availability and what happens if plans are developed which prove to be out of line with the eventual revenue situation? What are the capital implications of proposals and from where is the capital resource coming? Is it to be realised within Victoria, presumably by land sales, or are proposals dependent on DHSS/RHA capital allocations.

Needs: do proposals meet perceived needs, both in volume and quality? Arguably even more significantly, whose perception of need; and of the local users, the providers the RHA, the DHSS?

Accessibility: are services provided in the right place and in the right environment? What is the proper balance of care particularly between hospitals and the community? Is there a positive approach to continuity of care?

Acceptability: are proposals regarded as realistic by the providers and the community, including doctors, trade unions, CHC, politicians? Can they, in the real world, be negotiated.

Context: do proposals match those of other related organisations, including the RHA, the medical school, adjacent health authorities and appropriate local authorities?

Timetable: to what degree is the timetable for proposals itself a constraint? How rigid does the programme of implementation have to be?

SOURCE: *Evaluation of health services in Victoria: A strategic framework for the future:* Volume II, 1984.

(c) the closure of St Mary Abbot's Hospital would facilitate the development of a community model for priority services.

However, there were questions raised about the financial viability of this option—particularly as it would not sufficiently reduce the level of local acute services.

The other option which senior management wished to explore was Option D which proposed the closure of Westminster and St Stephen's

Hospital and the development of a new hospital on the St Mary Abbot's site. The attraction of this option was the centrality of the site in the Victoria District and the prospects that it would help to achieve the long-term financial targets of the Authority. Furthermore it would enable the provision of high quality hospital services.

However, the option was radical and risky as the document explained:

> It represents in political terms, a high risk option. There is an apparently unchallenged assumption in health planning circles, that one of the major sources in London's problems in relation to acute services, is that too many of its teaching hospitals have been rebuilt at an immense captial cost, too near to the centre of London, with its continuing downward trend of residential population.

The District Health Authority discussed the strategic framework at its September 1984 meeting and requested a further financial appraisal of the options in the framework. This led to a feasibility study of the option of providing a new hospital on the St Mary Abbot's site. The study concluded that a 670 bed teaching hospital would require a £43·6m capital investment and cost £33m per annum in revenue terms. The potential revenue savings were calculated at up to £14m per annum.

The St Mary Abbot's option gained a degree of support in Victoria during 1984/85 prior to the establishment of Riverside. However, major objections were raised. First, from a broader perspective it was not viewed as a very appropriate location because it was only a couple of miles away from both St Mary's Hospital, Paddington and Charing Cross Hospital, Hammersmith. Second, the net capital cost of £43·6m would have made large demands on the Region's already heavily committed capital resources and by building on the St Mary Abbot's site would have precluded the sale of a very valuable site. Third, the site was not very accessible and this could have led to difficulties in obtaining planning permission.

For senior management the preliminary appraisal of options in 1984 began to prepare the District for major changes in services. This message was reinforced by the merger with Hammersmith and Fulham. The St Mary Abbot's option had also helped to float the idea of a new teaching hospital which had revealed considerable enthusiasm from the consultant medical staff to a project of this nature. However, it was clear that obtaining a new hospital was a politically risky strategy in which the ground would need to be carefully prepared and a viable financial package created.

The alternative preferred option which would have maintained St Stephen's Hospital and the Westminster Hospital, but close St Mary Abbot's began to look increasingly vulnerable. When Riverside was established the need for two DGH-type hospitals in the Victoria part of the District was questioned. It was evident that the new District would have to recast its options to adjust to the different context.

THE REGIONAL STRATEGY

The establishment of Riverside coincided with the North-West Thames Regional Health Authority's preparation of their ten year strategy to 1994. The Region anticipated major changes in its overall pattern of services to meet a number of national policy objectives:

1. *The distribution of resources*

(a) To fulfil its RAWP target. The Region was the most over-target Region nationally and therefore expected its growth monies to be syphoned off to RAWP gaining Regions in the Midlands and the North.

(b) Within the Region resources were to be redistributed from central London Districts where the population was declining to districts outside London where the population was growing and services were still being developed.

2. *Changes in the use of resources*

(a) The Region aimed to reduce unnecessary admissions to hospital by increasing the use of day surgery and placing greater emphasis on the effective use of out-patient services.

(b) The Region forecast that with increases in efficiency and changes in local acute caseload, by 1994, 2,000 fewer beds would be required.

3. *Priority services*

The Region was committed to strengthening priority services in inner-city districts and the shire districts.

The Regional Health Authority therefore needed to mobilise £99m to achieve these service changes over the strategic period. In 1988/89 the Regional allocation was £870m which was projected to reduce to £844m by 1994 (at 1988/89 prices). The Region therefore needed to liberate resources from inner-London Districts. Riverside as the largest District with a budget of £130m was required to deliver £32m to Regional coffers. This reduction had three main elements. The first was an adjustment of £6m which reflected the closure of Bansted Hospital, a long-stay hospital which lay outside the District. Second, Riverside was judged to be over-provided for priority services (except mental handicap) and Riverside was £10m in excess of their 1994 target. The third element related to local acute services which were at least £16m above the level of funding anticipated to be available by 1994.

The Region faced a number of conflicting pressures. There was the overriding need to meet their RAWP target, yet achieve redistribution within the Region. The shire counties exerted considerable pressure to improve their resource situation for new developments. This was during the introduction of general management when the new general managers were trying to demonstrate that the changes had beneficial effects for their Districts. However, this money had to be funnelled out of inner-London and there were planning and political constraints to be overcome before Riverside could release their resources. The first step had been taken through the establishment of Riverside but although a new hospital had been mooted Riverside's strategy remained undeveloped. A new approach was required.

MULTI-SCENARIO PLANNING

Prior to the establishment of Riverside, Victoria Health Authority had been working with the King's Fund College to examine future service planning issues. Senior managers in Victoria recognised that large scale changes were inevitable in the future. The scale of these changes were magnified with the formation of Riverside. The use of outside expertise to help examine change was seen as vital particularly as the potential scale of change was greater than had been achieved to date in the NHS.

There was also recognition that the traditional option appraisal/cost benefits analysis approach was too narrow and failed to grasp the complexity of the environment in which Riverside worked, which was characterised by great uncertainty about the future. The financial appraisal carried out to determine the revenue costs of the proposed new hospital had used a modifed Exeter forecasting model but this needed to be adjusted to take into account outpatient, accident and emergency and teaching costs which were omitted from the model. These modifications were relatively crude and it contributed to the desire to explore alternative planning methodologies.

Similarly at the Region key individuals were supportive of a project to develop alternative planning methodologies. This reflected the desire not only to move away from fixed point planning but also to nurture Riverside to help them create a viable strategy which was the financial bedrock upon which the regional strategy rested.

The King's Fund College began to work with Riverside to help them review their acute services and to establish the criteria to use for this rationalisation process. The first step had been taken during the first half of 1985 to establish a data base which required linking the incompatible data from the previous Districts and generating new data on activity and workload.

The King's Fund College was developing alternative planning methodologies which tried to improve on existing approaches in the NHS. A nucleus of staff at the college had been associated with the Ottawa-Carleton Regional District Health Council project in Ontario, Canada in the late 1970s[1]. This project aimed to construct a planning system which avoided the traditional shortcomings of health service planning. In particular the inflexibility of these traditional approaches, with their insensitivity to the political environment and their emphasis on quantitative data which may not be available or sufficiently accurate, was avoided. Instead planning activity was conceived as a sequential decision making process where an attempt was made to keep future options open as far as possible. Consequently, short-term actions, other things being equal, were preferred which kept a large number of future options in order to maintain a greater degree of strategic flexibility.

This approach was premised on the assumption that although it was impossible to predict the future with certainty, it was possible to identify what the consequences would be if a particular view of the future occurred, and to use that information to assist the process of taking short-term decisions. This would help Riverside move towards the desired service pattern irrespective of the particular future which occurred.

This methodology had two discernable elements. First, there was the requirement to forecast alternative futures by examination of the future demand and supply for health care. Second, policy options had to be fashioned and assessed in the light of the alternative futures.

A planning team was set up which included the Director of Planning, a specialist in community medicine, a nursing representative and a member of the King's Fund Faculty. This core group met more informally with the District, the Region and the King's Fund representative to help formulate options which would be consistent with the alternative futures.

The planning group acknowledged that there were numerous factors which affected health care provision and, consequently, an infinite number of permutations could be assembled generating widely differing futures. However, it was concluded that the sources of uncertainty could be divided into two categories—demand and supply for health care. Equal significance was attached to supply and demand factors in

1. For a fuller discussion of this project see Best, G., Parston, G., Rosenhead, J. (1986). 'Robustness in Practice—the Regional Planning of Health Services', *Journal of the Operational Research Society*, **37**, (5).

analysing the future. Six areas were identified as of paramount significance:

demand for health care is influenced by

1. population changes
2. epidemiology
3. medical practice and technology

supply of health care is influenced by

4. health and social policy
5. resources
6. medical practice and technology

The group used a range of published data sources including OPCS and GLC data in the case of population projections and more localised regional/district generated data to predict future caseload in Riverside. The group was also dependent on individual members own interests and knowledge to help gauge the significance of each factor.

In the case of future population changes, OPCS data had been shown to be fallible in their projection of population size and structures in inner-London. The group focused on three issues. First, changes in the age structure of the Riverside population. Second, the predicted level of population in the future, and third, the anticipated changes in the flow of people seeking treatment in Riverside. These discussions raised issues which needed resolution between the District and the Region, the degree to which the Region would accept cross boundary flows and were willing to allow a cross charging system clearly impinged on the demand side projections of Riverside's alternative futures. This scenario approach therefore allowed a fruitful dialogue between the District and the Region, in which the exact element of disagreement was pinpointed and the difference resolved.

The epidemiological analysis focused on the changing pattern of morbidity and the impact of population change and social conditions on the future. The incidence of cardio-vascular disease and cancer which were the main cause of mortality were investigated and evidence suggested that morbidity from these diseases was static. The group examined future trends in the spread of AIDS and morbidity from psychiatric illness.

Change in medical practice and technology was examined from both a demand and supply side perspective. On the demand side, for example, it was concluded that advances in treatment procedures through the use of new techniques in radiology, would make fewer invasive surgery techniques necessary. Similarly, increased emphasis on preventative measures would sustain life longer but if morbidity increased expectations about the possibilities of medical intervention, this could result in increased demand. On the supply side, the experience of the spread of CT scanning has demonstrated the rapidity with which the supply of diagnostic techniques spread. The discussions on changes in medical practice and technology were very speculative, and the group concluded that in the next decade the most significant trends for future service provision would be in the trend away from inpatient admissions and the availability of new techniques in more local settings.

SUPPLY SIDE

The supply side analysis also examined, for example, the shifting health and social policy arena. The changing priorities and policies of government in relation to health care and the impact of the Region's strategic intentions and objectives were the most important variables considered. A final influence on the supply of health care would be the financial and manpower resource position of the authority. This required judgements about the future of the RAWP formula and the perennial issue of health service funding. The future manpower resources of health care had become an equally grave issue with unfavourable demographic trends accelerating existing difficulties in the recruitment market.

The result of these deliberations was a mosaic of information about the future. Each element of uncertainty categorised by supply and demand were combined in different ways to yield alternative pictures of the future. The alternative futures each had a demand definition (either high, medium, or low) and each had a supply definition (either high, moderate, or low). The demand definitions used a mixture of population projections and London Health Planning Consortium data weighted by a RAWP-type Standardised Mortality Ratio (SMR) calculation. For caseload supply side definitions and financial terms were derived from the DHSS RAWP model.

This led to the development of a matrix of alternative futures. However, a number were unlikely to occur. The case of a low demand high supply future is illustrative. The amount of resources spent on health care is finite with governments endeavouring to limit expenditure. Private health care will also only be developed where a demand has been identified. Consequently a state of high supply and low demand was a 'future' with little purchase on reality. The three futures selected to enable a reasonable definition of the overall directions of policy were:

Future 1: low demand and low supply

Future 2: high demand and moderate supply

Future 3: moderate demand and high supply

The planning team were then able to consider policy options for the future against the three futures outlined.

CONSEQUENCES FOR THE AUTHORITY?

The exploration of a different planning methodology during 1985/86 contributed to the achievement of change in the Authority. Senior management recognised the scale of the change envisaged, but no consensus existed in the Authority about the future configeration of acute services. The possibility of a new hospital on the St Mary Abbot's site had emerged, but although it commanded some support, the financial and political climate of the 1980s, coupled with the practical disadvantage of the option produced scepticism about the likelihood of a new hospital being built. Nonetheless, the establishment of Riverside—premised on rationalisation—had perhaps strengthened the case against maintaining both St Stephen's Hospital and Westminster Hospital which was the alternative preferred option of the Authority. An impasse existed with the Authority lacking clear criteria to decide which hospital to close.

This situation was exacerbated by the particular political complexion of the Health Authority membership. The merger had left a number of local authority councillors from Hammersmith and Fulham who were Labour party councillors and opposed to reductions in service. Conversely, Conservative councillors from Kensington and Chelsea were more supportive of service reductions. A number of members were also uncommitted. Consequently, the Authority had been unwilling to decide which hospital should be closed at the end of 1985. Senior management hoped that the alternative futures work would provide a set of evaluative criteria against which to judge future service plans.

Senior management also recognised that the future of the Westminster Hospital, in particular, was an intensely political issue due to its associations with the Palace of Westminster. Any evaluative criteria and options generated needed to consider the political viability of the strategy. To achieve change management could not simply leave the production of the strategy to the planning group. However, the planning activity could be used to legitimate whatever might emerge from the political negotiating process. The involvement of a respected organisation—the King's Fund College ensured that it would be more difficult to refute the strategy that emerged. Furthermore, it gave Riverside time to formulate their strategy with the added flexibility of being dispensed from fulfilling Regional and national planning time-tables. The Region granted Riverside this immunity to allow them time to formulate their strategy on condition Riverside would ultimately deliver the revenue savings they had agreed.

The planning project also enabled an informal and continuing dialogue between the Region and Riverside. The publication of the Regional strategy in October 1985 established the context for planning activity in Riverside. The Authority accepted the logic of the Regional strategy that inner city Districts like Riverside were relatively over-provided and had to release funds to enable developments to occur in the shire counties. Pragmatically Riverside recognised it would be futile to resist the funding reductions planned. The Region had an incentive to help Riverside achieve change as painlessly as possible. Consequently, the basis existed for a fruitful relationship between the Region and the District. Riverside therefore gained a reputation at the Region as a cooperative partner and this accumulated reservoir of good will was to prove valuable in the future.

Naturally, differences existed. The 1985 strategy had outlined a local acute bed target of 625 beds by 1994, a reduction from the 1986 level of 960 beds. The District disputed the basis on which the figure was compiled which they viewed as an arbitrary figure to sustain a finance orientated strategy. The Region did not view the bed target as immutable. They recognised that the number of beds was of limited significance without reference to the activity levels in those beds. The real concern of the Region was to ensure that the activity levels associated with the number of beds enabled Riverside to keep within their financial target.

The medical school were concerned about the 625 local acute bed figure because of the need to have a sufficient number of beds to provide adequate teaching facilities for their annual intake of 171 medical students which they calcuated as a figure of 685 beds.

Senior management had accepted the need for bed reductions but wished to retain enough local acute beds to ensure that two viable teaching hospitals could be maintained. The Region allowed the figure to rise sharply from 625 beds to 736 local acute beds, provided Riverside delivered the revenue savings after the number of sites had been reduced. This also enabled the District General Manager to return to the clinical staff having vanquished the proposal to reduce the bed target to 625.

An Approach to the Minister

During the breathing space provided by the planning project senior management wanted to explore the political feasibility of closing the Westminster Hospital but were constrained by the unwillingness of the Health Authority to act. Senior management were anxious to avoid a closure decision by default but this possibility was looming as Westminster lost services one by one making it increasingly vulnerable to closure.

Senior management were concerned that a review of obstetric services in early 1986 would result in a recommendation that obstetrics should be based at the Charing Cross Hospital. The campaign mounted against the proposal would then have been converted into a 'save the Westminster Hospital' campaign which management were anxious to avoid.

The January 1986 meeting of the Riverside Health Authority had discussed the merits of retaining services at St Stephen's Hospital and the Westminster Hospital. The Authority had deferred making a decision but were inclined to favour the retention of St Stephen's Hospital as the better of two unsatisfactory options. This preference was based on St Stephen's being a more appropriate hospital due to its character as a DGH with a well defined catchment area, its higher throughput of accident and emergency cases and its focus as a centre of priority services for the community. However, the possibility of closing the Westminster, as well as requiring a ministerial decision like the other options, was more difficult due to the political protection that the Westminster enjoyed. Previous Ministers had not been prepared to sanction the closure of the Westminster. The situation was complicated by Riverside's short-term programme which planned to transfer the services of the Westminster Children's Hospital to the Westminster Hospital. A plan which clashed with the longer-term aspiration to close the Westminster. Consequently, the District Chairman approached Mr Hayhoe, the Minister for Health in 1986 to discuss the future of hospital services in Riverside.

The meeting proved to be inconclusive and the Minister said he would not support any proposals which led to the closure of Westminster *or* St Stephen's Hospitals in the foreseeable future. He also indicated that the option to build a new DGH on the St Mary Abbot's Hospital site was not regarded as viable because of the problem of capital funding. Nonetheless the District was encouraged to place emphasis on the long-term option to close St Mary Abbot's Hospital.

Closure of the West London Hospital

The failure to resolve the long-term planning issues and the continuing work of the planning group on the alternative futures ensured that 1986 was dominated by short-term issues. The District faced financial difficulties with the requirement to effect savings of £3,940,000 in 1986/87 against an allocation of £123m which was a reduction of 3·2 per cent. This level of reduction was due to continue every year and needed actions which would release revenue on a longer-term basis rather than a short-term basis as ward closures implied.

The first measure considered was the closure of the West London Hospital in Hammersmith. It provided 139 inpatient beds for obstetrics, geriatric, and psycho-geriatric patients. It also housed a special care baby unit (SCBU). The Authority considered that none of the services were appropriately provided as the long-stay geriatric service was provided in an institutional setting rather than as part of a DGH service. Regional guidance indicated that Riverside had substantial over provision of maternity services in relation to the residential population. Consequently, the Authority proposed the closure of the West London Maternity Unit with no reprovision. The closure of the hospital was expected to release £2,783,000 revenue savings per annum.

The proposals generated an enormous wave of opposition. This stemmed from the reputation the hospital had for providing maternity services in an innovatory manner which met the wishes of the women it served. The degree of opposition which had been heightened by a pending by-election made management pause and review the strategy. Other considerations contributed to make the closure of the West London less attractive. First, the closure of the Westminster Hospital had at minimum become an issue for discussion in the District and this opened up the possibility that in future the hospital might be allowed to close. It was therefore not sensible to move the academic department of Obstetrics and Gynaecology to the Westminster and might precipitate future difficulties if they were then required to move again.

Second, if the closure of the Westminster was on the horizon this required an inducement to make the medical staff move from the Westminster. This point was made baldly in a Riverside Authority paper entitled *Future Rationalisation of Services at Westminster and St Stephen's Hospitals*, dated 11 February 1986:

> Many medical staff (and therefore the people who are directly influenced by medical staff) are susceptible to inducements to accept the closure of Westminster Hospital. The most obvious and effective would be the offer of a new hospital at either St Mary Abbot's or Brompton. It is not inconceivable, however, that this tactical approach could be successful if what was on offer was the replacement of existing Westminster-based departments at St Stephen's Hospital and the demonstration of commitment to making St Stephen's into a teaching hospital of comparable status to that which is currently enjoyed by Westminster Hospital.

It was therefore necessary to ensure that sufficient trade existed for a new hospital wherever that might eventually be located. The dominance of Charing Cross meant other specialities not at Charing Cross needed to be hoarded and then decanted to a new hospital. However, if the West London Hospital closed, coupled with the falling numbers of births projected, the obstetric workload would evaporate without the attraction of the West London, leaving the new hospital without obstetrics. This would make it difficult to attract paediatrics to a new hospital and the fragility of the plan would be exposed.

As the Authority meeting approached in January 1987, where a decision would be made, senior management decided to withdraw the plan with the agreement of the Chairman. This confounded many Health Authority members who had finally reluctantly agreed to back the proposal. This led to confusion within the Health Authority about the direction of the acute services strategy. It also entailed abandoning the main option to generate short-term revenue savings for the District. This raised the stakes for management as by jeopardising short-term savings it became imperative to deliver long-term savings which would require substantial reductions in acute services.

In February 1987 the plan to move the Westminster Children's Hospital to the Westminster Hospital met with a similar fate. It required £4·5m to be spent on providing improved facilities at Westminster and the Region were unwilling to finance the project. This was a veiled signal that the future of the Westminster was in jeopardy. It was apparent that after the withdrawal of the West London closure plan at the end of 1986 tinkering with the existing pattern of provision would be insufficiently radical to achieve the savings needed. As the possibility that the Westminster might close emerged, it became illogical to place new services at the Westminster Hospital and the plan withered.

Strategic Framework

During 1986 the planning group, having completed work on the alternative futures, began to link these futures to five basic policy options. This drew on the earlier strategic planning work in Victoria and developed the evaluative criteria to be used. The publication of the strategic framework had been delayed because of Regional concern that the document referred to hospital closures. They all included the reprovision of the services at St Mary Abbot's and the eventual closure of that hospital.

1. retention of all three District General Hospitals: Charing Cross, St Stephen's and Westminster.

Concentration of District General Hospitals on two sites:

2. Charing Cross and St Stephen's

3. Charing Cross and Westminster

4. Charing Cross and a new site in Riverside East

5. St Stephen's and Westminster.

Each policy option was described in terms consistent with the three separate and distinct views of the future which yielded a matrix of fifteen possibilities. However, the analysis of the options was in the context of the Regional strategic framework. The policy analysis also drew on the 'guiding principles' determined by the Authority which, for example, favoured Riverside residents.

The first option to retain all three DGHs had the advantage that it maximised accessibility for Riverside residents to DGHs. It also had least requirement for capital and involved no major hospital closures. However, it was only a viable option if resources allocated to the District were increased or reductions were made in the priority services. Neither course of action seemed likely and therefore support for the status quo position was waning.

The option to retain DGH services at Charing Cross and St Stephen's was viable but it had three main disadvantages. First, it did not deliver local DGH services for the population of South Westminster. Second, it required significant capital to enable services to be moved from the Westminster. Third, it involved the ultimate closure of the Westminster Hospital.

The third option to retain services at Charing Cross and Westminster had parallel advantages and disadvantages from the second option. It also involved significant capital expenditure and the eventual closure of a hospital, St Stephen's in this case. Furthermore, it diminished the accessibility of services for the population in Chelsea and South Kensington and there were also doubts about its financial viability.

The option to retain services at Charing Cross and develop a DGH on a new site in Riverside East revived the discussion in the predecessor Victoria Health Authority about a new hospital on the St Mary Abbot's site. It had the advantage of being supported in principle by the Medical School and the District Medical Committee. It satisfied most of the evaluative criteria derived from the guiding principles, although depending on the site location it could have disadvantaged part of the District's catchment population in terms of accessibility.

It had two major disadvantages. First, it needed substantial capital expenditure to build the new hospital and it was improbable Regional or national coffers would be available. Second, financial viability could only be achieved following the completion of capital work when revenue savings from the rationalisation of services would come on stream. This entailed the delay in realisation of District revenue targets until the end of the strategic period.

The most significant aspect of the option was the siting of the new hospital. There were three main proposals: redevelopment of the St Mary Abbot's site, the use of the existing St Stephen's, or finding a new site in Chelsea. The St Mary Abbot's option was no longer as favoured as during the deliberations of 1984/85. This was not least because of the potential value of the site and the recognition that any chance of building a new hospital would be dictated by the need to generate capital from within the District through land sales. Furthermore, the Authority was beginning to think about more radical options than would have been possible in 1984/85, when discussions about St Mary Abbot's had helped to raise the possibility of developing a new hospital and had sustained debate by neither favouring St Stephen's or Westminster. Nonetheless, in 1986/87 the debate had moved on and the problems of accessibility and its proximity to St Mary's, Paddington made it a less attractive option. Difficulties were also foreseen in obtaining planning permission.

The other possible location of a new hospital was on a site adjoining Brompton Hospital in Chelsea which was dubbed the Brompton option. The consultant medical staff were very supportive of the scheme and had been involved in finding a site in Chelsea which strengthened their commitment to the scheme. The site proposed was the Chelsea College of Science and Technology which was due to be vacated by the University of London during 1987. The attraction for the clinicians was the location which was close to the Brompton and National Heart Hospitals and the Royal Marsden Hospital. Imperial College was also only half a mile from the site. The clinicians felt there would be opportunities to develop close links between a new hospital, the specialist hospitals and the post-graduate institutes which would strengthen the new hospital as collaboration in research would raise its prestige.

Significant drawbacks existed to the scheme. First, the use of a site not owned by the Health Authority required a large initial capital outlay. Second, the time-scale was viewed as too long-term to achieve the necessary savings required by the Region. This was because the acquisition of land in the Chelsea area would probably have required compulsory purchase orders, which would have taken many years to achieve and would have been accompanied by the uncertainty about if the application would be granted. Finally, the proposed site was only half a mile from the existing St Stephen's site; which led the focus of attention for the new hospital to shift to the St Stephen's site.

The final option considered was the retention of St Stephen's and Westminster with the closure of Charing Cross. This option was rejected as it would have required a major closure in Charing Cross, where major investment had taken place. It was also becoming the natural home of high technology regional and supra-district specialties which made its closure inconceivable.

The strategic framework document concluded that the most flexible response remained the retention of all three existing DGHs which was the short-to-medium term policy being adopted by the Authority. Sustaining this policy only appeared to be possible through an improved financial situation or reductions in the level of priority services. The preferred policy option, therefore, sought to concentrate district general hospital services on the Charing Cross site and a site in Riverside East. This overlapped substantially with the most viable option which planned to place the new hospital on the St Stephen's site. Consequently, the preferred option and the most viable option were merged.

A new Hospital in the Making

Discussion of the strategic framework was muted as it did not outline one clearly favoured option and because it was anticipated that further work would be carried out on gauging the suitability of the preferred option. Nonetheless the statement of guiding principles led to some disquiet amongst medical staff who felt it implied a diminution of the importance of the teaching function in Riverside's hospitals. This was due to the emphasis on providing services for the residential population of Riverside which was in conflict with teaching hospitals practice of attracting referrals from outside the District.

As the spectre loomed of a possible two site DGH without the Westminster, anxiety about the closure of the hospital re-emerged. This would not be possible without ministerial approval. Consequently, senior management took informal soundings from the Department of Health about the political feasibility of closing the Westminster. It was evident that the support of the Westminster Hospital clinical staff and local MPs were essential if the Department of Health was to be persuaded of the merit of the case for closure. In addition the bulk of the District Health Authority membership and strong support from the Regional Health Authority membership was viewed as of paramount importance. Furthermore, if blanket opposition from the media emerged this was unlikely to enhance the projects chances of success. The Department accepted that a feasibility study should be carried out to examine the possibility of placing a new hospital on the St Stephen's site.

The study was carried out jointly by regional and district officers and was available in April 1987 for the May Health Authority meeting. Crucially it demonstrated that a new hospital could be fitted on to the St Stephen's site. The study assumed that maternity services would be provided from the new Westminster and Chelsea Hospital (as it was to be called) with a capacity of not less than 2,000 deliveries a year. This was considered by the Region to be the minimum viable size for a maternity unit and provision was made for fifty-four maternity beds and fourteen special care baby cots. Forty-six specialist paediatric beds were included.

Local acute bed provision was calculated by reference to the negotiations with Region over Riverside's bed target. In April 1987 there were 847 local acute beds available in the District. The medical schools calculation that 685 local acute beds were required for teaching contrasted with the Regional framework projection of 625 local acute beds in Riverside by 1994. The 'alternative futures' work yielded a median total of 736 local acute beds which was the basis used for the feasibility study. The deduction of 356 beds for Charing Cross left 389 local acute beds for the New Westminster and Chelsea Hospital. The study included plans for acute services for elderly people and for mentally ill people.

It was estimated that the development of the Westminster and Chelsea Hospital would enable the existing sites of Westminster Hospital and Westminster Children's Hospital to be sold. The St Mary Abbot's Hospital and West London Hospital would be sold following reprovision of services. The sale of sites was estimated at £39m. The cost of redeveloping the West Wing but leaving the East Wing intact was estimated at £34m with an additional £5m needed to develop community-based facilities to replace St Mary Abbot's Hospital.

Informal consultation on the feasibility study commenced after the Health Authority meeting in May. On 7 May the Regional General Manager, Mr David Kenny had received a letter from Mr Graham Hart of the NHS Management Board outlining the Department's views and emphasised the sensitivity of the closure of the Westminster Hospital:

> I am writing to confirm that we are content for Riverside to begin informal discussion on a 2-DGH option for the future of hospital services in Riverside, and in particular on the possibility of rebuilding the Westminster Hospital on a new site.
>
> There is one particular aspect which we should like you to consider at an early stage. This concerns the future availability of services in the vicinity of the Parliamentary complex at Westminster should the Westminster Hospital move. You have suggested that a health centre might be established in this part of Riverside to provide services for both those living in the neighbourhood, and for those working in it, but in association with full accident and emergency services and major in-patient facilities being provided by St Thomas' Hospital.
>
> We would be grateful if you would assess at an early stage this aspect of any proposal being considered and come forward with positive proposals for future services.

A number of views emerged from the informal consultation process. It became apparent that medical staff at Westminster Hospital would not be satisfied with the move to a revamped St Stephen's Hospital. They did not regard the plan as providing for a proper teaching hospital on the

St Stephen's site. This view reflected the traditional disdain the Westminster Hospital clinicians had for St Stephen's Hospital, because although it participated fully in undergraduate teaching it was not a fully fledged teaching hospital and its origins as a workhouse infirmary reinforced this impression. This potentially represented a serious difficulty in bringing the project to fruition.

In general medical staff accepted the principle of the concentration of acute services as did the District Medical Committee. The medical school's support in principle was tempered by the proposals falling short of their aspirations in terms of the inadequacy of certain academic facilities.

At the June Health Authority meeting the other possible site options for the hospital were discussed. The Authority accepted that work already completed on the 'St Mary Abbot's option' in 1984 and 1985 had produced sufficient information to make a further option appraisal unnecessary. The District General Manager reiterated that in addition to the costs of the developments and its viability, on a site only two miles from St Mary's, Paddington, there were doubts about the willingness of the local authority to grant planning permission.

In reviewing the prospects for the Brompton option it was apparent that a split site would be necessary using the Brompton Hospital (North) site which was due to be vacated in 1990 after the completion of the redevelopment of the Brompton, and the Chelsea College of Science and Technology site. However, the Chelsea College site was unlikely to be available prior to 1993 and would necessitate an expensive deep core design. The use of a split-site presented many planning difficulties which would have required detailed negotiations with the Planning Authority. The delays and uncertainty about if the scheme could be brought to a satisfactory conclusion and the potential cost of the scheme persuaded the Authority that the preliminary review of the Brompton site did not justify proceeding to a detailed feasibility study.

A second concern put the almost diametrically opposed view. While accepting the principle of the concentration of acute services on two district general hospitals the community units wished to see the new hospital having the character of a local community hospital, rather than be dominated by services and departments which derived from the commitment to ensure that the new hospital was a major university hospital.

The Authority accepted that there was sufficient support to proceed to the next stage of planning. This had two main elements. First, a revised functional concept for the proposed hospital which was to form the basis of the consultation documentation. Second, a further review of the strategic options to inform the option appraisal which would form part of the consultation document.

The Authority agreed, and work began on the revised functional content of the new hospital to take account of the criticisms levelled at the plan. The allocation of specialities to the new hospital accepted that the departments based at Charing Cross would not alter and the remaining specialties were placed in the Westminster and Chelsea Hospital. However, as the district and region planners worked in the Autumn to devise a functional content for the new hospital difficulties emerged.

St. Stephen's: from phased redevelopment to demolition

As a result of the debate generated by the feasibility study, senior management in collaboration with the Region and external surveyors advice prepared a report which examined in detail the site development options at St Stephen's. It was published in February 1988 and rejected a number of the assumptions in the St Stephen's feasibility study as follows:

1. Theatres required expansion not total replacement
2. ITU was adequate
3. X-ray required expansion not total replacement
4. A & E could adequately be expanded
5. UGC space requirements were minimal
6. A significant amount of accommodation could be located in the area now occupied by the Kobler centre
7. East wing assessed to be in reasonable condition
8. Rehabilitation required minimal expansion not total replacement.

A major recalculation of the new buildings on the St Stephen's site had to be undertaken. The inclusion of new theatres, a new ITU and cardiology facilities, not previously identified resulted in major increase in demands for space. Signals from the Region during the Autumn suggested that to meet the revised space requirements would overload the site and the architect was not confident that the revised space requirements could be included. Concern also existed about the condition of the East Wing. Despite only having been built in the 1960s a study undertaken on the East Wing in November 1987 suggested that £11·3m would need to be spent to bring the Wing up to a total suitable condition for its existing use.

A major development on the western part of the site in tandem with the continued use of the East Wing raised concerns about the quality of patient care in the redevelopment phase, due to the problems associated with dust, dirt, noise, and additional traffic. The retention of the East Wing also reduced the overall flexibility in the use of the site which led to a less than ideal design solution because a number of the existing buildings were poorly located. Consequently, during the latter half of 1987 two inter-twined processes led to the need to fundamentally reappraise the option to develop St Stephen's. First, was the over-riding imperative to make the new hospital acceptable to the Westminster clinical staff. This involved a series of delicate informal negotiations with the Westminster consultants to accommodate their aspirations for a fully fledged teaching hospital. Second, work on the revised functional content indicated that it was no longer possible to fit all the specialties into a refurbished St Stephen's.

A possible solution was the demolition of the whole of St Stephen's site and the rebuilding of a new hospital from scratch. The Region had a new Director of Estates from the private sector who argued this type of solution was becoming more usual as experience from new buildings in the City of London demonstrated. However, this solution had massive implications. It effectively doubled the project from the closure of not only the Westminster but in addition St Stephen's. This raised the issue not only of the financial viability of the plan nor of the acceptability of the solution in particular to the St Stephen's clinicians but also the massive practical problem of finding sufficient accommodation to maintain services during the rebuilding period. The most pressing problem was that Riverside had agreed to issue a consultation document at the end of January 1988 and yet it was only in October 1987 that it was decided that a refurbished St Stephen's was not viable.

Senior management knew that the January deadline for the consultation document could not be breached, yet there was real concern about the need to clear the whole St Stephen's site. There was a real danger that such a radical change in strategy decided in a short space of time would alienate and disorientate groups who had been nurtured to support the strategy. Nonetheless, senior management decided this was a risk that had to be taken and decided to plan the consultation document on the basis of the demolition of St Stephen's.

In November a small working party began to examine the options for the decanting of services during the rebuilding period. This involved establishing the capacity of Charing Cross, and Westminster and searching for beds in other NHS hospitals or the private sector. At a meeting with the Region at the end of November the District acknowledged they were still short of 100 beds. The main specialties involved were orthopaedics and gynaecology. Discussion took place with other NHS hospitals and the independent sector. Agreement was reached with the Royal Masonic Hospital for 60 beds for elective orthopaedic surgery. This was attractive to the orthopaedic division who were keen to separate cold admissions from emergency work because of the disruptive impact of trauma work on their elective admissions and the difficulties that staff shortages in the operating theatres had created. The gynaecologists were less keen about their services being split between sites because of concerns about safety. Consequently, a series of capital schemes were used to enable gynaecology services for Riverside East to be provided at Westminster Hospital in line with the twenty-eight beds to be provided in the proposed Westminster and Chelsea Hospital.

Work started in earnest on the consultation document in December with a Riverside plan which involved the demolition of St Stephen's. This was revealed in informal discussions in November and December. It immediately kindled opposition at St Stephen's which in turn made the Westminster consultants waiver as they did not wish to confront their colleagues at St Stephen's. All sides began to gear up for a bruising battle ahead.

The Westminster and Chelsea Hospital Proposal

The proposal commenced by summarising the context in which Riverside had to operate. A number of salient points were outlined: the relatively high costs of local acute services in Riverside which in part derived from the inappropriate distribution of acute services between six sites; the priority in the Regional strategic framework which required Riverside to reduce their volume of local acute services from 851 beds to 736 beds in 1994. This was coupled to a reduction of £18m by 1994 in the overall revenue allocation of £140m in 1987/88.

The authors argued that the proposals met the need to contract services through a reduction of 115 local acute beds but in addition substantially improved the physical environment for service delivery yet also yielded revenue savings by the concentration of acute services on two sites.

The central proposal was for a new main teaching hospital, which it was emphasised would be complementary to Charing Cross, and was to be sited on the existing St Stephen's Hospital site. It was designed to have a capacity of 665 beds and to be recognised for undergraduate medical education. It was also to provide services for elderly people for that part of the District which lay within the Royal Borough of Kensington and Chelsea and the City of Westminster. Similary it was to provide acute mental illness services for the catchment population within the Royal Borough of Kensington and Chelsea.

The inpatient services at St Mary Abbot's from long-stay elderly and elderly mentally ill were to be replaced by new more community-based facilities. The proposals therefore would allow the eventual closure of the Westminster, Westminster Children's, St Mary Abbot's and West London Hospitals.

To complement the Westminster and Chelsea Hospital attention was given to future provision of health care in South Westminster. Many members of Parliament who had constituencies outside London did not have easy access to a general practitioner and looked to Westminster Hospital's medical staff for their health care. Reliance on the Westminster Hospital was not solely from the Palace of Westminster. The perceived lack of adequate primary care facilities was reinforced by two consumer surveys undertaken during 1985. In 1987 the Kensington and Chelsea and Westminster Family Practitioner Committee's analysis[2] of GPs distribution found that eight of the eleven practices in the area were located to the west of Vauxhall Bridge Road.

It was proposed to establish a primary health care facility in South Westminster. It aimed to provide services beyond those of traditional health care by providing consultant-based outpatient clinics, collecting points for diagnostic specimens and X-ray facilities in the health centre. Nurse practitioners were also to staff a walk-in service at the clinic.

The design and construction of the hospital was to be revolutionary for the NHS in that the Authority planned to use fast track construction methods adopted from private office developments. In particular the use of a management contract rather than a main contract ensured a quicker project through parallel working on site and the use of five tower cranes instead of only one. It was therefore planned to develop the hospital in $3\frac{1}{2}$ years and in only one phase which reduced by two-thirds the conventional time to plan, design, and build an NHS hospital. This one-off design and rapidity increased costs. The NHS cost yardsticks would have a allowed a budget of £82m, while the cost of the estimated new hospital using fast track building methods was between £97m and £131m. Obviously, revenue savings would come on stream quicker and were expected to flow from the following changes in District services:

1. a net reduction in local acute beds
2. a reduction in the unit cost per patient
3. the opportunity to reduce the number of hospital sites.

It was estimated that if the revenue consequences of the new hospital were in the order of £35m, the net revenue savings were in the Region of £15m.

2 *The Outlook for General Practice in Kensington and Chelsea and Westminster*, Kensington and Chelsea and Westminster Family Practitioner Committee, 1987.

The document concluded by summarising the merits of the proposal as follows:

> The particular configuration of acute services proposed, maximises effectiveness of service delivery for the catchment population as a whole, while meeting revenue targets set for the District by the RHA. It also creates opportunities for improvements both for acute services in a major new hospital, and for priority care services in the nursing homes and health care facilities. The capital developments represent a unique opportunity to provide modern buildings for the health care of the catchment population of Riverside into the twenty-first century. This is only achievable if the comprehensive and radical proposals presented in this document are implemented.

Members discussed the consultation document at their January 1988 meeting. Members requested further clarification of the Region's objections to a phased building programme on the St Stephen's site. The Region therefore agreed to prepare a report outlining the site development options at St Stephen's. On the issue of decanting members were informed that the Region had agreed to pay reasonable decanting costs during the construction period. Finally, members requested information on the effect on waiting lists of the reduction in the trauma and orthopaedic bed allocation. The acute UGM maintained that throughput levels would be sustained by use of the independent sector and an increase in day care facilities would compensate for the reduction in inpatient beds. It was agreed that the document be issued for formal consultation for three months.

'Four Hospitals into One Might Just Go'

The issue of the consultation document at the beginning of February aroused immediate interest and concern. In total approximately 2,500 copies of the document were distributed to organisations and individuals. A flurry of activity surrounded its release with considerable media interest, which was predominantly hostile to the proposals emphasising the cost saving nature of the package. The *Evening Standard* proclaimed 'Health experts fight to keep hospital open' which focused on the closure of the Westminster Children's Hospital. However, more favourable pieces appeared in *The Independent* and the *Health Services Journal*, the latter guardedly headlining 'Four hospitals into one might just go'.

The reaction within the District was a complex mixture of: incredulity; disbelief that the plan would occur; pockets of fierce resistance; and support from influential individuals who had given their support to the plan either through genuine belief in its merits, or due to a pragmatic acceptance of the way the tide was running.

Anguish at St Stephen's

Senior management had always been aware of the potential difficulty of closing Westminster Hospital. However, the change of strategy, with the demolition of St Stephen's dramatically altered the St Stephen's reaction to the project and produced an unanticipated level of opposition. This was particularly worrying for management as there had not been sufficient time to cultivate support at St Stephen's before the release of the document. Debate then took place in the public domain making it harder for people to change their views without losing face.

Furthermore, the Health Authority request for further information on site options at St Stephen's revealed that many members had yet to be convinced of the merit in demolishing St Stephen's. The risk existed that if support haemorrhaged at St Stephen's, Westminster could follow leaving the plan in tatters. The lack of detail on the decanting arrangements in the consultation document left management vulnerable to criticism.

Concern at St Stephen's was particularly marked amongst those clinicians who did not have any sessions at the Westminster Hospital and therefore felt particularly vulnerable about the closure of St Stephen's. There was also a feeling that St Stephen's was going to be absorbed into a greater Westminster Hospital and the name of the hospital, excluding any reference to St Stephen's, seemed to confirm these fears. The relationship between clinicians at Westminster and St Stephen's had been frosty and neither side was sanguine about their forthcoming union.

The most fundamental disagreement with the proposals concerned the likely disruption of medical services to the community during the redevelopment period of three-to-four years. A group of consultants at St Stephen's commissioned N. Lichfield and Partners, a group of planning development and economics consultants, to examine the community impact of the disruption of services. The report summarised the St Stephen's consultants concern:

> They consider that the disruption to medical services would be severe. They furthermore consider that the disruption could be averted if instead of complete clearance for redevelopment there was phased demolition and rebuilding on the site.

The report examined the impact of the proposals and compared the Health Authority's favoured option with a phased demolition and redevelopment over seven years (the rehabilitation option). However, although the report backed its sponsors inclination for a phased redevelopment, the report was extremely cautious in its advocacy of this position. In cost terms analysis of the two options was limited. On operating costs between the two proposals it stated 'no estimates are available'. Similarly on capital costs it acknowledged 'the difference between the options is uncertain'. Its strongest prediction was that the number of patients treated as a result of redevelopment would be less than with the rehabilitation option. Yet even here conclusions were tempered by recognition that cross-boundary flows made it difficult to predict the impact on waiting lists. The final analysis was cautious:

> It cannot be said, however, that a clear conclusion emerges as to whether rehabilitation or redevelopment is the preferred option in the community interest.

Consequently the faltering tone of the report raised sufficient doubts about its conclusions that the report failed to gain credibility amongst medical staff and did not become significant in the deliberations over the proposals.

In addition senior management were advancing a 'there is no alternative' line and were using a study written by the Region: *St Stephen's Hospital site development options* to pursue this line. The report examined four major possibilities for site development and concluded in favour of total site demolition and rebuilding in a single phase because it would be quicker, therefore releasing revenue savings earlier and would result in a more satisfactory hospital.

The consequences for AIDS patients were also an area of controversy. The Kobler day centre for AIDS patients was to remain on the St Stephen's site during the construction of the new hospital. However, the centre was designed for outpatient and day centre care with the assumption of inpatient beds on site. The danger was that the AIDS patients would no longer wish to be treated at the Kobler centre and that unavailability or dislike of the Westminster would divert patients to St Thomas's or Charing Cross. The Authority weakly replied that the temporary location of inpatient services at Westminster Hospital would not put at risk the integrated concept of care that had been developed at St Stephen's because particular arrangements would be made to ensure that medical staff could move easily between sites.

A more intractable area of discussion was the impact on accident and emergency services of the closure of St Stephen's for three years during the rebuilding period. In January 1988 the Academic Department of Community Medicine published their investigation of patient flows for accident and emergency cases which examined the likely effects of:

1. permanent closure of Westminster Hospital's Accident and Emergency Department:

2. temporary closure of the Accident and Emergency Department at St Stephen's whilst rebuilding was taking place.

The report concluded that:

1. Temporary closure of the St Stephen's site would result in an increase in A&E workload of approximately 37 per cent at the Westminster and 22 per cent at Charing Cross.
2. Permanent closure of Westminster would result in an increase in A&E workload of approximately 35 per cent at St Thomas's and 5 per cent at St Stephen's.

It also commented on the planned closure of St James's Balham in August 1988: 'if that hospital were to close whilst a hospital was being rebuilt on the St Stephen's site chaos would ensue'.

Opponents made political capital out of the report and the above quotation in particular. However, the Authority acknowledged that resources would need to be injected into the Westminster Hospital which tempered opposition. In addition inter-Regional discussions were taking place to resolve the issue of St James'. More significantly, the thrust of the report and a further document from the Department of Community Medicine implied that the Westminster and Chelsea Hospital on the basis of the epidemiological evidence was too large and fewer beds would be sufficient. It consequently proved easy to undermine the position of the Department of Community Medicine as the notion that the hospital should be smaller won the Department few allies.

The Westminster Hospitals Development Fund

Although opposition had flared at St Stephen's the expectation had been that the most concerted opponents of the scheme would be based at the Westminster. Consequently, clinicians at the Westminster had been cultivated to support the project through the offer of a new teaching hospital. This led to a mixed reaction when the document was published. Strong loyalty remained for the Westminster Hospital but many of the younger clinicians in particular recognised the way the tide was running having witnessed the gradual removal of specialties from the Westminster, the most recent having been the decision to centralise oncology services at Charing Cross. The limited support afforded to the oncology department at the Westminster (who opposed the move) by the rest of the clinical body was a portent of the general grudging acceptance of the Westminster and Chelsea.

The most focused opposition came under the auspices of the Westminster Hospitals Development Fund. The fund was set up to oppose the proposals and had the central purpose of fighting for the retention *in* Westminster of the Westminster Hospital and the Westminster

Children's Hospital. It moved quickly, holding meetings at the House of Lords, and attracted to their cause Viscount Tonypandy as their President and a Nobel Laureate, Professor Dorothy Hodgkin as their patron. Lord Ennals, Secretary of State for Health (from 1976-9), became Chairman and he proved to be a valuable asset due to his proximity to the citadel of power where he could lobby for the fund.

The fund drew up alternative proposals which they submitted to Riverside in the hope that they would be considered on a par with Riverside's own proposals. The main elements of the fund's proposals were:

1. A new Westminster Teaching Hospital comprising 364 acute beds;

2. A slightly larger Westminster Children's Hospital, comprising 100 beds;

3. An academic building comprising all the requirements for the continued training of doctors and nurses. In addition this academic centre was to provide eight floors of convalescent beds, totalling 364 beds;

4. The retention of St Stephen's Hospital.

The fund maintained that the scheme could be self-financing through the use of land sales, but their estimates on revenue savings were vague. Senior management were sceptical about the funds proposal which argued that more beds could be provided on the Westminster site while reducing revenue costs. The proposals were not in tune with national policy in advocating increased levels of paediatric beds or the provision of convalescent beds in a hospital environment. However, it was not primarily the feasibility of their proposals which was the litmus test in terms of the amount of support they were able to attract, rather it was their approach which raised doubts amongst potential supporters.

First, the clinicians involved in the fund were not particularly senior in the medical hierarchy of the Westminster Hospital. Senior clinicians disliked being represented by these individuals which made them less willing to support the fund. The fund therefore failed to galvanise support amongst those individuals who could have leant weight to their campaign. Second, there was a perception that the fund was primarily concerned with the face of the Westminster Children's Hospital. This reduced its appeal as the paediatricians enjoyed an uneasy relationship with the rest of the consultant body. Management exploited this perception by arguing that the fund was solely interested in the fate of the Children's Hospital. Third, the fund proved insufficiently sensitive to the position of St Stephen's. They failed to understand the resentment and suspicion of the St Stephen's clinicians at the focus on the Westminster which was going to survive albeit on a different site. Consequently, the fund was unable to broaden its support beyond the confines of the Westminster. Fourth, a number of Westminster clinicians felt disquiet about the manner in which a signature appeal from former medical students at the Westminster Hospital had been used which reinforced doubts about the fund.

The impact of the fund was limited although could never be ignored by the Authority due to its links to the Palace of Westminster. The fund obtained a meeting with Kenneth Clarke and David Mellor in September 1988 where their proposals were considered. However, this reflected more on the political acumen of Lord Ennals than the strength of the fund's support. Ultimately the failure of the fund to obtain any public backing from the Westminster consultant body left its credibility in tatters.

If the situation at St Stephen's and Westminster were characterised by upheaval, in marked contrast the position at Charing Cross was relatively tranquil. Charing Cross had always been detached from the machinations about the future of Westminster and St Stephen's as they felt developments in Riverside East would have little impact on them. Two discernible views emerged at Charing Cross.

There was scepticism about the likelihood of the Westminster and Chelsea emerging but even if it happened, the new hospital was not viewed as a threat to Charing Cross's pre-eminence in the District as it increasingly gathered on its site a cluster of supra-District and Regional specialties. The planning for the new hospital confirmed this position as it had always taken the location of specialties at Charing Cross as immutable.

Charing Cross was not completely immune from the situation in the District which was deteriorating rapidly and had been exacerbated by the postponing of short-term remedial action in 1987. The Authority carried forward a budget deficit in 1987/88 and with the District's contribution to the Regional Strategic Development Fund required savings of £8·9m in 1989/90. Consequently, Charing Cross were eager that Riverside East's financial difficulties were resolved so that the District could be placed on a more solid financial footing.

The CHC Response

The Riverside Community Health Council were not prepared for the extent of the changes proposed in the consultation document, but immediately set up four working groups to consider the proposals. The CHC felt it faced a number of difficulties in representing the views of the public.

First, the CHC consistently complained about the lack of detail in the document and this led the CHC to ask for over 150 clarifications to the document during the consultation period. This reflected the rushed manner in which the document was compiled. Second, the CHC believed a three month consultation period was insufficient for proposals of such magnitude. The CHC's request for a six week extension to the consultation period was rejected which reinforced the view in the CHC that the proposals were dictated by financial considerations and were to be implemented regardless of the level of public opposition. Third, the CHC contained many diverse interest groups which made it harder for a unified position to emerge as different communities were affected by the proposals in different ways. Fourth, the only survey that the CHC had time to conduct reflected this diversity. A survey of GP opinion yielded such varied responses that the CHC found it impossible to draw conclusions. Finally many CHC members recognised the financial situation the Health Authority faced and had reservations about simply opposing the Health Authority position. As the CHC Chairman commented in his oral response at the Health Authority meeting on 26 May 1988:

> We know the financial constraints you were facing and made every effort to treat them sympathetically. Your task would have been easier if the health service were adequately funded and if the RAWP redistribution processes were working out as intended. It is not your fault that DHAs in Bedfordshire and Hertfordshire are also in deficit and finding it difficult to complete their expansion plans.

Nonetheless the CHC had overwhelming reservations about the proposals and formally opposed the plan. The CHC rejected the 115 bed reduction, were particularly anxious about accident and emergency provision doubting the ability of the Westminster to cope and mirrored the concern at St Stephen's about AIDS services. The CHC was also critical of Riverside's failure to mention the inevitable patient flow to St Thomas' Hospital.

The CHC managed to command significant media attention but ultimately as the District had the backing of the Regional Health Authority its influence was always likely to be of limited significance. This did not mean the Health Authority ignored the CHC. They would have preferred to gain their support, which some managers believed was possible despite the CHC secretary being implacably opposed, and a number of senior clinicians were despatched to the CHC meeting when the document was discussed, to put the Authority's view. However, the views of the CHC were peripheral compared to the importance of the ferment within the DHA itself.

Campaign for the Defence of Riverside

A host of other organisations commented on the proposals. The campaign for the Defence of Riverside (CAMDOR) was an offshoot of trade union organisation in Riverside. It was established prior to the publication of the consultation document in July 1987 to oppose the reduction of NHS provision in Riverside and latterly the Westminster and Chelsea project. CAMDOR had strong links with Hammersmith and Fulham Health Authority members and the local Labour MP, Clive Soley, who presented a petition with 50,000 signatures to Parliament opposing the closures.

CAMDOR's style of protest was initially direct with a series of road-block demonstrations pin-pointing the threatened hospitals. Towards the end of 1988 CAMDOR began to concentrate on the need for Riverside to gain planning permission from Kensington and Chelsea Borough Council with the aim of lobbying the council to refuse planning permission. This activity was assisted by the pressure group Planning Aid for London. CAMDOR's activity was very visible and they had a ready-made organisation through their roots in Riverside trade union structures. However, they faced a number of obstacles in waging a successful campaign.

First, the Health Authority had implemented a no compulsory redundancy policy. Although this did not prevent considerable discloation for staff and significant job losses, it drew the sting from CAMDOR's campaign as staff were not so directly threatened. Second, it proved harder to campaign successfully across the District than for an individual hospital, as people did not identify with the District as a whole. Finally, as the Health Authority was ultimately trying to persuade the Government about the merit of their proposals the opposition of a trade union backed organisation was unlikely to be a major impediment to their chances of success.

Neighbouring Health Authorities were naturally concerned about the impact of reductions in service on patient flows to their hospitals with West Lambeth District which contained St Thomas' Hospital the most vocal. The Kensington and Chelsea and Westminster Family Practitioner Committee welcomed the proposed developments in primary health care but wanted the character of a DGH to be retained in the new hospital. The London Borough of Hammersmith and Fulham opposed the proposal and deplored the finance-led nature of the proposed development. Westminster City Council also opposed the plans and in particular the closure of the Westminster Hospital. This could create difficulties in the future over the sale of the Westminster Hospital site.

Although a range of opposition groups were amassed against the proposals, the Health Authority had a number of powerful allies. The Charing Cross and Westminster Medical School were supportive of the plan. The medical school was largely reactive in its responses to Riverside's plans. Its primary concern was to maitain sufficient beds in the District to meet the requirements for medical education and the revised figure for local acute beds of 736 beds fulfilled their needs. The medical school also carried out clinical teaching not only at Charing Cross and Westminster, but also at St Stephen's, West London, West Middlesex and Queen Mary's, Roehampton.

Consequently, in one sense it was less concerned than other groups about the particular configuration of acute services because of the range of sites available. However, the medical school did not like being on so many sites because it raised costs and made internal communications more difficult. It was therefore supportive of the reduction in the number of sites and attracted by the prospects of a new teaching hospital. Although the medical school did not play a major part in the discussions about Westminster and Chelsea, the project could not have proceeded without their support.

The medical staff in Riverside formally supported the proposals through the District Medical Committee. The DMC chairman in particular played a role in countering opposition from disaffected groups of clinicians within the District. It was essential that the proposals were not seen as a purely managerial strategy to affect change. The support of the DMC not only gave legitimacy to the proposals but also undermined clinical opposition. This was particularly important in the public arena as when letters appeared in *The Times* in March 1988 and *The Independent* in September 1988 attacking the proposals, the response of the Authority was signed by the Chairman of the District Medical Committee.

As the consultation period drew to a close management reflected on the array of responses to the document, it now remained up to the Health Authority to frame their response.

The Authority Decides

Riverside Health Authority met on 26 May 1988 to consider the outcome of the formal consultation document and the commentary written by officers in response to consultation. They argued the proposals constituted the most effective way of reducing revenue expenditure while at the same time improving services.

Members had reservations about the impact of the proposals on neighbouring districts and wanted assurances that the project would proceed in its entirety before reductions in service outlined in the consultation document were contemplated. After discussion the Health Authority Chairman proposed the following motion:

> That the proposals detailed in the consultation document should be adopted by the Authority and that the Authority will not commence the decanting of clinical services from St Stephen's Hospital until it has secured assurances from the Regional Health Authority that the total project will proceed.

This motion was passed with thirteen votes in favour and three votes against.

The proposals were then referred to the Regional Health Authority for a decision. They agreed the proposal at their meeting of 9 June 1988 and referred the proposal to the Secretary of State for a decision.

During this period a great deal of activity was taking place. At the Region the Approval in Principle submission was being drawn up which was the detailed planning submission for the Department of Health. It identified the Regional strategy to achieve greater equality of access to local acute services and develop priority services by 1994. It outlined the requirement to match patterns of service to population trends and it high-lighted the inefficient fragmentation of services in the provision of services in the District. Detailed appraisal of the options re-iterated support for the Westminster and Chelsea Hospital project.

At district level work continued on a number of fronts. There was a need to translate the no compulsory redundancy policy into a viable strategy given that there would be an overall reduction of 650 jobs as a result of the project. It was believed this would not create difficulties due to the historically high levels of staff turnover in London Hospitals and the shortages of staff in particular specialties. Experience gained from the closure of Banstead Hospital in 1986 was used where change had been facilitated by the use of a staff bureau.

The purpose of the staff bureau established at St Stephen's Hospital was to assist managers to get the right people into appropriate jobs in the new organisation and to counsel staff about their future. In the main this worked successfully but two caveats are necessary. Firstly, tensions existed between district and unit staff, as unit staff wanted to pick and choose staff in a manner that was not always compatible with the no compulsory redundancy policy. Consequently, unit managers felt at times that staff were foisted on them. Secondly, the attention to the needs of staff at St Stephen's led to a relative neglect of the needs of staff at the Westminster Hospital. However, staff at the receiving hospital were also experiencing great change and had anxieties about the transfer of large numbers of staff from St Stephen's.

Decanting arrangements were also being drawn up. This involved almost seventy enabling schemes to help transfer services from St Stephen's Hospital, and to reorganise services at St Mary Abbot's Hospital. Schemes ranged from a £2,000 scheme to re-site the St Mary Abbot's Hospital Library to a £1·3m scheme to furnish a hospital block to provide forty-one beds. This was to enable services at St Mary Abbot's Hospital to be concentrated on one half of the site releasing the other half for land sales. Other work included negotiating with clinicians about the interim arrangements, devising a residential accommodation strategy and ensuring satisfactory public relations.

Apart from the agreement of the Secretary of State the most critical hurdle that still faced the Health Authority was obtaining planning permission from Kensington and Chelsea's Planning Committee to build the Westminster and Chelsea Hospital.

Kensington and Chelsea had an ambivalent attitude towards the project. They regretted that it had proved impossible to sustain all three District General Hospitals within Riverside. They lent cautious support to the project as they wanted a hospital within the Borough, but had reservations about the scale of the development in the middle of a residential area of Chelsea. The Region took informal soundings from Kensington and Chelsea who raised questions on the size of building in particular. This led the Region to defer their planning application which was due for consideration at the September 1988 meeting of the Kensington and Chelsea's Planning Committee.

The Committee was lobbied to approve the plan with Conservative councillors facing the possibility of opposing a plan which the Health Secretary, Kenneth Clarke, seemed set to approve. The District believed that if planning permission was refused a successful appeal could be lodged. However, this would have lead to a lengthy delay and jeopardised a good relationship with the Borough whose support was necessary for the crucial sale of the St Mary Abbot's site. Consequently, concessions had to be made, in particular one floor of the new building had to be removed. This increased the size of the new hospital's footprint but the Planning Committee all voted for the hospital plan to proceed.

A final decision now rested with the new Secretary of State for Health, Kenneth Clarke. There were mixed feelings within the Authority about the prospects for the plan's approval. A number assumed that the Region and a select group of individuals would never have invested so much effort nor relied so heavily on Riverside releasing revenue for the Regional strategy unless tacit approval had been gained from the Department of Health to close the Westminster Hospital. However, other staff felt that the delay in making the decision, and adverse publicity during September and October coupled with a change of

Minister had left the decision in the balance. The deliberations of the Health Service Review further complicated the issue.

On 22 December 1988, Riverside were informed that ministerial approval had been granted.

CONCLUSION

Riverside have embarked on an audacious programme of re-organisation in the District which has proceeded rapidly from conception to execution. Other health authorities who face similar predicaments with shrinking populations and budgets have been watching the experience of Riverside intently. Bloomsbury have recently launched a plan to rationalise services and build a new teaching hospital arguing this is the only way to remain financially viable; similar proposals have emerged in Parkside. Other cities are not immune from this process. In Birmingham, plans have been drawn up to close at least eight hospitals and amalgamate two health districts into one.

The closure of a hospital or hospitals always generates controversy regardless of the merits of the case for its closure because of the ties that staff and the wider community have developed with the institution. Yet the 1980s have witnessed closures of famous hospitals, even in the face of vigorous campaigns opposed to closure. This raises questions about the nature of the management of change in the NHS.

In Riverside a number of factors contributed to the achievement of change. The establishment of the Authority itself provided new opportunities to change service provision as the combination of two health authorities enabled the self-sufficiency assumptions of each former health authority to be examined and services to be centralised on fewer sites. The combination of the medical schools reinforced this momentum for change. Consequently from 1984/85 onwards management has been creating an atmosphere that portrayed change as inevitable, but was careful to avoid specifying the changes that were anticipated. This was until a coalition of support had been built to ensure the changes would occur regardless of the inevitable opposition that would be spawned by any plans to close a hospital.

This strategy was a clear departure from the rational planning approach which health authorities pursued in the 1960s and 1970s. This assumed that if the most rational planning solution was devised based on objective information of patient flows, transport patterns, population changes, and financial viability, ultimately people could be convinced of the merits of a plan even if it included unpalatable elements notably hospital closures. Belief in this type of approach had become frayed during the 1970s due to recognition that planning was not a purely technical process but was also intrinsically political and that future uncertainties jeopardised plans made years in advance.

In Riverside, management believed that achieving change was essentially a process of political negotiation and that building a workable consensus was of greater importance than the actual details of where services were to be located. This process involved identifying key groups and individuals and ascertaining their conditions for supporting change. It involved being pragmatic about the particular service that would evolve rather than adhering rigidly to formal planning criteria.

However, the success of this type of approach is dependent partly on its covert nature. Management had to adhere publicly to the formal planning process and concepts for three reasons. Firstly, if management had admitted that their favoured solution was no more rational or appropriate than others, this would have undermined their credibility and their arguments that no viable alternative existed. Consequently, new avenues of debate which they did not wish to pursue would have been opened up. Secondly, it could have jeopardised the support of many powerful interest groups who would not have wished to have it acknowledged that their support was due to private benefits rather than 'the public good'. Finally, it would have raised wider issues about services, as critics might have concluded that plans were drawn up to satisfy producer rather than consumer needs.

Management identified the key groups who would be needed to sanction change. The closure of the Westminster Hospital was clearly going to need the support of the Department of Health due to its proximity to the Houses of Parliament. Therefore, if no support was forthcoming from these quarters the prospects would be bleak. Furthermore, as the idea of the new Westminster and Chelsea Hospital emerged, the agreement of the Secretary of State would be required and in turn the Treasury would need to be consulted on the cost of the scheme. Hence in early 1986 when the Health Authority first discussed the retention of St Stephen's or the Westminster the District Chairman approached the Minister for Health recognising not only that decisions on the future of hospital services would require ministerial approval, but also that no previous minister had been prepared to countenance the closure of the Westminster.

The Region was a key actor in any proposed changes and the District recognised that without Regional support it would not be possible to bring their plans to fruition. The Region was nationally the highest above its RAWP target and therefore faced a period of financial retrenchment, but this was not to be evenly distributed across the Region. Instead the inner-London Districts with historically generous levels of provision but declining populations were expected to free-up resources to support developments in the shire counties.

It was the magnitude of change in Riverside's case and their centrality to the success of the Regional strategy that necessitated Regional support in helping Riverside bring about change. The District did not view the Region as an adversary, judging that the reduction in their resource level was in the main justified and that a more satisfactory outcome would result if they worked cooperatively with the Region to affect this reduction. Consequently, as Riverside established a reputation of being helpful and delivering on their promises, regional officers allowed management more room for manoeuvre than they allowed other authorities. A notable example of this approach was the decision to absolve Riverside of the need to submit a District Strategic Plan in 1986.

At District level a different gloss was put on the relationship with Region. It was useful for management to be able to legitimate decisions by recourse to arguments about change being imposed from above. This was a useful tool in gaining acceptance for unpalatable changes, for example, the local acute bed numbers, but at the same time allowed senior management to gain victories with the Region (an upwardly revised bed target) and appear to be gaining the best outcome for the District.

Internally a number of groups needed to be persuaded of the merits of the proposed changes. The potentially most powerful dissenters were likely to be the medical staff at the hospital earmarked for closure. Management moved on a number of fronts. First, the medical advisory machinery was reformed in order to try and shape it into a form which would be more supportive of managerial objectives. Management tried to shape the District Medical Committee (DMC) so that it was not dominated by any particular hospital and therfore could be viewed as reflecting a corporate view across the District enabling management to argue that medical committees at individual hospitals were inevitably partisan and that only the DMC should be taken seriously. The DMC had started to forge this corporate voice by preventing the committee being totally dominated by the Charing Cross Hospital, by ensuring a consultant at the Westminster Hospital was the first chairman. Nonetheless, this did not significantly reduce the influence of the Charing Cross Hospital as it still provided the dominant voice in the District. The DMC therefore tried to neutralise clinical voices which were opposed to change and was important in delivering clinical support for the strategy.

A second managerial strand in cultivating clinical support was the incentives offered to clinicians in accepting hospital closures. The rebuilding of St Stephen's plan which was favoured in early 1987 was abandoned because it was not sufficiently attractive an option to persuade the Westminster clinicians to accept the closure of the Westminster. It was only the creation of a new teaching hospital that would be sufficient to ensure that the bulk of the Westminster clinicians would support the plan.

A third strand was the manner in which debate within the Health Authority was channelled towards the achievement of management objectives. The decision-making process was tightly controlled with senior managers refusing to accede to demands for the establishment of committees to carry out the planning activity. Instead a small number of individuals were coopted to undertake various planning activities. This also helped the authority to argue that no viable alternative plan existed and this was a position sustained throughout the consultation period and beyond.

An additional important factor in helping to bring about change was the role of the King's Fund College and the use of multi-scenario planning. First the use of an academic body helped to legitimate the necessary changes because Riverside could appeal to the neutrality and objectivity of the advice they were gaining from the King's Fund as a vehicle for change. However, the nature of multi-scenario planning is that it does not close off options but rather views planning as an evolutionary process based on a series of short term incremental decisions. This provided senior management with maximum flexibility to adapt the strategy to the political circumstances pertaining in the District in order to fashion a workable consensus.

However, once it was judged that a sufficient coalition existed to achieve support for the Westminster and Chelsea Hospital project the malleability of multi-scenario planning (and consequently the risk of alternative options emerging) was abandoned and instead management argued 'There is no alternative'.

The viability of the strategy and its success was heavily dependent on the value of land sales. In particular the large St Mary Abbot's Hospital site in the heart of Kensington was central to the viability of the plan. It was estimated that sale of half of the St Mary Abbot's site and the Westminster and Westminster Children's would yield over £40m. The intention was that the land sales would be sufficient to cover the capital costs as it was clear that finance would not be forthcoming from the Treasury. However, the land sales have not proved to be sufficient for two reasons.

First, to win support for the scheme extra facilities had to be provided. The most significant change came from the redevelopment of St Stephen's Hospital, estimated at £34m, to the establishment of a new hospital costed initially at between £97m and £131m. However, the estimated cost of the new hospital and associated developments has continued to rise to a figure approaching £173m—a change which reflects poor capital costing and indexing, exacerbated by the rising costs of labour in the building industry in the south of England.

A final difficulty has been the fall in value of the land being sold, reflecting not only the fickle state of the property market but also a change of heart by Kensington and Chelsea Borough Council who have not allowed as many residential units to be built on the vacated half of the St Mary Abbot's site as originally planned, hence reducing the value of the land sales. The consequences are that the Region could ultimately have to use funds from the Regional capital programme to sustain the project.

For the District the more immediate problem will be its commitment on the revenue side. This commitment to funnel over £15m per annum into the Regional Strategic Development Fund is immutable as, without this flow, the Regional policy of developing facilities in the shire counties will not be achievable. The whole rationale for the Region of developing the Westminster and Chelsea Hospital to facilitate reducing Riverside's budget would fail without this release of resources. The degree to which the new hospital will save revenue is not clear as no good methodology exists for costing new facilities.

The White Paper: A Further Complication

The White Paper will add a further dimension to the equation, as in future hospitals will be providers of care, selling their services to purchasers rather than automatically receiving allocations as at present. In the post-White Paper era, workload levels in hospitals, units and departments will depend on contractual obligations to purchasers, from within and outside the District. This will increase uncertainty. Riverside have adopted an ironically inflexible strategy, perhaps saddling themselves with an expensive new hospital just as the chill winds of competition and capital charges raise questions about the project.

Only safeguards agreed by Region (and, by implication, the Department of Health) can ensure that patient flows fit the planned provision of services in Riverside. This will mean the regulation of competition.

CHAPTER 3

Case study: Northville Western

THE ORIGIN OF NORTHVILLE WESTERN

Northville Western Health Authority (NWHA) came into existence in 1982 with the abolition of the Area Health Authority which had been responsible for planning services across the whole city. The Area Health Authority had been unable to produce a strategic plan that satisfied all parties in Northville. In particular it had proved difficult to reach agreement on the provision of acute services across the city and this situation had been exacerbated by the growing rivalry between the two teaching hospitals in the city. Attempts to resolve these differences by establishing one health authority were resisted by the rival camps, centred around the teaching hospitals. Consequently in 1982 the city was split vertically in half creating two authorities covering the west and east of the city. The creation of the NWHA and the requirement for districts to produce their own strategic plan rekindled the debate about the provision of acute services in the city.

Description of the District

Northville Western Health Authority has a resident population of 361,000 (OPCS 1981 census) covering the western half of the city and Wharfetown, a market town in the north of the district of 12,000 population with its own hospital services. There are additional pockets of population to the west of the city. There are considerable cross-boundary flows between the two health authorities and outflows to the neighbouring authorities to the south-west of the city. The Authority in 1984 was providing services from eleven hospital sites on a revenue budget in excess of £70m. The main sites and their position in the District are illustrated simply at Appendix 1. The dominant hospital (A) was the teaching hospital for the District located in the centre of the city but on a crowded site hemmed in by developments on all sides and housed in predominantly Victorian buildings of poor functional suitability. A new wing (Hospital B) had been added on the site catering primarily for the specialities of Obstetrics, Gynaecology and Paediatrics.

Hospital C which was located outside the authority's boundaries in Northville Eastern Health Authority (NEHA) was predominantly hutted accommodation of very poor quality. Hospital D is situated on the North-Western outskirts of the city while the hospital in Wharfe-town (Hospital E) was on the northern perimeter of the district. The main hospitals relevant to this study are listed in Table 5.

TABLE 5. *Hospital provision in Northville Western Health Authority with bed numbers and main specialities, 1985*

Hospital	*Bed Numbers* (1985)	*Main Specialities*
A	657	General Medicine (152 General Surgery (124) *Regional Specialities* Neurology (17) Cardiology (23) Neurosurgery (24) Plastic Surgery (5) Thoriacic Surgery (26) Nephrology (13) *Area Specialities* Rheumatology (6) Opthalmology (23) ENT Surgery (24)
B	276	Paediatric Medicine (31) Paediatric Surgery (29) Gynaecology (184) Obstetrics (96) Special Care Baby Unit (36)
C	346	Geriatric Medicine (156) General Medicine (72) General Surgery (49)
D	154	Radiotherapy (154)
E	195	General Medicine (46) General Surgery (55) Orthopaedic Surgery (22) Geriatric Medicine (156)
F	848	Mental Illness: All categories (848)
G	235	Geriatric Medicine (156) Chest Diseases (26) Mental Illness (32)
H	58	Convalescent
DISTRICT TOTAL	3,030	

SOURCE: Northville Western Health Authority, DHA Strategic Plan 1985

The Management structure of the Authority was altering dramatically at the beginning of the review process with the implementation of the Griffiths report and the appointment of district and unit general managers. Five units of management were established on the basis of geographical and functional planning responsibilities. For example one unit contained Hospital C and district wide planning responsibilities for services for the elderly. A six-person Management Board reported to the District General Manager but did not involve the Unit General Managers who had their own Unit General Manager forum. The extent to which these two separate bodies were able to link up was to be important for the success of the review.

The professional advisory machinery had two strands. Faculty represented all NHS clinicians in Northville Western Health Authority with an executive Steering committee which represented Faculty via the District Medical Officer to the District General Manager. Faculty itself had twelve separate functional divisions (i.e. paediatrics, dentistry, etc) and geographical divisions representing particular hospitals or groups of hospitals. The second strand comprised a separate scientific advisory function (SSEC) which had four divisions (clinical science, radiotherapy, radiology and pathology) which also reported through the District Medical Officer to the District General Manager.

Shaping the Future

In 1983 Northville Western District Health Authority began preparing their first strategic plan. The District Administrator in June 1983 prepared a discussion paper on the strategy for hospital services in the District which was tabled at the District Management Team. The immediate catalyst for the report had been a management of change workshop attended by the District Administrator where he realised that the changes facing the District were so far reaching that there was a need to move beyond the crude mechanics of bed reductions and changes in use of hospitals to the involvement of staff and members in shaping the future. The District Administrator was keen to find out whether and how key individuals in the District perceived problems and to generate a debate on overcoming them. The District Administrator outlined this task in shaping the future as:

> To seek a consensus on current problems and future goals, provide the framework for shorter-term operational planning and closure changes—of—use proposals and facilitate the production in 1984 of a ten year strategic plan under the NHS Planning system.

For management, the Authority faced three serious predicaments. First, was the serious and deteriorating *financial* situation with a gross deficit of £1·4m 1982/83. This situation was not new, in 1975 the Area Health Authority had taken emergency action to correct an over spend of £300,000. The situation worsened after the 1982 re-organisation with the opening of the new wing, (Hospital B) and the District being in excess of its RAWP target. National policy which imposed efficiency savings and underfunded pay awards accentuated the financial difficulties facing the District.

Second, the *distribution* of institutions, services and patients across the District was viewed as unsatisfactory. Ten per cent of hospital beds were unused and unstaffed which led, because they were scattered across the District, to an inefficient use of physical and financial resources. For example, geriatric beds were poorly distributed leading to elderly patients occupying acute beds with access to investigative, rather than rehabilitation facilities. This created a situation in which there was regular dislocation of cold elective surgery at Hospital A preventing the planning of clinical services and compounding the variation in activity and workload across the District.

A third difficulty was the fact that published norms, adjusted for teaching and supra-district specialities implied that the District had 100-120 acute beds in *excess* of what should have been required to meet its requirements. This situation had clear implications for the District's revenue position.

The District Administrator elaborated a number of options which included the closure of either Hospital C or Hospital E due to the opening of the new Hospital B. The Authority adopted a less radical option which involved re-defining the roles and relationships of the existing units:

1. Hospital C was to form part of a multi-site District General Hospital and was to change its role to cater for rehabilitation as well as rheumatology, orthopaedic, and other elective surgery.

2. Hospital E in Wharfetown was to serve the North of the District and needed major redevelopment. It was to have limited numbers of beds for elective surgery and medicine but an enhanced role for the provision of inpatient geriatric services.

3. Accident and emergency services were to be based at Hospital A which was also to have the main concentration of acute services and certain regional specialities.

This document began to generate discussion of the District's difficulties through the construction of an agenda for future change. It also signalled to the Regional Health Authority the intentions of the District. An issue which the discussion document did not explore in any detail was the condition of the estate, yet it was becoming clear that if there were to be bed reductions and hospital closures not only the distribution of services but the condition of those facilities would be an important element in the sifting of acute services.

Reviewing the Estate

The immediate impetus to comprehensively review the estate was the publication of HC(83)22 the Ceri Davies report which required health authorities to carry out a survey of their estate and assess the cost of maintenance. Estate control plans were also to be prepared and notional rents to be introduced. The Region devised a questionnaire, which supplemented by site visits helped build up a profile of the pattern of provision and utilisation of estate resources.

In line with the guidance set out in HC(83)22, the estate data base provided the following information on all the property managed by Northville Western Health Authority;

(a) a description plan and aerial photograph

(b) the notional rent

(c) an indication of the existing use

(d) a summary of the full property assessment which included

i functional suitability

ii space utilisation (including an assessment of spare capacity)

iii a systematic record of the condition of the stock

iv a broad assessment of energy performance

v an assessment of compliance with statutory requirements

The exercise was undertaken by a four person team consisting of regional officers from the Estates Department and planning officers from the District (one of whom had a nursing background). They spent nearly sixteen months carrying out the survey using the DHSS building notes for guidance to establish if the buildings were suitable for the practice of alternative forms of modern medicine. A Steering Group helped to devise the functional characteristics criteria. For example, on space utilisation each area was classified as:

Category 1—empty or grossly under-used, or

Category 2—under-used, or

Category 3—adequate, or

Category 4—over-crowded/over-used, or . . . ?

The final report which incorporated the results of a Condition Survey carried out by a firm of Chartered Surveyors was considered by the DHA in June 1984. It suggested that the cost of restoring the estate to a sound condition over ten years would be £35m (Table 6). The survey confirmed District and Regional Managements impression that many of the District's hospitals were old and inadequate comprising, in the case of Hospital A, buildings dating from the 1860's and in four other hospitals 'hutted ward' accommodation operating well beyond its original planned life.

The survey had certain omissions in terms of its future value to the Review team. The survey did not consider whether departments were in the correct place either internally within a hospital or externally within the whole District. This was a consequence of the survey being geared to individual departments rather than taking an overview of the whole site.

Furthermore the data was categorised in a manner specific to the Authority preventing comparisons between different authorities.

The survey was seen as valuable at district level as it provided a source of information to facilitate the planning process rather than relying on totally unstructured subjective impressions. It also enabled a dialogue to be established with the different units about future provision of services. The District also used the survey to request additional funding from the Region due to the inadequacies revealed, but this request did not come to fruition. The units were less sanguine about the survey being both sceptical about its impact on the funding situation yet anxious that it might be used by district officers to impose solutions not favoured by clinical interests particularly at Hospital A.

TABLE 6. *Costs of bringing hospitals and other buildings up to a defined reasonable standard by 1994*

Hospital	*£m*
Hospital A	9·87
Hospital C	4·19
Hospital D	1·66
Hospital E	2·32
Hospital F	9·46
Hospital G	3·31
Other Hospitals (4)	4·55
TOTAL	35·36

SOURCE: *Estate Management and Condition Survey Report*, Northville Western Health Authority, 1984

The Preparation of the 1985 Strategy

Discussion on 'Shaping the Future' had revealed important dimensions of managerial and clinical thinking in the District. First, it had become apparent that it would be very difficult to close Hospital E. The process of closing the maternity unit at the hospital had provoked strong opposition from a community who were witnessing closures of other services in neighbouring authorities. The need to be sensitive to this community's feelings influenced the 1985 strategy as it was to impinge on the 1987 review. Second, support was beginning to emerge from clinical staff for the closure of Hospital C and management believed medical support could be cultivated for its closure if there was the lure of increased beds at Hospital A.

Third, management recognised that hospital services were being delivered from too many sites and had hinted at the need to reduce the number of beds in Shaping the Future but were cautious about grasping the nettle. Northville Western Health Authority had won the battle to remain separate from Northville Eastern as they were reluctant to reduce the influence of the Authority by bed reductions. This was despite the Region's wishes (supported by the university and the local authority) to prevent two separate districts emerging. It was also a turbulent period for the Authority, which was embarking on the restructuring assocated with the Griffiths proposals.

The 1985–94 District Strategic Plan was the first strategic plan prepared by the Authority. It was modelled on *Shaping the Future* proposing the concentration of acute services at Hospitals A and E with a changed use for Hospital C. The plan was a compromise trying to nudge the Authority in the required direction while maintaining the consent of medical staff. At the same time the strategy contained high aspirations for future developments but lacked specific details as to how the strategy was to be achieved. This was acknowledged in the plan:

> In view of the overall financial position, the ability of the Authority to fund the developments outlined in the strategic plan will be limited by the extent to which it can achieve cost improvement programmes . . . unless an understanding can be reached with the RHA on the service needs in this District and the means by which the additional resources required to enable it to meet those needs identified, the majority of the proposals contained in this document will remain little more than statements of objectives with little prospect of implementation during the period covered by the plan.

The Regional Response

Regional Health Authority guidance on the preparation of strategic plans had been unchanged since their 1978 planning guidelines. A Regional strategic plan was being prepared but this was published after District strategic plans had been received in March 1985 and incorporated into the Regional Strategy during Summer 1985. The Region was entering a period of transition. Difficulties over the appointment of their Regional General Manager delayed his arrival until Autumn 1985. This signalled a period of restructuring with the amalgamation of the capital planning and service planning departments and the appointment of a new director of corporate planning in January 1986. In short, 1986 was to be a year when the Region was looking inwards towards its own needs rather than towards providing a sense of direction for the districts.

Historically the relationship between the Region and both Northville Districts had been difficult. Although the Region recognised that the Northville Western District faced severe difficulties due to their poor building stock which inhibited efficient clinical practice there was a belief that management was too reactive and not prepared to manage the clinicians. Instead it was felt the Authority tended to lobby the Region for increased resources when the District already exceeded its previous tranche of resource. Yet there was an ambivalence on the part of the Region to tackling the problems of the District because of a reluctance to antagonise powerful teaching hospital interests at Hospital A which had links with the Department of Health. Consequently the District Administrator felt he received confused signals from the Region on their intentions.

The Region submitted their strategy to the Department of Health in the Autumn of 1985 who rejected it for three reasons. First, the capital and revenue assumptions were unrealistic. Second, the strategy failed to tackle the implied acute bed over-provision in the Region. Although the Region had begun to prepare guidance on bed reductions for districts they were not mandatory targets but guidelines and did not have the required effect as they failed to give districts clear signals about Regional priorities. In addition to this the Department of Health was beginning to quicken the pace on its culling of acute beds. Finally the strategy failed to tackle the aspirations of the two teaching districts and the lack of investment in replacement hospital stock in Northville. The Region was asked to recast its strategic plan by 30 June 1987. This made necessary a review by the districts of their strategies. The importance of Northville in the Region, with the complicating factors of a medical school and ageing hospital provision, made Regional involvement in the review of both DHA's propitious.

On 1 October 1985 the Authority had their annual review meeting with the Region which coincided with the Regional General Manager's first day in post. The Region asked the District to recast its strategy within the resources likely to be available. The District Chairman and Administrator reacted forcibly stressing that it was unrealistic to contemplate a District strategic capital programme which did not address the acknowledged deficiencies of building stock until the next century and argued that the Regional capital allocation of £8m for the District over the next decade was inadequate. The District Chairman requested that the Region join with them in a joint approach to the Department of Health for more capital to break the impasse. This request was rejected by the Region.

Breaking the Deadlock: The Establishment of the Review

The Regional General Manager had been left in no doubt about the strength of feeling in Northville Western and was sympathetic to the poor conditions of building stock prevailing in the District. The need to tackle the problems facing Northville Western was reiterated by a strongly worded letter from the District General Manager[3] on 4 November 1985, which conveyed members alarm at being told the District strategy had been rejected and expressed the view that:

> Given the acknowledgement by Region over several years of the inadequacy of the buildings in Northville, the Regional strategic plan itself is believed to be grossly inadequate.

Pressure on the Region to take some action was also coming from heightened press interest in the state of Hospital A. The local papers carried a wave of stories in December 1985 which suggested that there was a crisis facing Hospital A and quoted the £10m suggested in the condition survey to carry out essential structural repairs. The papers reported the lack of regional finance available and the decision not to back Northville Western's suggestion of a joint approach to the Department of Health.

The Region needed to counter the impression that it was neglecting a leading teaching hospital which the District Chairman had described as the 'Jewel in the Crown'. The Region suggested establishing a joint Working Party to address the problems of the age and condition of the building stock in the District and to look at alternative costed solutions.

The decision to establish a Joint Working Party was accepted by the District. For senior Management there was a degree of satisfaction that the Region had been forced to recognise the needs of the Authority. Clinical staff were sceptical of the review bringing positive outcomes but were persuaded by management that if the District did not cooperate with the exercise the Region would not be willing to invest necessary capital in Northville Western.

The Region broadened the exercise to include Northville Eastern Health Authority and the University. It had been considering a recommendation from the Regional University Liaison Committee that a Joint Working Party of the University and the two District Health Authorities be established to:

> Identify those factors which affect the ability of the Northville DHA's to maintain reasonable standards and facilities in relation to their responsibilities for the support of clinical teaching, the provision of health care and a suitable environment for research and help coordinate any steps which might have to be taken to mitigate the effects of any further reduction in the university's recurring grant.
>
> Regional University Liaison Committee, November 1985.

The Region decided to also incorporate the university review into a single review of the General Hospital strategy. This was clear recogni-

3. The District Administrator was appointed District General Manager in the Griffiths reorganisation.

tion of Hospital A as a major teaching hospital with a central role in the delivery of services in Northville Western Health Authority. However incorporating the University also enabled the Region to postpone some of the difficult issues to be resolved with the university, for example the joint funding of clinical posts, because the review was unlikely to dwell on these specialist issues. The Dean of the Medical School became anxious about the opportunities being given to the medical school to participate.

The Regional decision to undertake a similar joint planning exercise with Northville Eastern Health Authority was aimed at developing a cohesive plan for services across the whole of the city. This served to increase the complexity of the planning task facing both Districts. The Region needed to establish clear guidelines on areas of responsibility for each District if service duplication was to be reduced and clear guidelines on which issues should be resolved locally between the Districts and which issues would be decided by Region.

The historical legacy of the relationship between the two Districts suggested that reaching agreement on the distribution of services which would lead to gainers and losers would be a difficult task. Hospital A had traditionally been the dominant teaching hospital in the city evolving through its establishment as a voluntary hospital to incorporation into the NHS. Northville Eastern had established a teaching hospital (Hospital 1) which was viewed by clinical staff at Hospital A as inferior to their own hospital.

This was due its evolution into a teaching hospital from its inception as a municipal hospital. It frequently catered for geriatric patients which Hospital A were reluctant to admit being of limited interest for teaching purposes. However in more recent years the fortunes of the two hospitals have altered with Hospital 1 becoming a full teaching hospital in 1970 with a steady influx of resource from that date. In the 1980s context of declining availability of resources competition for resources between the Authorities has intensified with neither likely to have the propensity to make sacrifices which would benefit the other hospital.

In January 1986 the Region and District General Manager agreed Terms of Reference for the exercise as follows:

The Joint Working Party was to:

1. Produce a comprehensive statement of objectives for general hospital services, incorporating District, teaching, research, regional specialities and 'tertiary referral' roles;

2. review the present provision of general hospital services, (including regional specialities) and the condition, suitability and location of the building stock from which they are delivered against the agreed strategic

aims and objectives for the District, and for Northville as a whole, including the discharge of the DHA's responsibility for the provision of clinical teaching and research facilities;

3. prepare programmes for change over the next five and ten years, so that services are provided within accommodation which is of an acceptable, defined standard, correctly located and accessible to the population served;

4. attach a priority rating to the various elements in the programmes, so that implementation of the proposed changes can be phased to match the resources made available;

5. reconsider the DHA's District Strategic Plan in the light of this review;

6. make recommendations to both General Managers for consideration by the RHA and DHA, as necessary:

The Working Party was requested to take into account revised resource assumptions issued by the Region, revised Regional policies on Regionally co-ordinated specialities the need to reduce acute beds in the Region and the needs of the university in maintaining clinical teaching and research. The Authority had to submit their District Strategic plan by 31 March 1987.

Setting the Wheels in Motion

Northville Western Hospital Authority formally endorsed the Terms of Reference in February 1986 and accepted the incorporation within the review of the study proposed by the university. The Regional Health Authority likewise endorsed the initiative. The first task facing the District General Manager was building a team that could carry out the task in the limited time available. He believed there was need for the full time commitment of a senior officer to coordinate the planning effort reporting to him, supported by a multi-disciplinary panel of professional staff. In addition detailed statistical, epidemiological, financial, and estate information would be necessary. Finally machinery had to be developed whereby the professional advisory bodies could contribute to the development of policies and priorities.

The District was not too well placed to fulfil this brief as it faced a severe shortage of staff particularly in the finance, community medicine, and information disciplines. This position was exacerbated by the departure of the Head of Planning leaving a new post as head of corporate planning and administration to be filled.

The key central post of the Project Leader needed to be filled by an individual who knew the District well and who was not viewed as partisan to any particular unit. This led to the appointment of a member of the planning department as Project Leader. He ostensibly worked to the head of corporate planning but as this individual arrived in the District in August 1986 new to the NHS he wished to settle into the post before taking an active role. Consequently throughout the review the District General Manager worked closely with the Project Leader, meeting once or twice a week to discuss progress.

The first few months from March until September 1986 was taken up deciding how the review was to be carried out and liberating individuals from other work to enable them to join the multi-disciplinary panel which was to support the team leader. This process was sluggish because until the Head of Corporate Planning took up his post the team leader could not devote all his time to the review process.

A special project team was established under the Project Leader which became known as the Joint Review Support Group. It was envisaged this Group would support the Project Manager in his main objective of providing senior management and Authority members with clear recommendations for action to achieve strategic change supported by evidence from research studies and the advice of clinical and other professions. The Support Group was not therefore to act as a planning group but was instead to test out the implications of policies brought to it acting in a 'think tank' capacity thereby helping to shape the planning agenda and ultimately to help present the plan.

The composition of the Group was shaped by the Terms of Reference and was decided by the District General Manager and the Project Leader. They were striving to achieve a group which worked well together as a group, were technically competent and who had an analytical bent yet were sensitive to the environment in which the review was being conducted. The composition of the Group and lines of managerial accountability are shown in Table 7.

The Regional representative had a slightly different role as she was entrusted with promoting the Regional perspective indicating their support or anxieties about particular plans and monitoring District plans for the Region. The employment of a health economist was seen as valuable in gaining a more objective and informed overview of the proposals. It was also believed that the employment of an academic would strengthen the District's case in negotiating with the Region. The involvement of the Deputy District Treasurer, although delayed until January 1987 due to the departure of the previous post-holder, was invaluable. The rejection of the previous strategic plan for financial reasons led to great emphasis on producing an affordable strategy. The Deputy District Treasurer therefore allowed immediate feedback on the cost of different options. Finally the University representative acted as a two-way link between the University and the Medical School.

TABLE 7. *Composition of the Support Group and Managerial Lines of Accountability*

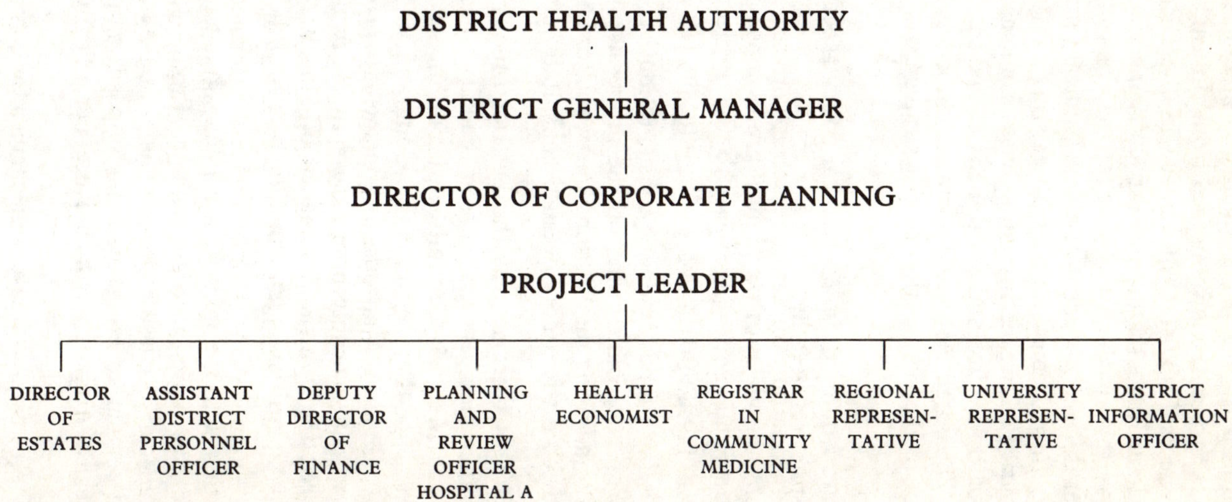

The District General Manager was keen to involve clinicians in the preparation of the strategy and wanted a mechanism to consult them quickly, informally and in a manner which ensured that a clear unambiguous corporate view emerged from clinical staff. The complexity of the medical advisory machinery in the District and the large number of consultants that attended Faculty meetings made it inappropriate to use this machinery. However the District General Manager stressed that the establishment of a new Clinical Group did not remove the need for formal consultation with existing advisory bodies.

The Clinical Policy Steering Group was established in April 1986 as a sounding board for ideas and to offer advice and comments on emergent proposals. The intention was to enable clinicians to make a central contribution to the preparation of the strategy. Its terms of reference were that:

The Group would advise on medical policy aspects of the review of general hospital services by:

(a) seeking the views of the clinical professions on service objectives and priorities and conveying these to the Project Leader or other members of the Support Group as appropriate;

(b) reviewing proposals under consideration by the Working Party and as appropriate commenting on the proposals on behalf of clinical professions or advising the Working Party and/or District Management on the need for further more detailed consultation.

The Group's Chairman was the District Medical officer and there were nine other members drawn from Faculty, the University, SSEC, and the local Medical Committee. From management the Project Leader attended, the Registrar in Community Medicine and the Acute Unit General Manager responsible for Hospital A because the review was inextricably bound up with the future of that hospital. This mirrored the clinical dominance of Hospital A consultants on the Group which discouraged consultants from other hospitals becoming involved.

Consultation with the Unit General Managers and District Management Board was more informal, with the Project Leader and District General Manager discussing developments as they arose. The Project Leader had regular meetings with his opposite number in Northville Eastern Health Authority which were periodically attended by the Region.

In addition to establishing the mechanics for carrying out the review the Project Leader needed to decide on an appropriate methodology for the review. The terms of reference were sufficiently broad to theoretically enable a wide spectrum of approaches, from a purely rational comprehensive approach, to a purely pragmatic approach.

The former rational/comprehensive approach would commence from the medical needs of the population and arrive with a series of options that would fulfil these needs. This process would involve four stages:

1. the collaboration and use of epidemiological evidence to measure the need for services;

2. the evaluation of competing clinical interventions to respond to the need;

3. defining targets for the provision of facilities and services based on agreed models of intervention; and,

4. evaluations of a range of options for achieving the agreed options.

At the other end of the scale, pragmatism would involve an incremental approach which moved from the current pattern of provision to a new level of provision by trying to grasp opportunities (accommodation, etc) which were available in the foreseeable future. This approach would involve three stages:

1. establishing a target for services and accommodation based on 'norms';

2. identificiation of realistic and readily available opportunities for meeting targets for accommodation; and,

3. selective evaluation of the advantages and disadvantages of the available opportunities and testing the norms.

The comprehensive approach was rejected because it would have been impossible to compile the epidemiological evidence and complete the other stages of the process in the time available. This type of approach would probably have led to unaffordable, idealistic solutions as the process would have ignored the current pattern of provision in the city being service driven rather than capital orientated. Consequently the emergent strategy would not have been affordable nor acceptable to the Region.

Conversely the pragmatic approach would seek to move to a new pattern of service by examining regional guidelines, targets, and accommodation presently available. This type of approach was adopted. The choice for the District was in a sense illusory being limited not only by the time and managerial resources available but through a series of regional constraints on bed numbers and finance. This dicatated that a pragmatic approach was adopted but sufficient flexibility was available to graft on elements of a rational comprehensive planning model.

Nonetheless the danger existed that focusing on resources available and existing provision could result in a capital led strategy which was not sufficiently based on service needs.

Establishing the Boundaries of the Pragmatic Approach

The pragmatic approach required recognition of the constraints that would shape the strategy. Foremost were the age specific bed targets outlined by the Region in June 1986 imposing an acute and geriatric specialties bed target for Northville Western of 1,260 beds a reduction from the previous figure of 1,447. This single piece of information dominated the review process and served as the framework for elaboration of the strategy.

In 1984 the Regional Community Medicine Department began to examine the overall provision of acute and geriatric beds across districts. The aim was to move away from the use of norms because these were usually based on bed usage. However, the Region argued that the use of beds was heavily influenced by the number of beds available. Consequently studies were undertaken in five districts which examined bed usage between 1980–82 in district acute specialities and geriatric medicine but then applied an age specific weighting. The Districts were chosen because they did not contain teaching hospitals or significant amounts of regional speciality work. A number of assumptions were added into the equation including that overall occupancy would be at least 85 per cent and turnover interval on average two days or less. Finally pointers from known achievers in the Region and high performers nationally (i.e. lower rates of inpatient provision) were used to encourage districts to emulate these reductions. This arithmetic was suggestive of a reduction from a RHA total of 13,527 acute and geriatric beds in 1983 to a figure of 12,136 beds by 1994.

In January 1985 the Region offered guidance on bed reductions from the strategic planning period which requested Districts to examine their policies on allocating beds and to reduce them in line with the Region's thinking. However district strategic plan submissions in 1985 totalled 13,285 beds by 1994 in acute and geriatric specialities. The Region in redrafting its strategic plan had been set a Ministerial review task to reduce these levels of provision and a new target (T2) of 12,300 beds was proposed for the Region by 1994. For Northville Western this represented a reduction from 1,440 to 1,260 beds by 1994 in the geriatric and acute specialities. In June 1986 the Region informed Districts that the targets were to be achieved by 1994.

There were a number of different reactions to the imposition of the bed target in the District. At first the full implications of the targets were not perceived and the targets were not immediately challenged.

Management did not view the target as immutable and were suspicious of the manner in which it had been constructed. Attempts to prise more information from the Region on its completion led to greater frustration as there was reluctance by regional officers to accept responsibility for the targets and an unwillingness to reveal the detailed calculations to the District. This fuelled the suspicions of senior district officers that the calculations were essentially bogus constructed simply as a means to legitimate a Department of Health directive to reduce bed numbers in the Region.

Management also were aware that clinical staff would never accept the bed target if management could not satisfactorily explain the manner in which the figures had been calculated. In order to win credibility with the clinicians the Project Leader had to be seen to be fighting the Region on the target to defend the District's beds. If the Project Leader had not asked the Health Economist on the support team to spend time refuting the basis of the T2 targets the fragile support lent by the clinicians to the review process may have evaporated. The clinicians particularly at Hospital A were extremely concerned about bed reductions because there had always been an element in their psyche which was most interested in maximising bed numbers and the influence associated with this.

Paradoxically while management continued to try and refute the T2 target and to increase the resources associated with it the target proved a powerful catalyst for change in the District. Although since *Shaping the Future* there had been hints at bed reductions management had never felt in a strong enough position *vis-à-vis* the clinicians to drive through these changes. The externally imposed target deflected blame onto an external agency. Furthermore in the context of the tight financial framework the T2 target was a necessary adjunct to bringing the District back into balance. As one senior manager candidly explained:

> the T2 target was like God, if he hadn't been there we would have had to invent him.

The financial situation facing the District which had a £2·5m deficit was acute and a central objective of the review was to produce a strategy that was affordable to ease the District's financial difficulties. However the review was not embarked upon specifically to address revenue funding and the District General Manager was concerned that if the review was used to rectify financial problems it would fundamentally affect the character of the review, the nature of regional involvement and could jeapordise clinical cooperation. Nonetheless the review could not ignore the pressing financial problems facing Northville Western and the District General Manager made it clear that the review team would need to make finance sensitive decisions.

A complicating factor was both the initial absence and conflicting mixture of signals from the Region on finance available. The District assumed that the Region wouldn't have established the Review unless it was sympathetic to the injection of capital into the District but critically the amount of capital available was not specified. Regional officers acknowledged that 'there was not a district capital framework'. Instead districts were asked to submit bids which would be considered by the Region. The District had reservations about this approach as they felt they had little idea of how large the capital cake was and the size of the slice they were likely to obtain. In a period of great upheaval at the Region they wished to keep the districts at arm's length to enable the Region to have maximum room for manoeuvre in its negotiations with the Department of Health over the new regional strategic plan.

There was greater clarity on the revenue position. The Region had adopted a financial framework for strategic planning which broke expenditure down by broad client group. The main categories being non-psychiatric, mental illness service, mental handicap services, community health and ambulance services. The objective was to encourage districts to spend resources in care group terms thereby moving towards achieving regional priorities by taking notes of the finance allocated to each care group and trying to move towards the target allocation. Additional allocations included financing regional specialities, teaching commitments and the Medical Physics service.

The model targets for each group were devised on a RAWP style weighted population basis except the non-psychiatric allocation which used a planning population basis, i.e. a weighted crude population. This in particular provoked debate about the efficacy of the total. This model produced a figure of £92m revenue for the District in 1993/94 but there was no indication for districts of the pathway to their 1993/94 revenue totals.

There was widespread criticism of this approach because it encouraged districts to front load their strategies with heavy revenue commitments which tapered to meet the revenue target by 1993/94. However formulating strategies in this manner meant bridging finance was required in the early years of the strategy. This finance proved not to be available to the extent required.

The Region argued that the approach improved flexibility encouraging district's to adopt a responsible attitude. Furthermore the Region believed that until it had seen the District strategies it could not decide the most appropriate allocation of resources and in respect of the bridging finance the Region could not have predicted the deterioration in its own financial position. Consequently the review team were clear that the strategy had to help rectify the financial imbalance the District suffered but there was uncertainty over the amount of capital available to establish a more rational pattern of provision which would curb the revenue imbalance.

Political constraints

In addition to the constraint of the ubiquitous bed target and the financial situation a series of more subtle political influences were acknowledged but the potential impact on the review was opaque. There existed a powerful lobby in Wharfetown which had made management cautious about changing the role of Hospital E in 1985. The strength of feeling in Wharfetown, a small market town of approximately 12,000 residents arose from the desire of the town to retain their own identity and remain separate from Northville. The town had achieved this by having its own local council and Hospital E was a symbol of this independence. Although the hospital was deteriorating and consisted mainly of temporary building stock, it was viewed as a valued resource by the local community. A slim majority for the Conservative MP in the town, who was being challenged strongly by a local Liberal councillor, ensured a high profile for discussions over the future of the Hospital.

In the winter of 1986 speculation escalated of an imminent general election in early 1987. The scene was set for the future of Hospital E to become a major political issue with the local politicans vying with each other to appear the most supportive of a future for Hospital E.

An additional potential political issue concerned the absence of hospital provision in the south of Northville in either District. The south of the city is poor, reflected in high morbidity compared to the affluent parts of North West Northville and statutory services are not well developed while general practitioner facilities are inadequate. HAA figures showed very low rates of referral to neighbouring districts to the south and south west of the city. The Labour controlled City Council and prominent Labour MPs had been vocal in the past on the need for improved provision in the south of the city.

The Review Team also needed to devise a strategy that recognised the teaching and training responsibilities of the District. The university had schools of medicine and dentistry which took 160 medical and fifty-four dental students each year amounting to a clinical student population at any time of 450 medical undergraduates and 200 dental undergraduates. There were also two schools of nursing for general and psychiatric nursing and five paramedical training schools for diagnostic radiography, therapeutic radiography, physiotherapy, orthoptics and a speech therapy school based at the polytechnic. The needs of these training establishments was highlighted in late 1983 when Hospital A was threatened with withdrawal of recognition for nurse training because of the low ratio of trained to untrained nurses and the inadequacy of arrangements for acute medical admissions. A similar situation arose in physiotherapy, when the Chartered Society of Physiotherapy threatened the withdrawal of training recognition because the existing school buildings did not come up to the standards set by them. For the medical school the central issue was that there was a sufficiently large hospital close to the university to provide adequate facilities for clinical teaching and research.

A myriad of national and regional policies needed to be taken into account when trying to establish a framework for the review process. The District had responsibility for nine regional specialities and five area specialities (Table 8) and as the review covered both Districts there was a need for guidance on the integrated provision of these services. The Region was undertaking a review of regional specialities. The District expected to produce an outcome similar to other regional reviews which had advocated the reduction in the number of sites from which regional services are delivered. Regional guidance was to assume a status quo position on service levels. This gave the District cause for concern as the future location of regional specialities could have a major impact on the other acute services. As one regional officer admitted 'The Region should have taken a stronger lead, the problem was no advice was given'.

TABLE 8. *Regional specialities and Area specialities present in Northville Western District Health Authority*

Regional Specialities	*Area Specialities*
1 Neurology	ENT specialities
2 Neurosurgery	Dermatology
3 Cardiology (approx 50%)	Opthalmology
4 Cardiothoracic surgery	Rheumatology
6 Plastic Surgery	Units for the younger disabled
7 Nephrology	
8 Paediatric Surgery	
9 Neo-natal Intensive Care	

SOURCE: Northville Western DHA District Strategy 1987–94, March 1987

National policies on the developments of community care which had figured prominently in the outline regional strategic plan were likely to squeeze the money available to the acute sector. Similarly government policies to increase efficiency through the implementation of cost improvement programmes created a climate where financial stringency was necessary. National guidance on optimal size of hospitals and the condition of the estate needed consideration. The District itself faced major demographic changes, although the population of the District was static the composition was changing with a doubling of the population over seventy-five forecast by 1994. This required major development in geriatric and psychogeriatric services.

To summarise, until September 1986 effort was concentrated on establishing the review process itself. The Clinical Policy Steering Group was set up after discussions with the professional advisory bodies. Nominations were being received from clinical staff. The Project Leader had been appointed and he was gathering together a Support Group to help carry out the review task. The decision had been made to adopt a pragmatic approach to the review and work had begun on deciding exactly what this entailed and how these tasks would be allocated between different members of the Group. The state was set for the review process to start in earnest.

The Strategy in the Making

Informed policy discussion with the Clinical and Support Groups required the collection of data on services in the District. It was only through this process which tried to arrive at a comprehensive picture of the District and the performance of those services, that problems could be identified leading to the search for solutions. A difficulty in this context was the role of the information department in the District. It was not highly developed nor integrated into the planning department and at that time was fully committed to the implementation of the Körner proposals. Consequently it tended to look outwards serving the needs of the Region and Department of Health but less able to support the planning efforts of the Review Team.

A valuable source of information came from a series of ten papers prepared over the summer of 1986 by an Assistant Regional Principal at the Department of Health. The paper titled 'Northville where are we now?' examined existing performance indicators of both Districts and the potential and means for improved future performance. The overall approach concentrated on improved bed management reasoning that it was not possible to plan for the future unless the current position was known.

The first paper examined the demand for the service using hospitalisation rates as a proxy. It found that Northville Western's rate was well above both the England and Regional figures. In terms of bed usage measured by throughput the Authority failed to achieve the Regional or English average, nor did it compare favourably with a comparable teaching hospital cluster. This information was used to gauge the effect on waiting lists if empty but staffed and available beds were used. The effect of achieving a maximum turnover internal of no more than two days was considered. The effects were measured in two ways:

1. where a waiting list existed, additional discharges/deaths that would be possible were calcuated.

2. when there was no waiting list or where it was possible to eliminate it, the number of beds that could be removed was calculated.

The second part of the process reviewed length of stay. Where the District's length of stay was not at least equal to the average length of stay of the comparator group then it was possible to calculate both the number of additional discharges and deaths and/or the beds that could go if the average length of stay could be achieved. The final element of the process considered the level of day case work undertaken. A finance paper argued that the use of the three approaches (turnover interval, length of stay, day cases) could lead to significant cost improvements.

The Project Leader explained the bed management approach at the first meeting of the clinical policy Steering Group on 31 July 1986 and the scope it offered to increase the number of patients treated or to reduce bed numbers. There were difficulties in gaining acceptance for this approach. First, for many of the clinicians it was the first time they had been presented with this type of information and they may have felt threatened by the potential which management had to monitor their work and not to be reliant on clinicians for their information. Second the clincians criticised the data arguing it was lacking in terms of both accuracy and consistency of definition. For example, the Region in compiling its statistics did not recognise day case work which created anomalies. The information was considered to be of too general a nature to come to definite conclusions about reducing bed numbers. Finally doubts were expressed about the validity of comparative data with Districts that did not share similar characteristics of clinical organisation, demography and epidemiology.

To resolve these objections it was agreed that the Registrar in Community Medicine would join with the Project Leader to produce more disaggregated data. The Committee of Physicians agreed to a review of the need for clinical facilities in the medical specialities. It was envisaged that these discussions would lead to the development of a process for using existing statistics as a basis for determining the need for such facilities which would then be applied to other clinical specialities by the Review Team and the clinicians concerned. This information was prepared for General Medicine and Geriatric Medicine in the District between 1983–85 and a similar document was then prepared for the surgical specialities and Gynaecology.

It was during this period that the Support Group began to start work.

It met every Thursday in an informal manner concentrating in the early months on discussing key issues rather than carrying out detailed planning work. The first meeting of the Support Team on 25 September 1986 discussed the expected outcomes of the review, how the outcomes were to be achieved and tried to identify a way of starting the planning process. The Project Leader explained that the work already carried out had aimed to:

(a) provide more information about current services policies, practices, activity, workload, resources, etc;

(b) establish a process for discussing targets for clinical facilities with medical staff.

The planning processing had therefore not really started. He presented a key issues paper (Table 9) which aimed to open a debate on what the key issues and underlying problems that needed to be resolved were. The aim was to move discussions beyond identifying symptoms to underlying pathologies.

The Support Group spent October and part of November identifying and defining the problems. This involved allocation of specific tasks and brainstorming sessions. This process had three dimensions:

(a) the collection of quantifiable information

(b) the collection of qualitative information

(c) Group discussion and presentation of papers at the Support Group meetings.

The first stage had been started off by the 'Northville: Where are we now?' series and had subsequently been built on by the Registrar in Community Medicines more detailed examination of specialities. The Deputy Project Leader pursued the work she had begun in preparing the estate data base. This involved preparing a series of statements on provision across the District which included community services, clinical facilities, day hospital places, nursing home beds, clinical undergraduate teaching resources and private/local authority residential homes. At the conclusion of this process (which was broken down by care group as appropriate) the Review Team knew:

(a) the services in the District and their location;

(b) the condition of the buildings and their functional suitability;

(c) activity levels.

In accordance with the pragmatic approach use of the T2 target levels of provision taken with the information on the estate helped to establish

TABLE 9. *Key issues paper presented to Support Group, 25 September 1986*

Key Issue	*For Investigation/Assessment/Analysis*
1 Acute and long stay bed base.	Hospitalisation rates and the underlying reasons and justification for these.
	Possibility for distribution within the District.
	Bed requirements.
2 Supra Districts services by two Health Districts (inc NWHA).	Desirability and feasability of rationalisation.
3 Teaching facilities.	Desirability and feasibility of rationalisation.
4 Collaboration with the private sector.	Possibilities for provision.
5 Policy for distribution of revenue funds.	Effects on acute hospital services of development of community based and other priority services.
6 Diagnostic and scientific.	Possibilities for concentration services on fewer sites and likely impact of technological advances.
7 Non-clinical services.	Scope for rationalisation.
8 Self sufficiency in provision of services.	Possibilities.
9 Outpatient services.	Desirability and feasibility of rationalisation.
10 Day hospitals.	Role.

SOURCE: Northville Western DHA, 1986

the nature, scale, and significance of problems arising from the delivery of hospital services. It was through establishing an agreed list of problems that work on solutions could begin.

A further piece of quantitative work which revealed suitability for locating hospital services was the work carried out on travelling times. This examined the length of time taken to reach a particular hospital by a certain mode of transport. This analysis demonstrated the ease of access to particular hospitals and was able to make comparisons through the use of isochrons whose circumference delineates equal travel time areas.

The information was collected from the Regional Passenger Transport Authority but was complicated by the impending deregulation of the bus service and the upheaval to routes this would create. It was not clear the effect this would have on the future accuracy of these isochrons. The Transport Authority stated their willingness to consider new routes to serve for example a new hospital and therefore suggested that sites should not be excluded for consideration on the basis of lengthy travel time. Rail travel was briefly examined but was not seen as being particularly relevant for travel to the city's hospitals except for patients from outside the District.

The extent of car ownership was of greater significance and affected the weighting assigned to the accessibility survey. The information was a significant variable in deciding where to locate services.

Broader information on socio-economic factors was explored but was not used for planning purposes. The Jarman index revealed to some degree inner city social and economic deprivation and resultant high morbidity but the information from the Jarman index and OPCS sources was not sufficiently precise or disaggregated enough to guide planning decisions at sub-district level nor dramatic enough in its likely consequences to justify further work in this area.

Quantitative information was supplemented by qualitative information. This included strong feelings about the large number of hospital sites and their disparate locations raising questions about their future viability. The condition of buildings and the effect on the quality of care were also continually mentioned. The Support Group started discussions by generating hypothetical scenarios about specific major changes. Questions included discussing what would happen if Hospitals C, E, etc, closed and this was based on discussions about what the District was doing well and badly.

The work undertaken by the Support Group to define problems also included collaboration with the university in a fact finding exercise to identify problems experienced by the main academic clinical departments. The university also undertook an informal review of curriculum requirements, which was used as a general framework for assessing the critical mass of teaching beds to be provided on the main DGH site.

By November a clear picture was emerging of the nature of the problems facing the Districts provision of acute hospital services. This was to provide the basis for examining opportunities for solving the difficulties through capital investment and rationalisation. The main problems were summarised as:

(a) The recurring imbalance between service commitments and financial resources.

(b) The spread of the general hospital services in the District over a large number of sites fragmenting and duplicating clinical services on and between sites.

(c) The age of hospital buildings in the District, few of which had been built in this century, hardly any of which had been built in the last 30 years and some of which were constructed of temporary building materials. This gave rise to overcrowded wards and congested sites.

(d) The uncontrolled and haphazard way in which these sites had been developed.

(e) The location of hospitals with relation to the populations they serve more than half of the hospitals in the District being either outside its boundaries or barely within them.

The Support Group assumed that given the nature of the problems any strategy emerging would involve major change. As a norm based approach was adopted due to the centrality of the regional bed target and the attempt to validate this target through the review of clinical workload carried out by the Registrar in Community Medicine, the logical next step with the information the support team had obtained was to marry the estate data base information with the T2 target to move towards a strategy for rationalisation.

An integral part of the assessment of the potential of the existing estate to provide for acute ward hospital beds within the District was the categorisation of existing stock into three categories:

1. Economic efficiency—the optimal size of acute hospital wards is twenty-eight beds because at this size, average unit costs are believed to be at a minimum. Analysis of the existing acute bed stock identified a number of wards as being less than 'ideal' on the grounds of economic efficiency.

2. Functional suitability—this criteria was used to assess the degree to which existing acute bed stock met the functional requirements of acute medicine. Problems identified included limited accommodation, overcrowding, structural deterioration and safety and fire regulations. Consequently, a number of wards were identified as being less than ideal on the grounds of functional suitability.

3. Wider issues of viability—this criteria was used to assess wards which were unsuitable due to the isolation of location or the insufficient number of wards on one site to justify the continued use of the site for acute hospital purposes.

The application of these criteria to the existing bed stock led to division into two parts:

(a) ideal acute beds;

(b) less than ideal acute beds.

This showed a marked deficiency in ideal wards. The consequent identification of an acute bed gap led to the examination of measures to improve the less than ideal bed stock and pursuit of other options, for example building new facilities, use of the private sector or changing the purpose of existing accommodation.

Tackling the Region

The Support Team could not suspend their work until the differences with the Region had been resolved. This required them to use the T2 bed target and the financial model as guidance while simultaneous attempts were made to refute the validity of these figures. The District had dual aims. First it needed to demonstrate to its clinicians that it was trying to increase the beds available to medical staff by providing a detached critique of the T2 bed target. Second it wanted to increase the revenue available to the Review Team of the general hospital strategy by chipping away at the anomalies in the financial model in order to squeeze more resources out of the Region. The Region's secrecy concerning the compilation of the bed target fuelled the District's suspicion that the Region was hiding information and acted as a spur to further endeavour in this area.

The first criticism of the T2 bed target concerned the adjustment the Region made to Northville Western's catchment population to reflect major cross-boundary flows. The Region assumed neutrality in flows between Northville Western DHA and Northville Eastern DHA. However certain other major flows inwards or outwards were counted as the Districts catchment population was increased (for inflows) and reduced (for outflows). As the financial model was in the RAWP format and therefore dominated by population, adjustments in population due to cross-boundary flows had major financial implications.

The District believed the data the Region was using was very historical based on 1981 OPCS data and did not adequately compensate the District for its cross-boundary inflows. The 1981 OPCS data was criticised because it was compiled in the summer when the large student population of the city was absent. Furthermore its extrapolation of growth rates in different age groups proved to be inaccurate. The 1985 data the District used showed higher cross-boundary inflows than was recognised by the Region.

The District was critical of the model financial target because it excluded a number of pertinent factors. The District has been assigned sixty beds for tertiary referrals but the criteria used to define a tertiary referral were unclear. They were also omitted from the financial framework. The District argued that a tertiary referral by definition reflected a more complex case which would require more costly treatment. Similarly radiotherapy outpatient costs were well in excess of the average outpatient cost which the Region was using to fund the service and therefore extra funding was required. The outcome of these discussions were mixed. The District managed to obtain extra target funding for tertiary referrals and outpatients but the negotiations over the T2 target became deadlocked. The District therefore accepted the target in the interim and as the March 1987 deadline approached the figure became immutable.

Relations between the District and Region were strained by press reports that emerged at the end of October of substantial new investments of £9m in Northville Eastern District Health Authority at Hospital 1. This alarmed the Northville Western consultants and caused the District General Manager to write to the Regional General Manager on 28 October in the following terms:

> It is a great pity that an apparently quite public display of this possible major scheme was made without any prior notification to us at a time when the Joint Review is at a critical stage of its development. We have, for example been telling our consultants that major capital proposals will not be firmed up except in the context of the Review.

The reply from the Region served to reassure the District as it hinted at a similar sum being made available to Northville Western for redevelopment of Hospital A. However, the ability of the two parties to work jointly was undermined by the lack of trust and uncertainty about possible negotiations that were taking place with Northville Eastern without the District's knowledge. The distrust was exacerbated by the essentially competitive nature of the strategic planning process.

This situation was not eased by regional officers not assigning a senior officer to the Group. She was not viewed by district officers as carrying sufficient authority for the task. It was not clear what was expected of her and consequently she tended to act as a delegate rather than a representative of regional perspectives. Consequently when questions arose about regional policy these had to be referred back to more senior officers causing delay and frustration for the Support Group.

There was also disquiet amongst the Review Team about the position of regional specialities. The Support Group believed very strongly that policy in relation to such services could have a significant impact on strategy for general hospital development in Northville. The Project Leader believed that while the initiative had to rest with the Region the District could make a contribution in two ways:

1. giving advice on the specialities which should be subject to a review of policy within the context of the strategic review;

2. providing information, both subjective and objective about the perceived strengths and weaknesses of current policies.

There was considerable delay in establishing a clear position from the Region and they were slow to respond to the proposals from the District. In December it emerged that the Region wished to delegate the responsibility to the Districts. This prompted the Northville Eastern District General Manager to write to the Director of Planning at the Region on 3 December 1986 expressing concern:

> When the Review was established it was acknowledged that a key aspect would be the future pattern of provision in relation to the Regional specialists in Northville, particularly where services were duplicated between the two Districts. The clear understanding within the Districts was the Regional officers would be taking the lead in deciding on the future siting of these services and I am, therefore, disturbed to learn that my clinical colleagues have been led to understand that this is a District responsibility.

The issue was not satisfactorily resolved in that the District's were told to plan on a status quo basis and to await the outcome of the regional review of these specialities.

The Service Brief

By mid November 1986 sufficient progress had been made to enable the Project Leader to prepare the service brief. This took stock of progress to date and drawing conclusions from this information outlined an agenda of possible options for detailed examination and discussion. The service brief elaborated on the assumptions underlying the planning process. This reiterated the pragmatic approach which set targets for all facilities and gave primacy to the establishment of future bed requirements. It stressed the need to derive these targets from the review of clinical workload but in the absence of this review being completed the T2 target would have to be used as a proxy. The linkage of the T2 target to the condition of the estate had defined the scale and nature of the problems facing the District. It had emerged that 1500 general hospital beds were likely to be required.

The Project Leader argued that this was suggestive of a two site solution of a main teaching hospital of circa 1000 beds plus a second district general hospital of 500 beds which would allow a roughly equal distribution of District beds between two sites with a concentration of area and regional specialities on the main teaching unit site. Department of Health guidance on hospital size made a one site option unacceptable. Conversely the total bed requirement was insufficient to justify an economical three site solution.

The Brief discussed possible locations for a two site DGH, Hospital A was a useful site due to its central location, proximity to the medical school and continuing capital investment. However it also possessed many old buildings which in the long term would need to be replaced and was a congested site with limited prospects for expansion. Hospital C and G were ruled out for DGH purposes due to their location. Hospital C being outside the District but insufficiently distant from Hospital G was on the periphery of the DHA. In addition their infrastructure was in poor condition.

Hospital E was in a relatively suitable complementary location for serving the Northern part of the District if Hospital A served the south. However there was an urgent need to replace the obsolete and unsuitable, hutted wards. There was also a question mark over the capacity of the site and its ability to accommodate new DGH type developments. Hospital D was well located to serve the North of the District. The existing building stock was almost wholly committed to the regional radiotherapy service and DGH type facilities would have complemented these services.

Option 1 Two site DGH
Hospital A partially redeveloped and partially upgraded
Hospital E redeveloped

Option 2 Two site DGH
Hospital A partially redeveloped and partially upgraded
Hospital D developed

Option 3 Two site DGH
Hospital A partially redeveloped and partially upgraded
Greenfield site purchased and developed

It had not been difficult to identify solutions. The condition survey and estate data base had brought into sharp relief the poor condition of the estate particularly at Hospital C and E. The location of many of the hospitals in neighbouring authorities on the perimeter of the District at a time when regional philosophy was geared towards District self sufficiency excluded a number of sites for development although not Hospital E. The possibility of a second DGH had also been under discussion for a number of years. For may observers in the District the most novel suggestion was the possible development of Hospital D. This option had been raised and was being vigorously advocated by the Acute Unit General Manager, who presided over this patch.

It was necessary to further define the roles of the two DGH's with regard to the distribution, by speciality, of inpatient beds and supporting services in order to begin to test their feasibility. This could have been done by two different methods, either:

(a) establishing through consultation with the medical profession criteria for such allocations; or

(b) the Support Group could have developed hypothetical alternative models for critical assessment by the medical profession.

The Clinical Policy Steering Group was invited to:

1. comment on the initial views of the Joint Review Support Group with regard to the selection of available courses of future action.

2. advise on criteria for comparing these.

3. advise on the possibilities for future distribution of beds and other facilities between future proposed DGH sites.

This agenda proved to be too daunting a task for the Clinical Policy Steering Group to tackle. As the Support Group increasingly fashioned the strategy the Clinical Group atrophied creating a vacuum in clinical policy which was unlikely to remain vacant for long.

The Clinical Policy Steering Group: A Body in Search of a Role?

As its name suggested the original intention was that the Clinical Group would lead planning activity by deciding on future models of service and the location of specialities; and would strongly support the Project Leader and the Support Group by supplying them with relevant information. As its name suggests the Support Group was never envisaged as being the Steering Group for the main planning activity. The reversal of roles occurred because it quickly became apparent to the Project Leader that the Clinical Group was not capable of fulfilling its role and therefore the Support Group had to step into the breach.

From its inception in April 1986 it had difficulty defining the task it was required to perform. Clinical staff were sceptical about the review leading to positive outcomes and were cajoled into becoming involved because senior management argued if the District did not cooperate there would be no prospect of the Region making monies available. They were also wary of becoming involved in a process that could lead to reductions in bed numbers. Consequently the Group was floundering because it did not have a clear sense of direction and this situation was aggravated by the Group not forging links with the clinicians it sought to represent.

The first meeting of the Group discussed the bed management

approach and obtained agreement that the Registrar in Community Medicine should carry out more detailed work on assessing the need for beds, outpatient sessions, and day case places through workload analysis. The need to review Regional specialities was also raised. At the end of November the service brief was considered by the District Management Board. The proposal that 1000 general hospital beds should be based at Hospital A and 500 should be based at a second DGH was considered appropriate. However, it was felt that Hospital A might be able to function effectively as a single site DGH with more than 1,000 beds supported by one or more smaller hospitals. Hospital E was considered unsuitable for DGH development because of its remote location which would be inconvenient for teaching functions. The suggestion that Hospital D be developed received considerable support because it as not remote from centres of population and bringing the regional radiotherapy centre within a general hospital would benefit both the centre and other specialities. A caveat was the difficult access route to the hospital. Finally it was thought there might be merit in examining options for a three site DGH and a greenfield site.

Consequently four options remained:

1. a single site DGH
2. a two site development based at Hospital A and Hospital D
3. a two site development based at Hospital A and a greenfield site
4. a three site option.

The Group continued its deliberations throughout January and February 1987 and began detailed discussion concerning the distribution of district, area and regional specialities between Hospital A and a new second DGH. It was during this period however that the latent tensions between the Clinical Group and the Support Group and the wider clinical body began to emerge.

In the early period of the review the Clinical Group were willing to accept in general terms the direction of the review and it is possible that they viewed the review as a paper exercise of little significance. However as the review moved towards the March 1987 deadline the proposals generated by the Support Group were more specific and the superficial consensus of the early period evaporated. The implications of the review for medical staff was also becoming more apparent.

During February it became clear that the endorsement of the Support Group's suggestions by the Clinical Group was not acceptable to the wider body of consultants. At a Faculty meeting on 16 February a clear preference for a one site DGH emerged which had been discounted by the Policy Group. This dissonance reflected the lack of communication between the Clinical Group and members of the Faculty. Members of the Clinical Group did not fulfil their constituency role and failed to act as representatives for their colleagues. Instead of adopting a corporate approach they tended to act in defence of their own particular interests.

A further difficulty for the Clinical Group was their uneasy relationship with the Support Group. Due to the complexity of the issues and the uncertainty over their role the Clinical Group had difficulty generating ideas and increasingly responded to the Support Group who were carrying out the detailed planning work. As the pace of the review quickened the Clinical Group were left behind and they became frustrated at being asked to endorse policies they had not suggested and which they had reservations about. The Clinical Group became suspicious that the Support Group was witholding information from them and placing obstacles in the way of their favoured strategy. Consequently they did not take responsibiity for decisions as they felt little real influence over them and backtracked when it was clear that Faculty favoured a one site option.

The Clinical Group was chaired by the District Medical Officer who had a difficult task balancing the needs of the review process and the need to maintain the cooperation of the clinicians. He tried to protect the Clinical Group from exposure to all aspects of the Support Group's work as he believed they were moving too quickly in terms of the magnitude of change to sustain clinical support. Circumstances made the clinicians wary and the Chairman began to lose the confidence of the staff who believed he was siding with the planners. This exacerbated the difficulties of the Clinical Group which was unable to function effectively.

The Group was unrepresentative in its membership, being dominated by consultants from Hospital A. It was only during February 1987 that it was suggested representatives from the other hospitals should be included. There was reluctance by medical staff to become involved as they saw the dominance of Hospital A consultants and the likelihood that they would have a limited impact on its proceedings. The composition of the Group and their uncertainty about their role led to no clear unambiguous advice emerging. The absence of a clear clinical policy served to encourage political manoeuvring between clinicians and managers and made it more difficult for the strategy that emerged to gain favour.

The University Response

The university was entering an uncertain period due to the reductions in university grants committee expenditure on higher education. Despite these reductions the university had no plans to change the scale of services it provided even though economies were likely to lead to the freezing of vacant medical posts in medical teaching departments. Paradoxically the greater incentives to seek external financial support may have led to expansion of university activities in parallel with retrenchment. Consequently the university was not in a position to predict the effect of these developments on its service requirements from Northville Western.

In general terms it was vital for the university that a hospital of sufficient size continued to exist near the university. This was to fulfil the requirements for a minimum number of patients for each speciality with the appropriate support services to provide a viable teaching base. Additionally it required accommodation, equipment and manpower resources to sustain required clinical teaching and research.

The university favoured the continuation of Hospital A as the dominant district general and teaching hospital. This implicitly reiterated their preference for one District Health Authority in Northville with services provided at Hospital A and Hospital 1. For the above reasons it was opposed to any diminution of Hospital A's range of facilities and instead was attracted to the idea of a single site DGH based at Hospital A where all teaching could be concentrated. The university recognised the practical difficulties of this position due to the congestion on the site. Despite this they were generally unwilling to contemplate the release of any unused land on the university site to facilitate new development at Hospital A. It acknowledged the possible need for a second complementary hospital which was preferable to a three site option viewed as less desirable for teaching purposes, but was anxious that the hospital should offer easy access from the university site. Furthermore there would need to be detailed discussions with the university concerning the optimal distribution of services between the two hospitals.

The Service Brief enabled the Support Group to gauge the feelings of the District concerning the emerging strategy. The response indicated general support for the idea of the two site DGH but detailed work was needed to determine the implications of this in terms of manpower and finance, the distribution of specialities between the sites; and the choice of sites. An undercurrent of dissent from a two site option remained and this emerged during the deliberations of the clinical policy Steering Group from February onwards.

The manpower strategy was allied to the decisions being taken concerning the role of the estate. It was essentially an approach which ensured that the manpower information provided accurately illustrated the staffing implications of the proposed strategy. The process had five main stages:

1. Assessing the existing allocation of manpower resources to ward based services. This involved an analysis of the manpower establishment by occupation and grade across the District.

2. An analysis of the existing manpower resources allocated to support services.

3. An assessment of the manpower required to meet the model of care outlined in the strategy, differentiated by speciality.

4. An analysis of the necessary manpower resources to enable adequate levels of support services to be provided to fulfil the strategy.

5. The production of a district-wide balance sheet which illustrated the effect of the strategy and confirmed that in terms of manpower availability and revenue consequences the strategy was achievable.

Predicting the need for manpower was complicated by a number of national initiatives and the historical legacy of understaffing in the District. Government policy which introduced mandatory competitive tendering for support services from 1983 had a marked effect on reducing the level of manpower required for support services through the twin processes of labour intensification and capital deepening. For example, changes in the technology of the catering industry through the use of cook chill systems has served to centralise the preparation of meals reducing the need for separate kitchens at each hospital. Changes of this nature clearly impinged on the necessary manpower requirements for the strategy.

Alterations to manpower levels were not confined to support services. The Government's report on medical staffing levels 'Achieving a balance' also required careful consideration. More difficult to predict was the likelihood of the Government approving the changes advocated for nurse training in the Project 2,000 proposals. At local level the District had a legacy of low staff levels and a poor ratio of unqualified to qualified staff; resulting in threats by the ENB to remove training status in 1984.

This triggered attempts to raise staff levels and change the ratio of qualified to unqualified staff. This process gained a new sense of urgency as the possibility of a new hospital would break the old staffing levels found in the old building stock. The stragtegy also implied a change in the skill mix due to the expansion of geriatric services which had been neglected in the District and the expansion of community services requiring increases in paramedical and nursing staff. Shortages existed in these areas across the Region and anxieties existed at District level about the intertia of the Region in adopting initiatives to increase the numbers of staff in these key areas. This raised major questions about the viability of district strategies as a consequence of skill shortages across the Region.

Detailed work was also being undertaken on the location of specialities across the District. The attempt to involve the clinicians in this process via the information prepared by the Registrar in Community Medicine had limited success due to the difficulties alluded to earlier in the clinical policy Steering Group and the reluctance of the clinicians to accept the accuracy of the data or to meaningfully discuss bed reductions. Consequently the Support Group had to carry out this work using more informal channels of communication with the clinicians and general managers. A particular focus was the role of the new Hospital B which had vacant accommodation because the costs of bringing the whole structure into use had been prohibitive. The use of this space would enable Hospital A to free up in the order of 100 beds which in turn could allow transfer of surgical beds from Hospital C opening up the way to its closure in 1994.

The decision on which specialities should occupy Hospital B is indicative of the manner in which the Support Group decided on the allocation of specialities. A paper by the Project Leader in December 1986 outlined the suggested criteria to be used for assessing the suitability for locating specialisms at Hospital B:

(a) self containment

(b) independence from other specialities

(c) association with paediatrics/obstetrics/gynaecology/dentistry

(d) relief of present accommodation problems

The decision on the number of hospitals depended upon the resolution of a number of issues, including whether or not:

1. The individual hospitals should provide a general range of services to a defined catchment area, specific services to the whole District to complement each other or a combination of both.

2. The teaching services and/or regional specialities and/or district/area specialities should be split between sites and if so in what proportion.

3. Individual clincians should work from more than one site.

4. The separate sites should deal with specific sources of referral for inpatient admission.

5. All hospitals should have outpatients departments and if so how should specialities be allocated between them.

In early February 1987 a seminar was held for members which detailed progress to date and requested that they consider three issues in particular.

(a) the uses of the empty space in Hospital B.

(b) the overall distribution of general hospital facilities within the District.

(c) proposals for phase two development of Hospital A.

The document rejected a one site DGH by quoting the national policy guidance—*The Future Pattern of Hospital Provision in England on Large Hospitals.*

> Experience has shown that a large degree of concentration on a single site may itself have serious disadvantages. Communications of all kind within the hospital become more complex and difficult as does management. Patients and relatives as well as staff find the hospital too impersonal. It often suffers from physical disadvantages such as distance between different departments and the need to provide air conditioning to internal areas with high energy requirements. It is sometimes supposed that one building is cheaper to run than two of equivalent functional content but this may not always be the case.

It was noted that the Clinical Group had expressed qualified preference for two sites but had not discounted a one site option if the potential disadvantages could be overcome. Within a two site option their preference was for a large unit of around 1,000 beds with responsibility for clinical teaching and specialist services but retaining the general medical and surgical service relating to a specific catchment area. A smaller unit of around 500 beds would provide for mutually interdependent services such as rehabilitation, rheumatology, the younger disabled and cold orthopaedics together with a general medical and surgical service related to a catchment area.

The suitability of existing sites was the other major factor in deciding on the future provision of general hospital services. The role of Hospital A and the adjacent Hospital B was the dominant element in planning the strategy due to its teaching hospital functions, central location and proximity to the medical and dental schools. The congestion of the site coupled with the age of some of the buildings required substantial investment in the site. Furthermore the lack of car parking facilities was acute. Nonetheless it would have been possible to develop the site to 1,000 beds and it therefore seemed essential to the Support Group to retain the site as the main DGH/teaching hospital in the District particularly bearing in mind the desire of the university not to fragment teaching facilities across too many sites.

The suggestion that Hospital A remain the dominant hospital in the District at around 1,000 beds led to the consideration of the location of the second site. The manner in which the site would be developed to allow it to become a complementary hospital and not be overshadowed by Hospital A was a crucial issue and proved to be a source of friction with the clinicians at Hospital A who were wary about the development of a hospital which could divert resources from Hospital A and in the future prove to be a rival. Hospital A clinicians were reluctant to allow developments which would dissipate the revitalisation of Hospital A because of their desire for the hospital to return to preeminence in Northville over Hospital 1.

Hospital E was not considered suitable for development for three reasons. First, it was situated on the northern border of the District and would not therefore be suitable for serving the South of the District. Second, its building stock was in poor condition and in particular the obsolete and hutted wards would need to be replaced. Third, an initial assessment had demonstrated that the site was not large enough to accommodate a 500 bed DGH. Consequently it could only be used if a three site option was adopted.

Hospital C was also considered unsuitable for development due its location close to Hospital A making it difficult to serve a separate catchment area. Furthermore the hospital was located in Northville Eastern and traditionally drew most of its patients from referrals by Northville Eastern General Practitioners. The development of Hospital C would have exacerbated these tendencies and potentially challenged the viability of particular Northville Eastern Hospitals. The condition of the estate was poor with many of the hutted buildings at the end of their useful life and the structural frame of the building corroding to a fatal degree. This precluded the site being developed unless there was a rapid and large capital injection.

Hospital D was gaining support for development. It was well located to serve the North of the District being situated in an area of expanding population. There was a wish to reduce the isolation of the site which was almost wholly committed to the regional radiotherapy service in contrast to good practice across the country. This created negative connotations for the site amongst local people which management wished to reduce. This could be achieved by the development of general hospital services which would complement the existing service. Politically the powerful lobby at Wharfetown might have been partially pacified by the development of the complementary hospital in the North of the District. The buildings were also in relatively good condition.

However the development of the site would not be without difficulties. The site was not flat and the hospital could only be reached via a narrow lane not suitable for buses or large volumes of traffic. It was also poorly served by public transport.

Finally the possibility of using a greenfield site in the North of the District was still under active consideration. Members were essentially supportive of management thinking and as only six weeks remained until the plan had to be submitted to the Region it was essential that work started on developing and quantifying the action plan to move from general intentions to a costed and timetabled development strategy. In the interim the District General Manager issued a discussion paper for informal consultation by 17 March at the latest, which mirrored the proposals outlined in the paper sent to members discussed above except left the position of Hospital E more open by suggesting the possibility that it could be the site for 250 beds as part of a three site option.

The Race for the Line

The Project Leader believed that to finalise the strategy and develop an action plan it was necessary for the Support Group to spend a week without interruptions and the diversions of other work away from the District. The aim of the week was to crystalise the options by putting all the information together and arriving at the most suitable options given the service objectives. This process was facilitated by the use of micro computers where a bed modelling programme had been developed and the presence of the whole Support Group for the week enabling immediate professional input and group decision making. The 'time out' week was also attended by officers from the Region and Northville Eastern Health Authority who were finalising their strategy.

A joint planning session held at the beginning of the week between the two Authority's considered in detail issues of joint concern between the Authority's. Members of the Support Group were allocated specific tasks involving the analysis and presentation of information on resources of manpower, estates and finance necessary to fulfil the plan. By allocating tasks to people who were already familiar with the ideas being tested and concentrating on major issues an inchoate action plan had evolved by the end of the week. A presentation for officers of Northville Western was held at the end of the week. The five Unit General Managers were present in addition to the District Management Board. The discussion confirmed support for a two site option and removed a one site option from consideration. A three site option was less favoured but remained in the running.

By obtaining feedback from senior management and having received members views at the seminar held for them in the middle of February, this allowed the Support Group to spend March concentrating on the preferred option of the District Health Authority. However a lot of energy was to be needed in convincing other parties of the merits of a two site option. In particular Faculty's preference for a one site DGH expressed at their meeting of 16 February during the Support Group's time out week was an ominous portent of future developments.

The decay of the clinical policy Support Group and undercurrents of clinical opposition to the strategy acted as spur to management to attract other allies to their cause. The Community Health Council (CHC) was a potential opponent of management plans which needed to be courted. The influence of CHC's has often been viewed as limited because of their distance from the management process, the difficulty of obtaining independent information/advice (because of their dependence on information derived from management) and their ambiguous role as both proponents and opponents of management due to the need for a continuing relationship with management. Nonetheless management have to consult the CHC over closures and Northville Western's management knew that they would have a better chance of selling the strategy to the clinicians and in particular to the Region if the strategy received the CHC's blessing.

The CHC had not participated in the review or expressed its position during 1986 due to the absence of a CHC secretary. The new CHC secretary recognised the importance of the review and during January/February 1987 arranged a number of public meetings attended by CHC members and health authority officers to inform the public of the Health Authority's thinking and to gauge public reaction. The CHC was divided with members drawn from Wharfetown strongly opposed to any diminution in the importance of Hospital E. There was concern at the lack of provision in the South of the city and the absence of plans to rectify this position.

The issue of accessibility was assigned a high priority and therefore considerable support was expressed for a three site option. Support for a three site option also lessened the discomfort felt by CHC members in supporting closures of hospitals. This was particularly acute as the Authority was consulting on the closure of two hospitals in the North of the city. They were influenced by arguments that a three site option would not help the District to shift such large amounts of funding from acute to priority services as a two site option and would not necessarily be more accessible, bearing in mind the radial transport networks in the city. Management and clinicians also emphasised their view that hospitals of 250 beds were not viable. The CHC eventually capitulated and backed a two site option.

An additional complicating factor in the preparation of the action plan was the forceful views expressed by the Chairman of the Health Authority. A new Chairman had been appointed in 1986 from a private sector background and with no previous contact of the NHS. The approach of the Chairman was contentious. In particular he sought to adopt a dominant position in decision making and was anxious to apply his private sector dictums to the deliberations of the Authority. A number of senior officers became disenchanted with this approach believing he usurped their authority and that his interventions were not sensitive to the culture of the NHS.

This difference in style impinged on the way in which the review process operated. The Chairman's view of the review process was different from senior officers interpretation of the review. The Chairman emphasised the capital planning aspects of the review focusing on the future of individual buildings which proved difficult to reconcile with the service planning approach favoured by officers. A logical extension of the capital planning approach was the Chairman's perception of the review as being in distinct chunks. For example, the role of Hospital A was one issue and the role of Hospitals D and E in the North of the city was a separate concern. The Chairman favoured separate individuals taking a lead role for each sector which prevented an integrated approach to service development. The final source of disagreement concerned the timetabling of developments in the District strategy with the Chairman insisting on a detailed timetable with target dates for completion of new developments in the near future. A similar difficulty arose over the use of empty space in Hospital B. The Chairman wanted to finalise the proposals even though consultation was still taking place. These edicts failed to acknowledge the planning realities of the NHS where plans take a number of years to come to fruition. Ultimately senior officers had to accept the structure imposed by the Chairman but this soured the relationship with him. If the relationship with the Chairman was proving difficult undercurrents of discontent from clinical staff were to vex management for the closing weeks of the review.

It is easy to exaggerate the degree of clinical opposition to a two site strategy. It was predominantly confined to a number of consultants at Hospital A. However the inability of the clinical policy Steering Group to function effectively and retain the confidence of clinical staff allowed a number of powerful clinicians to seize the initiative and campaign vigorously for a one site option based at Hospital A with in excess of 1,000 beds. Faculty at their meeting of 16 March 1987 reiterated their wish for a single site DGH. This caused the District General Manager to write to the Regional Quantity Surveyor on 19 March 1987 in the following terms:

> As you know our strategy is being prepared on the belief that providing significantly more than 1,000 beds on the Hospital A main site is neither desirable nor feasible. However, there is a view among some medical staff in the DHA that this is not supported by hard evidence.

The DGM requested information based on the broad costs of various single site DGH's.

The Registrar in Community Medicine and the Deputy District Treasurer prepared a paper entitled 'Obstacles to the Development of the Hospital A site above 1,000 beds.' This argued that developing more than 1,000 beds on the Hospital A site precluded the use of a nucleus template design because nucleus design has a maximum of three storeys and their would be insufficient space without whole scale demolition of the nurses home. The alternative would be to build a high rise building but this had a number of disadvantages:

1. inability to use the nucleus design with consequent loss of savings in planning design time and other advantages with the design.
2. capital and revenue costs rise steeply with the height of buildings.
3. congestion of the site and associated car parking difficulties.

It was not possible to convince all clinical staff of the disadvantages of a one site option and this precipitated a crisis meeting of the Clinical Policy Steering Group where non-medical members were excluded. It was decided to meet the District General Manager with a view to adopting new consultation procedures with Faculty. This signalled the final demise of the Clinical Policy Steering Group.

Marketing the Strategy

The review of the General Hospital services which was intended as a joint review between both Northville Authorities was published separately under the auspices of the District Strategic Plan. The strategy was presented to the District Health Authority on 31 March 1987 and the District General Manager summarised the approach adopted in the strategy:

> The strategy for General Hospital Services is based on a concept of two hospitals which together meet the needs arising both from the local community and from the District's role as a teaching and referral centre. Hospital A would be the main district hospital and teaching centre with the only Accident and Emergency Department and those highly specialised services requiring full clinical and diagnostic support. Planning and site constraints restrict its size to not much more than its present total bed

complement particularly if the wards and departments in the existing buildings are to be improved.

The function of the second complementary hospital, Hospital D would need to be integrated closely with Hospital A including full participation in the Bed Bureau and with joint consultant appointments in many of the specialities. It would need to be of sufficient size to attract staff and services of reasonable calibre and might provide the main base perhaps for some services such as rheumatology, rehabilitation and elective orthopaedic surgery, but it should not be so developed as to compete with Hospital A as a second comprehensive District General Hospital. The detailed clinical and operational policies for both hospitals will need to be discussed with the professional advisory bodies once the RHA's acceptance of this general approach has been secured.

In arguing for capital investment at Hospital D to rationalise non-Hospital A services and cease reliance on unsatisfactory buildings at Hospitals C and E where many of the present structures have a very limited future, the Authority must continue to urge the RHA to provide for that major investment at Hospital A which was absent from the original Regional Strategy for the period 1994.

Complementing the two site strategy was the plan to bring Hospital B into full use by December 1989 at a cost of £29·3m and phase 2 of Hospital A redevelopment a further £14·7m. Funding was expected from the Region and the Department of Health with the District anticipating land sales of about £3m predominantly from the closure of Hospital C in 1994. The strategy with a £52·4m capital injection needed to fulfil the plan for the development of general hospital services was approved by the Authority and went out for consultation.

The objection raised by lobbyists in Wharefetown had been anticipated but the reaction of other parties including clinicians, the city council and the CHC were harder to predict. The issues that emerged from the consultation process included the role of Hospital E, the absence of provision in the South of the city, the choice of specialities to be accommodated in Hospital B and the continuing expression of support for a one site DGH.

The Wharefetown parish council vigorously campaigned against the general hospital strategy because of the threat it posed to the future of Hospital E. The council objected to having to travel eleven miles to Hospital A and commented on the lack of parking facilities available. Concern was expressed at the drift to centralisation of service implied in the strategy. Furthermore the spectre of closure for the hospital had implications for the local economy as the District Health Authority was the largest employer in Wharfetown. Management had attempted to accommodate this lobby by siting the new general hospital at nearby Hospital D. This proved not to be sufficient so management left the possibility that the hospital could continue to be used for geriatric provision. In addition to this although a three site option was not favoured, at the option appraisal stage Hospital E was included as a possible site for a 250 bed general hospital.

The city council was suspicious of the District's quest to reduce the number of hospital sites viewing it solely as a cost reduction exercise. The council supported the retention of general hospital services at Wharefetown. The council was particularly anxious that no provision was planned for the south of the city. They argued that the deprivation and lack of facilities in the south merited the development of services. The Community Health Council also was concerned about this situation. The strength of feeling in the south of the city was reflected by the submission of a 3,200 signature petition from residents in the south calling for a 250 bedded hospital. The local Labour MP also lobbied for a hospital in the south.

The Support Group had decided against locating a hospital in the south of the city for three main reasons. First the transport system in this area of the city was poorly developed and bus routes ran radially into the centre of the city. Consequently to reach a new hospital in the south would require a journey into the centre of the city and out again for residents in the south of the city. Second, this situation was exacerbated by the motorways which carved up the south of the city and prevented formation of natural communities for a proposed DGH. Finally the corollary of poor transportation East to West was that adequate transport networks existed to the centre of the city enabling residents from south of the city to reach Hospital A within one hour. Nonetheless the Authority as a sop to feelings in the south promised some community developments in the south of the city.

The response from clinical staff was mixed. Strong support remained for a one site DGH located at Hospital A. However other clinicians were satisfied with the two site option because Hospital A was to remain dominant, the only disquiet being the role of the second hospital which many clinicians did not want to develop as a complementary hospital but rather wanted it to become a satellite of Hospital A. The question of which specialities were to be located in Hospital B also generated a vigorous debate.

To summarise, despite the turbulent weeks prior to the March 1987 deadline the Support Group managed to prepare a strategy on time which was approved in principle by the District and Regional Health Authorities. The closure of hospital services always engenders opposition and this was the case in Northville. However in the immediate aftermath of March 1987 the Support Group had reason to be pleased with their achievement in devising a strategy that the majority of parties in the District could accept. Subsequent events were to demonstrate the vulnerability of the strategy to rapidly changing circumstances. That is a different story.

CONCLUSION

Change and the Environment

Senior management in Northville Western Health Authority were confronted with an unfavourable context for change. For management to achieve change it is not solely the nature or scale of the change to be achieved and the actions taken by the key actors which determines or influences outcome. Managerial actions are affected by the environ mental context, and different contexts differ in their receptiveness to change.

In Northville Western Health Authority the environment was not conducive to change. The Authority had a legacy of unsatisfactory planning activity which had left the provision of acute beds in the city unresolved after the 1982 reorganisation. In addition the pressure to form one health authority for the whole city had been resisted because of the inevitable rationalisation this would have brought in its wake. However this meant that, when the Region cajoled the Authority to reduce bed numbers, there was less scope for merging services painlessly than if the exercise had been conducted across the whole city.

Crucially each District recognised that reductions in particular specialities would effectively allow the rival authority to become the sole provider of those services therefore enhancing their position and justifying continuing resources from the Region. A vicious circle could be instigated, with resources from Region diminishing cumulatively as—ironically—targets for rationalisation were met. Consequently the rivalry between the Districts inhibited change unless the Region took a strong lead.

Current Service Provision

Northville Western Health Authority had an inappropriate pattern of provision on which to base its future. General hospital services were located on nine sites which fragmented the delivery of services. These sites had been allowed to develop in an uncontrolled and random manner, which resulted in poor inter-departmental relationships militating against the efficient practice of medicine. Severe shortages of beds at Hospital A existed alongside significant numbers of unused and unstaffed beds at other hospitals. Hospital provision was predominantly ageing: few of the main hospitals had been built this century, and the more recent additions were frequently hutted accommodation designed as temporary provision. Finally, the location of hospitals in relation to the populations they served was unsatisfactory, as more than half of the hospitals in the District lay outside or on the perimeter of the District boundary.

Constraints upon Change: Clinician's Attitudes

However, this state of affairs did not lead to a widespread recognition of the need for radical change. A precondition for successful change is building a consensus within the organisation for change. This was, however, lacking in Northville Western for a number of reasons.

Firstly, although environmental pressure such as financial stringency can act as a catalyst (and indeed the financial situation was a key factor in bringing about change), the dominant clinicians in the District viewed the environmental pressures, be they financial targets or Regional bed targets as external to the way they worked. They were reluctant to recognise that they were partly responsible for the impasse in the District. Consequently the difficulties of the District were seen as due to the foisting of unfavourable policies on the District and therefore had to be combatted by fighting those external agencies, particularly the Region, to lift the financial restraints. Therefore it proved difficult for management to develop legitimacy for change and win the support of clinicians.

Secondly, the clinical body was dominated by clinicians in Hospital A, which prevented the development of a corporate clinical view of what was best for the whole District. The large number of hospitals (some facing closure) were primarily interested in their own future. These divisions were reinforced by the existence of five management units largely based on geographical location. Consequently, Hospital A clinicians were dominant and tended to evaluate policy options in terms of their impact on Hospital A. This led to hositility to the concept of a second, complementary hospital which surfaced in the closing stages of the review.

Thirdly, there was widespread cynicism about the Review process. Planning activity was viewed with suspicion by the clinicians, who believed it had never led to any gains for the District in the past. In the unfavourable financial situation, they believed the only outcome was likely to be further service reductions. Therefore there was little desire to be involved in the process or to follow its proceedings closely. In addition power within the District did not only reside in formal hierarchies but was vested in particular key clinicians who had little involvement in the formal management structures. Eventually this led to frenzied activity by Faculty in February as senior clinicians realised that the review was 'for real' and that therefore they needed to take seriously its deliberations.

Management Strategy

This unfavourable climate had been exacerbated by the cautious management approach which had prevailed in Northville Western Health Authority. This meant that management had been reluctant to spell out the degree of change the District faced. For example the 1985 District Strategic Plan failed to make explicit the necessity for bed reductions which management realised were on the horizon. Instead the strategy contained high aspirations for developments which the document itself acknowledged were probably unobtainable. Consequently, clinicians, were not sufficiently prepared for change and an aspirational strategy with no immediate tangible outcomes negated any belief in planning clinicians might have entertained. Management therefore did not effectively communicate with clinicians, which created difficulties in gaining support for change.

The establishment of the Joint Review was analogous to setting up a Royal Commission at national level. It was needed to get the Region out of a policy vacuum and enabled the Region to be seen to be doing something. The Joint Review got the Region off the hook of immediate action, enabling it to argue that it was responding to the concerns raised by the Authority which had been fanned by unfavourable press coverage at the end of 1985. The Region, with a new general manager and the rejection of its Regional Strategic Plan, was in no position to make policy decisions on the provision of services in Northville. Therefore the Joint Review provided an important breathing space for the Region.

Northville Western management viewed the establishment of the review as overdue recognition of the particular difficulties they faced. It was potentially complicated by the inclusion of Northville Eastern in the review remit. However, this did not impinge greatly on the review as neither District had an incentive to work cooperatively and the Region failed to offer guidance, for example on Regional specialties, which would have allowed a common understanding between the two Districts to emerge on matters affecting the whole city.

The Review process was carried out in a pragmatic way in the sense that it took account of existing service provision rather than searching for solutions which ignored the constraint or starting point of the existing service pattern. However, the pragmatic label can disguise the extent to which management's approach was actually grounded in a 'rational planning' model of decision-making. Although not unaware of the political dimensions of any plans, the support group did not view the marketing of any plan as their primary function. Instead they adopted a technocratic approach to the planning activity compiling information on functional suitability, access, clinical workload and other factors to establish options which would improve the delivery of services, yet achieve the redistribution of revenue and bed rationalisation sought by regional strategic targets.

As a result there was a separation of the conception of the plan from the management task of 'selling' the plan to interest groups and devising an implementation strategy. This is not to argue that other groups were not consulted but their views had limited influence on the proposed options.

This situation prevailed for a number of reasons. Firstly, it stemmed from the approach adopted by the support group which essentially assumed that if a rational solution was devised based on sound information, ultimately the logic of the plan would be vindicated and the perspectives of sectional interest groups would be seen as simply that and dismissed. Secondly, the medical staff themselves were reluctant to be involved in the process. Management wanted a medical representative on the support group but this was declined. Thirdly, as the planning activity quickened and the March deadline loomed, it became increasingly difficult to consult widely and keep clinicians fully informed of progress.

Clinical support was essential for the achievement of change. This was complicated by the medical advisory machinery in the District which prevented a single voice emerging to represent the medical perspective. Management tried to overcome this problem through the establishment of the Clinical Policy Steering Group. However this body never clearly established its role and was ultimately not prepared to take responsibility for its tepid support of management plans when it became clear this was contrary to the views of some powerful colleagues. The group lacked some credibility partly due to the choice of chairman who did not enjoy the confidence of his colleagues. This reflected the difficulty that district medical officers had in gaining recognition for their work amongst their clinical colleagues.

Management also did not have much to offer the clinicians to ensure their support. Although a rationalisation of services, might have eased the financial difficulties of the District—helping the bulk of clinicians —this type of incentive was distant and not immediately obvious. The dominance of Hospital A, however, made the development of a second site unpalatable as there was a wish to avoid the development of a potential rival for resources and also in order to compete with Hospital 1 a desire to concentrate resources on one site at Hospital A. Management were unable to offer clinicians any incentives to support their approach relying on only a general belief in the validity of the plan.

Management had difficulty in gaining the initiative in the debate over strategy. This stemmed from the legacy of reactive management in the

District. The implementation of general management with the aim of shifting from a professional ethos to a management ethos had an uneven impact across the NHS. In Northville Western it proved difficult to overcome the entrenched power of the clinical staff. Senior management were not helped by the role played by the Chairman of the Health Authority. The relationship between the Chairman and the District General Manager had a crucial bearing on the District as working together they can exert considerable leverage on policy in an authority. In Northville Western the Chairman and the District General Manager were unable to work in tandem due to the insensitivity of the chairman to the manner in which the NHS worked. This severely weakened the District General Manager who not only faced a powerful body of consultants but lacked support from the Chairman.

Information Problems

Management also faced difficulties in persuading clinicians of the validity of reducing beds because of the inadequate information available in the District. The information on Performance Indicators was criticised by clinicians because it excluded day case work. In addition, the information was at a very aggregate level and needed to be broken down into specialties to yield useful information for planning purposes. Clinicians, reluctant to accept management's case, were able to attack their arguments by pointing to the inaccuracy of the data.

This was particularly important in connection with the T2 bed target. This target was not accepted by the clinicians who were sceptical about the manner in which the figure was compiled. Management had to be seen to be combatting the Regional target yet at the same time were using the T2 target as a catalyst for change, a situation which was not always easy to reconcile.

The Region's Relationship with the District

The role of the Region was central to the successful outcome of the Review. Historically the relationship between the District and the Region has been a cool one and there was a lack of trust between the two parties. This was accentuated by the announcement of extra funding for Northville Eastern to develop facilities at Hospital 1 in October 1986. This alarmed management in Northville Western who had no prior warning of the announcement. It damaged management's credibility as they had been telling their own clinicians all decisions of that nature would be decided within the context of the joint review.

The District spent a lot of energy on a critique of the T2 target, but the rejection of the Regional strategy because the Regional bed numbers were too high suggested the Region was unlikely to shift its stance on his issue. An adversarial relationship was established with the Region which was not conducive to gaining Regional support for change. However, the Region itself was in disarray during 1986 and unable to give the necessary lead to the Authority on a range of key issues including the financial framework for the Review, the future of regional specialties and the durability of the T2 bed target. It was this lack of guidance that left the District with conflicting signals about the willingness of the Region to fund developments to help rationalise services in Northville Western. This ambiguity led to Districts bidding for resources which the Region was unable to provide leaving the Regional strategy in tatters and the future of Northville Western uncertain. This position could be complicated by the likelihood that Hospital A will become self-governing under the White Paper reforms. This would jeopardise the planning activity undertaken in the District and reinforce the fragmentation of services which Northville Western was trying to remedy.

APPENDIX 1

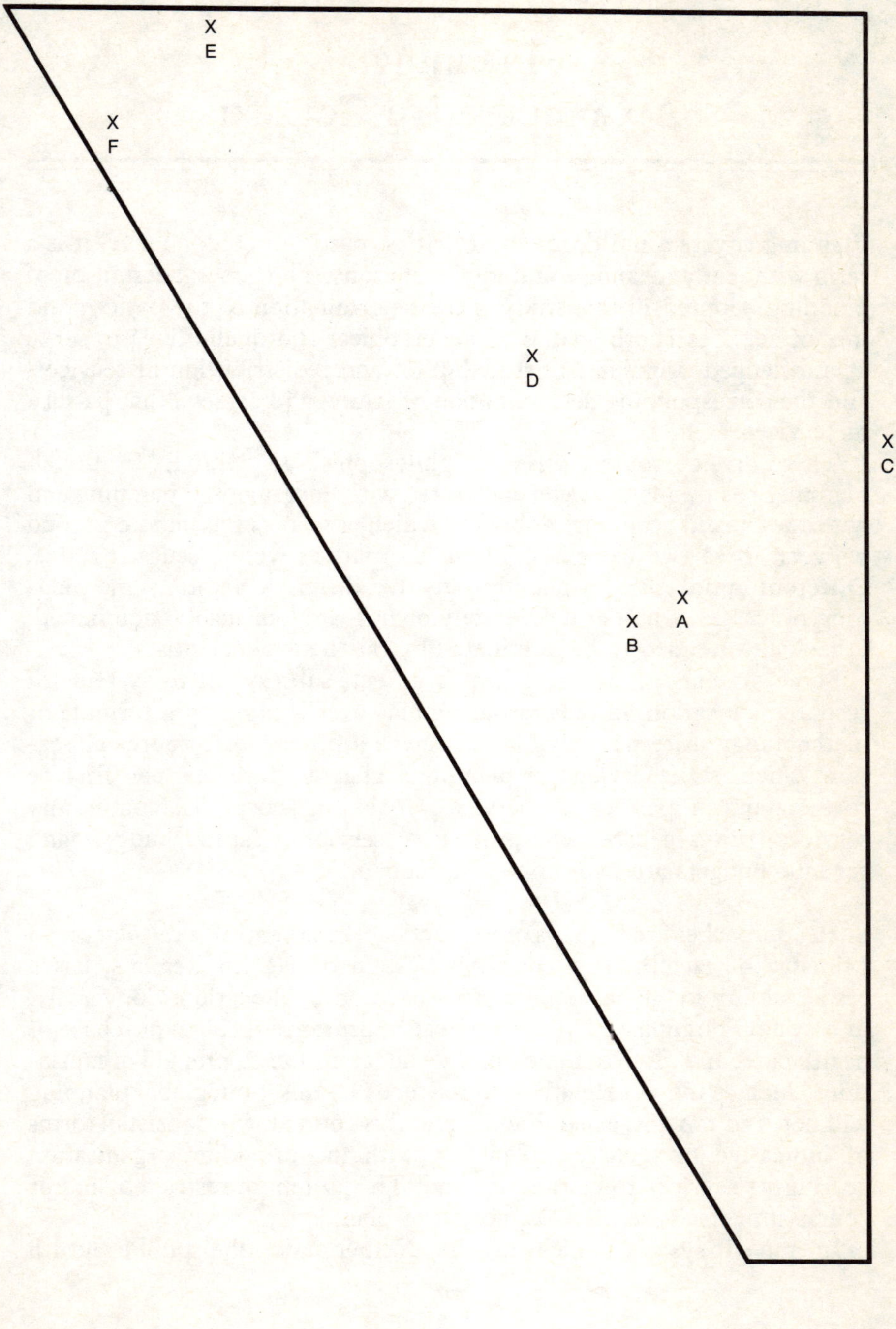

CHAPTER 4

Planning: A Comparative Context

Planning covers a multitude of activities; partly in consequence, it is a term with many meanings and interpretations. The general definition of planning adopted in this study is the determination of the pattern and mix of services (both spatial or geographical and qualitative) to serve acknowledged principles of distribution and redistribution of services, and the corresponding determination of strategy to achieve that pattern of services.

There are, of course, different philosophies of planning. 'Rational' planning has frequently been contrasted with 'incremental' planning and with the 'mixed scanning' approach which is seen as the middle ground between these two extremes. These alternatives were discussed above. Different approaches to planning involve different actors: some planning processes, whether deliberately or not, are 'politically' dominated; others are intended to be dominated by the 'neutral scientists'.

Some systems of planning are, in effect, subservient to systems of resource allocation, in that resources may be allocated by a formula or methodology. Alternatively, one can have a process of resource allocation which is subservient to planning. That is, decisions can first be taken about a pattern of services, including hospitals, community services, primary care, and preventive services. Capital budgets and revenue budgets are determined subsequently.

Such approaches are perhaps only practicable if a central body, whether a Ministry of Health or a country's system of Health Regions, has a responsibility for global planning and/or resource allocation. Conversely, in a system dominated by private health insurance, private purchase of health care, and (for example) private subscription to prepaid organisations, such as the US Health Maintenance Organisation, global planning will not, and can not, exist. Planning, in this context, will consist in forms of indicative or technical planning, with the providing organisation gearing its services to market demand. This is a more restricted, and or course universally applicable, notion of planning.

In mixed systems, such as the Netherlands, the public health insurance system and private health insurance schemes are the main sources of income for providing institutions and hospital facilities. Yet even there, as in West Germany and other European countries, national planning structures have been instituted which attempt to influence the pattern and distribution of services beyond that which would be determined purely by a purchasing market. Thus, in such mixed systems, one can distinguish between the insurance system, the overall financing system for providers, and the planning system as it affects providers.

These systems combine elements of a global resource allocation system with a market system. For example, following recent changes, the new budgeting model for Dutch hospitals came to include:-

1. A fixed component related to the number of inhabitants in the hospital's catchment area (25 per cent of the budget will be allocated on this basis);

2. A 'semi-fixed component' based on the number of specialties and beds of the hospital (35 per cent of the budget allocated by this factor); and,

3. A variable component—based on negotiations between the hospital management and the local insurance companies and sick funds dealing with the hospital—related to the number of patients to be treated in the following year.

This approach is not wholly unlike the system of resource allocation operating in Britain from the late 1960s until 1976, when Health Regions were reimbursed on the basis of population, facilities and activity. This approach was a 'half-way house'—not as systematic as the later RAWP system but more objective in attempting to gauge need than merely relying on historic patterns of provision.

It is interesting to note that, in the Netherlands, despite the existence of a public-private mix in financing, there is (still) a strong element of public planning. That is, a hospital cannot merely maximise its budget by selling itself in the market place, whether to payers, insurance companies and sick funds. Furthermore, payment can be prospective rather than retrospective, or merely reimbursing costs.

This reflects an international trend to see planning very much in terms of cost control. In consequence, loose methods of reimbursing hospitals have not been able to achieve it, and prospective reimbursement of hospitals based on global fees for types of case treated has developed. This has occurred for example even in the United States via the 'Diagnosis Related Group' (DRG) policy which is effectively a regulatory prices policy when each DRG is allotted a 'reasonable cost'.

In Britain also, determining the costs of treatment through various experiments with patient costing, a DRG type of costing and at the more aggregate level specialty and hospital costing have been developed: hitherto with a view to use in the planning process, and increasingly after the White Paper of 1989 and National Health Service Bill of 1990, with a view to use by hospitals which seek to market themselves in a more competitive environment.

This trend has been, arguably, at the expense of the school of thought that advocates comprehensive health service planning: which is charged with measuring the need for different types of services and redistributing resources across countries and across Regions where necessary. However, in practice, it is not surprising that lofty goals will often not be met. In the United States, for example, there was a move up to the late 1970s to incorporate a form of planning into what was largely a private system. Hospital development programmes after the Second World War such as the Hill-Burton Act of 1946 were followed by the Regional Medical Programmes Act 1965, the Comprehensive Health Planning Act of 1966 and, allegedly more significant, the National Health Planning and Resources Development Act of 1974 (Paton, 1990). However, planning has not been global: it has been capital-based planning; it has been voluntaristic rather than mandatory, increasingly into the 1980s; and, it has been diverted from 'public health' goals by provider coalitions at the level of the planning agency (the Health Systems Agency).

Both proponents and opponents of planning have been disappointed with results: planning has been discredited, and a renewed faith in competition has emerged instead. In the US, competition has replaced planning as the 'great white hope' for controlling costs and then—say those interested in greater equity—extending access to care by the poor. But neither has succeeded in so doing. This has raised a lively debate about whether profit-seeking health care institutions are cheaper and more cost-effective, or the reverse, and whether access to health care is easier or not. What has happened, both in the United States and Netherlands, is that, planning has developed into a restrictive activity, with resources development and redistribution very much downplayed in recent years (Kirkman-Liff, 1988).

There are thus a number of dimensions on which planning can be categorised. It can be comprehensive or incremental. It can address capital budgets, revenue budgets, or both—perhaps through a merging of the two. Indeed a major problem in health planning systems has often been that planned revenue budgets have not been consistent with implications of planned capital budgets. Thus we have had the phenomena of new hospitals without budgets to run them; or at the other extreme, revenue budgets with no meaningful services on which they can be spent.

In practice planning ought to be linked closely to resource allocation: again if it is not, one can find Health Regions or Districts receiving budgets through the resource allocation process acording to different criteria from those on which they are intending to develop services. Naturally again this is implying a global responsibility for a central planning system. An alternative, increasingly advocated in Britain, is to employ a central resource allocation system based on population-weighted need for health care (however defined), but then to allow the receiving Health Districts to determine their own service mix and to buy services from and sell services to each other on market principles (Enthoven, 1985). A publicly financed NHS, with financing separated from provision through a system of competing providers, is a unique experiment, as yet in an embryonic stage.

Competition or Planning?

One can identify 'competition in the market' and 'bureaucratic planning' as opposites in health care systems. In the Netherlands recently, the Dekker Commission has advocated increased competition between insurance companies and sick funds on the financing side, and decreased planning and increasing reliance on competition on the provider side. However, this is still expected to co-exist with the basic hospital planning law (the WZV law) instituted back in 1971.

In Britain, the recent White Paper (Department of Health, 1989a) has advocated a number of competitive measures on the supply side of health care: primarily, a system of trading for clinical, medical, community, and even preventive services between Districts within the National Health Service; optional budgets for general practices above a certain size to pay for the hospital care of their patients; and, provision for hospitals and indeed community units to 'opt out' of health authority control and act as independent providers albeit still NHS institutions. Arguably, facilities in the 'self-governing' category would be subject to minimal planning (accepting an obligation to provide 'core services' to their local catchment populations), and would act as economically free institutions allowed to raise money on capital markets and determine their own budgets and basis for 'profit'. Thus, the language of the business plan and the concept of marketing are rapidly being introduced in the British National Health Service.

However, this does not imply that planning will no longer be relevant. District Health Authorities will still receive budgets based broadly on their population's needs. It is then up to Districts to guide potential providers as to appropriate services and appropriate location of services. The fact that there may be competition in providing these services does not alter this fundamental fact. Furthermore Regions, above the level of the District, may be required to give guidance—or even mandates—as to the Region-wide distribution and pattern of services, to prevent unnecessary duplication or wasteful competition, i.e. to indulge in indicative planning at the very least and comprehensive planning at the most. Thus, to see a simplistic distinction between competition and planning may be naive.

This is especially so when one considers the broader dictates of public health, and moves away from a fixation with hospitals, as planning systems often tend in practice to have. Systems based on recognition of the global need of populations must have a capacity for making decisions as to, for example, the priority which preventive services will have in the aggregate as opposed to curative services; or as to the priority which community care will have when competing for scarce resources with acute budgets. Therefore, initial planning by Regional and District Authorities, whatever the health system is necessary.

It is dangerous to compare idealised theories with their real world opposites: for example, idealised competition compared with real world planning, warts and all; or real world competition, warts and all, compared with idealised planning. Rhetoric coming from political convictions tends to obscure this plain fact. Accepting insights from both philosophies may be useful. For example, *simulating* markets whereby primary care physicians refer patients for secondary care according to consumer choice as well as their own priorities, to allow modelling and construction of a planning system to situate facilities in line with such referral patterns, may be a promising means of proceeding. Thus health authorities can combine a strategic role yet avoid a heavy handed or bureaucratic top-down approach.

Indeed, in looking at the respective merits of either competition or planning, it is important to avoid over complexity or over-bureaucratic means of achieving one's aims. For example, if the catchment populations served by health facilities do not closely mirror the health Authorities which receive the resources, there will be problems about reconciling reimbursement for patients living outside the Authorities with reimbursement for patients within the Authorities' boundaries. Bureaucratic systems of so doing, as with some elements of pre-1991 subregional resource allocation in Britain, may develop perverse incentives. Hence the argument for the internal market. Similarly, one must exhibit caution in implementing competitive solutions which may, at the end of the day, be more bureaucratic to police than the bureaucratic systems they are intended to replace.

Variants of Planning

Technical variants of planning have changed and developed over the years. There is a continuing movement away from norms-based approaches, which are now seen as simplistic and inappropriate, as they deal with inputs rather than outputs or even outcomes from health care systems. A public health focus on health status and improvements therein presumably should be identified with planning systems which lay stress on outcomes to be achieved (health status) rather than inputs such as numbers of beds or even outputs, such as numbers of services delivered.

Planning for bed norms, a variant of capital planning, has been replaced in the British National Health Service with variants of service planning and planning for client groups. Broadly speaking, service planning accompanied the 1974 National Health Service reorganisation, and attempted to unify hospital and community health services (many of which had previously been the responsibility of local government). However, Regional based service planning was often comprehensive in theory but weak in practice on how objectives were to be met. In 1979, the emphasis moved to a devolved management-based planning approach within the District, in response to the view that planning had hitherto been a bureaucratic and remote activity.

Sophisticated systems of planning have been developed which attempt: to use local and national sources of data on morbidity and social deprivation; model the willingness to travel and normatively-defined i.e. acceptable distances to health care in different specialties; and model that distribution to locate facilities which will combine need and equity with economy. The umbrella of a publicly financed, publicly provided health care system makes these technical approaches possible.

However, other variants of planning have existed in other countries, although for example, the United States planning system in its short-lived heyday was described by one commentator as 'negative regulation' rather than planning. The implication is that, rather than active public control, there is reliance on indirect incentive. The Netherlands' system combines public planning with decentralised reimbursement of hospitals and other facilities. As in so many respects, European systems often have forms of planning which are stronger than in the US, yet weaker than in Britain.

As a generalisation, the most promising avenue for future coordination and development of planning policies geared to meeting public health objectives and need for health care in particular, is the reconciliation of certain competitive incentives with the overall goals of planning. For example, Diagnosis Related Groups can be instituted as a pricing system, which then forces hospitals to become more efficient and competitive, yet which may also allow global planning authorities such as Regions or Districts to cost out the desired service mix and geographical distribution of services. Health Maintenance Organisations in the United States, subject to certain caveats, may help the task of increasing efficiency on the provider side of health care, and therefore aid state and federal governments in enrolling dependent populations in HMOs, populations hitherto excluded from regular health care.

At the broadest level, no technical solution can exist to determine the strategic choices between, for example, acute and curative medicine and preventive and promotive health care. Analysis can help, and specific research can, for example, outline tangible health benefits of preventive health programmes; for example, anti-smoking programmes, which are allegedly very effective when employing the cost per Quality Adjusted Life Year approach. Yet, at the end of the day, social and political choices are bound to inform planning choices and health priorities. The most promising way forward, achieving the greatest consensus, appears to be two-fold: firstly, to stress changes in health status (whether for populations or for individuals) as the unit of achievement; and, secondly, to reconcile planning with more sensible economic incentives for providers, as the means to achieving improvements in health status.

CHAPTER 5

Case Study:

Resource allocation–need planning and competition in the NHS

INTRODUCTION

The White Paper *Working for Patients*, published in February 1989, proposed radical changes for the provision of health services (Department of Health, 1989a). Along with subsequent Working Papers (Department of Health, 1989b and 1990), it also proposed changes in the means of resource allocation to Regional and District Health Authorities from the Department of Health. Naturally such changes affect the nature of planning in the NHS in a fundamental way.

It is important to consider, firstly, how need for health services has been assessed in recent years and, secondly, how the provision of services has been related to such need, with a view to tracing the significance of present changes. In Section I the main policies affecting resource allocation are summarised, both at national level and in allocating monies from Regions to Districts. In Section II, competition and planning—and how they affect resource allocation—are discussed in the context of the White Paper. Examples of different policies for reconciling planning and resource allocation in different Regions are then reviewed in the main section, Section III.

SECTION I

The Complex Mosaic of Policy Issues

Resource Allocation and Planning

Resource allocation is of course merely one step on the road to the provision of services. Whether or not it is compatible with planning, within NHS Regions, is a major concern. There are different approaches to reconciling resource allocation with planning:

resource allocation-led approaches, which distribute money to Districts, thereby providing budgets out of which plans must be financed;

planning-led approaches, which lead to a more activist Regional role in instituting Region-wide plans for the provision of services, with resource allocation then following; and,

competitive strategies, increasingly to the fore after 1989, which seek to develop provider markets with District Health Authorities as the main purchasers of services from a variety of providers. This still requires resource allocation to Districts' *resident* populations, and so can be considered more 'resource allocation dependent' even than in the past, when allocations were often to Districts' planned *catchment* populations.

Competition

The rationale for competitive approaches as opposed to planning approaches is often thought to be as much a consequence of incompetent planning in the past as of the merits of 'textbook' competitive theory. This issue is implictly raised below, when planning is discussed with reference to policy in different Regions. The aim is to provide a brief review of Regional policy in different Regions, in Section III below.

There is now a widespread perception that, for political reasons at least, 'planning' has been superseded in the NHS by 'competition', a trend evidenced in other countries such as the United States and the Netherlands.

Capital Policy

There are now attempts to incorporate more sophisticated policies of capital allocation and capital accounting into the NHS, which have a significant effect upon resource allocation and the distribution of resources to authorities. Both in the past and still to a certain degree in the future, the separation of capital allocations from revenue allocations has been and will be a source of controversy. In a genuine market, of course, decisions on capital investment are taken by the provider to be justified along with running costs by the anticipation of revenue and profit. This may be true in the NHS too, but providers within the NHS (directly managed, not self-governing) may be regulated as to their access to capital to a great degree. In any case, the calculations as to how much to allow to *purchasers* to cover revenue and capital cost are still likely to be done separately. This is because there will not be a real capital market in the NHS; nor will there be freedom for purchasers to 'pay for' unregulated capital investment by providers.

In the past, capital-led approaches (which are often similar to planning-led approaches, since the primary purpose of the provision of capital is for the development, rationalisation or refurbishment of services) have often been distinguished both in theory and in practice from *revenue-led* approaches through which Regions have either allocated resources or mandated the provision of services.

Capital policy which is not reconciled with revenue policy can lead to services being developed without revenue to run them (hence the evolution in the past of the so-called 'Revenue Consequences of Capital Spending' (RCCS) policy to ensure that *revenue* was available for capital development.) Divorce of capital and revenue considerations can also mean the availability of revenue money without services upon which it can be efficiently and effectively used. Overall, such a divorce makes it difficult for authorities to make rational decisions as to whether to spend their money on revenue or capital or both.

One way of solving the dilemma is for capital and revenue budgets to be merged completely in allocating budgets to health authorities post-White Paper, allied to a policy of charging providers for capital. The Authorities would then be allowed to choose how to spend their global allocation and providers would make rational decisions on investing. 'Opted out' hospitals would have powers to operate in capital markets; for directly-managed hospitals, the Region would have to be the banker. Charges for capital could then be used to finance new developments to providing units, who would charge purchasing Districts a price for services which covered all costs (See Figure 1 below). Thus rational option appraisal would be possible.

Need

Meeting the need for health services has spawned complex debates concerning resource allocation, planning, and more recently various competitive strategies. A major area of investigation has of course been the construction of a formula to measure the need for health care. The RAWP committee in 1976 advocated that the best surrogate for need in health care, i.e. to measure morbidity, was the Standardised Mortality Ratio (SMR). The best review available on this topic is by Bevan and Mays (1987).

At the end of July 1988, the Review of RAWP Committee recommended, following an interim report of December 1986, that the SMR was no longer the best direct correlate of need on a one-to-one basis (NHS Management Board, 1988). Incorporating research which sought to identify need for health care in terms of the usage of health services and which argued that social deprivation was important in

FIGURE 1

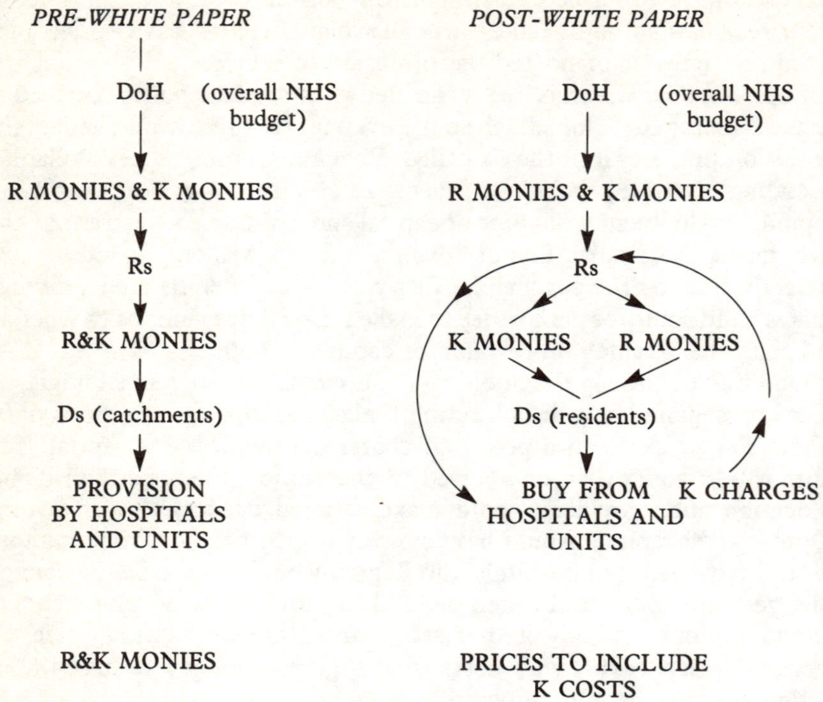

NOTE: Overall the money in the system is the same but there is now a distinction between purchasing and providing. A circular flow of capital from Regions to providers is financed from the policy of capital charging, additional to the flow of purchasing funds.

predicting that need, the Review of RAWP recommended that the Jarman Score (UPA8) be incorporated into the resource allocation formula. The SMR would still be employed but instead of being correlated with need on a one-to-one basis it would only represent 0·44 (i.e. 44 per cent) of the overall component predicting need. Thus a major import of the recommendations of the Review of RAWP was to reduce the significance of the SMR.

However, it was ambiguous as to whether it was being argued that the rest of the component measuring need would be taken up by the social deprivation factor. This controversy was heightened when the 1989 White Paper seemed broadly to accept the Review of RAWP recommendation to belittle the SMR (rounding off its new significance to 0·5 rather than 0·44) yet said nothing about whether or not a social deprivation factor was to be incorporated.

Later resolution of the same issue led to the square root of the SMR being adopted nationally, with no additional measure of social deprivation. This incidentally reduced the flow of funds away from the South-East of England. Some comentators had suggested that employing the particular social deprivation gauge of the Jarman Score was merely a complex methodological means of repatriating money to London, which was thought 'politically' necessary when the RAWP Review was beginning in 1985.

This has now been achieved by more direct political intervention to replace—or rather amend—the RAWP formula. Perhaps more important however than the incorporation of a new formula at national level is the criterion used by Regions in their formulae to allocate to Districts. Approaches have varied from Region to Region in the years since 1976.

Some Regions, having at first copied national RAWP and therefore replaced 'bidding' with formulae, have begun to move away from a formula approach. Broadly the new approaches combined strategic planning-led models with 'political' bidding processes. Following the 1989 White Paper, the new capitation approach to allocating resources both from the Centre to Regions and from Regions to Districts (heralded as a departure from RAWP, but embodying many similar principles) was at first thought likely to bring uniformity in the formulae for allocation from Regions to Districts. However, already Regions are diverging in approach—both to the technicalia of the formula, based on divergent gauges of need, and in the degree to which Regions wish to put Districts quickly on their 'resident targets', leaving all inter-District business to the market place. This is a contentious area involving high gainers and big losers, as well as the unpredictability of the market. Districts may choose to trade, or ironically to provide as much as possible themselves.

Overall, the post-White Paper system of resource allocation has kept the essence of RAWP at the national level, with three main changes:

1. cross-boundary flows are directly paid and contracted for;

2. targets are achieved vey quickly, at the *national to Regional* level; and

3. the formula is simplified, with only one application of the weights for usage and need, instead of separate formulae for different services; and the standardised mortality ratio is diminished in importance as a measure of need.

SECTION II

Reconciling Resource Allocation with Service Provision

Planning or Competition?

Considering the allocation of resources from Regions to Districts (on a formula basis broadly following the RAWP approach of 1976 (DHSS, 1976), before and after 1989, a number of options have existed *in theory* for Regions. They are:

(a) Implementing a sub-Regional version of a national RAWP-type or post-RAWP approach fairly straightforwardly.

(b) Amending the national formula for use at sub-Regional level.

(c) Keeping a formula approach of some sort, but allocating on the basis of catchment populations rather than Districts' resident populations. (In practice, post-White Paper regulations will prohibit this.)

(d) Keeping a formula approach of some sort, then instituting a system of market trading between Districts. This entails abolishing the indirect bureaucratic reimbursement of cross-boundary flows from one District to another (patients living in District A who are treated in District B) and instead instituting a system of direct cross charging by Districts. This can be done on an *ad hoc* basis or on the basis of agreed contracts for particular services in particular specialties.

It is in the abolishing of bureaucratic reimbursement of cross-boundary flows, and the movement instead to direct charging, that the 1989 White Paper recommendations 'abolish RAWP'. The only other senses in which they could be considered to do so lie in the changing of the system by which target allocations (i.e. the theoretical long-term monies Regions and Districts should get) are converted into actual allocations, and the simplification of the formula. A RAWP-type formula however remains.

In allocating from the centre to Regions, targets will be reached immediately after 1991. However, given the political and managerial impossibility of getting all Districts on target straight away (some would lose hugely and immediately—especially inner-city Districts) there is still a system for moving from actual to target allocations over a period of years, although not necessarily on the same principles as before, when Regions allocate to Districts.

(e) Encouraging as much District self-sufficiency as possible, following the allocation of resources to Districts. This is naturally the antithesis of the Government's proposals for 1989—but may be an unintended result in some areas of the country, as Districts deliberately contract with providers within their own boundaries, for political or other reasons. Not the least of these reasons may be the difficulty of enforcing contracts across District boundaries; the difficulty of reconciling in-patient care in a distant District with subsequent out-patient care in the patient's home District; and the desire to respond to popular demands for services to be provided locally, demands which tend to cut across political party boundaries.

In practice Districts are forming into *consortia*, to enable them to be 'mini Regions', planning for self-sufficiency provision to a great extent under the guise of competition.

(f) The next option is the one *thought* to be most squarely off the agenda as the result of the White Paper—abandoning resource allocation-led systems of service provision and moving to what has become known as *Regional Strategic Management*. This can vary from an *ad hoc* and 'political' form of planning to a very sophisticated attempted means of reconciling efficiency, equity and provision of services to those groups and geographical areas most in need. Naturally, Regional Strategic Management (or planning, by which it is variously known) on the latter basis is an exercise in comprehensive rational planning, and therefore subject to the pitfalls of over ambitiousness and insufficient recognition of 'politics'.

However, just as it would be naive to picture planning in its ideal theoretical state as opposed to its real world state, its would similarly be naive to consider the text book advantages of the market only and not the subversions of the market which frequently occur in the real world, especially in the field of health care, long considered to break many of the conditions necessary for the working of an efficient and effective market place.

The essence of Regional Strategic Management is that hypothesised need for services by different groups in different areas within the Region is modelled by reference to usage of services once an attempt has been made for control for existing supply. Next, specialty by specialty, unit by unit, a picture is built of the ideal distribution of services given current and feasible catchment areas and distances patients are willing to travel. Next the ideal mix and distribution of services is then compared with what exists at present. A strategy of 'getting from here to there' is then required. This may involve proposed amendments to existing habits which determine the consumption of care, including acceptable travel times and similar factors. Finally, a feasible plan for the redistribution of services, normally involving closures as well as redevelopments, is outlined.

The approach has been criticised for its derivation of the need for services not on account of its ignoring equity (for indeed a major aim of the policy is to increase equity by looking at which groups have hitherto been excluded from services, or which have 'under consumed' services according to predictions of their need) but because predicting need from existing patterns of usage is considered both conceptually and practically imperfect.

It should be noted that resource allocation formula which seek to employ usage of services (discharge rates whether or not modified by length of stay) as indicators of need are open to the same criticism. It could of course be argued that the pure use of Standardised Mortality Ratios, while not 'contaminated' by existing patterns of usage, suffer from not necessarily being related to experts' or patients' criteria of need in different specialties. This naturally relates to the debate as to whether a high death rate implies a high usage of services. It has been suggested that in the specialties where consumption of health care is most salient, that this is in fact so. However, the debate continues. Resources are only allocated to Districts, under Regional Strategic Management, after an ideal pattern of usage of services without reference to District boundaries is assembled, and Districts are therefore fairly incidental in the working of the model. The criticism therefore can arise that the lack of involvement by Districts can prove a politically difficult factor (see below).

Cross-Boundary Flows: Pre-White Paper

Considerations of the nature of the formula apart, there has been a wide consensus that RAWP has achieved its aim nationally, and that the *principles* of RAWP are applicable sub-Regionally. Given the smaller populations involved however, there have been both methodological and statistical problems in using RAWP sub-Regionally (Paton, 1985).

The major problem has occurred when Districts have treated a lot of patients from outside their boundaries, and/or exported a lot of patients from within their boundaries for treatment in other Districts. The cross-boundary flow in other words has been salient. The problem here has been the creation of perverse incentives for District management. Cross-boundary flow patients were not reimbursed out of the District's RAWP allocation, but at the national average specialty cost for that specialty.

Thus the amount of money a District gets for treating a patient from outside its boundaries will very likely be different from the amount of money it gets for treating a patient of its own. In some cases this leads to an incentive to import patients; in other cases it leads to an incentive only to treat a District's own patients.

The issue is complicated further by the fact that the cross-boundary flow has only gone into the future *target* allocation, not the actual current allocation for the District. Therefore, a District may do work for other Districts and only have theoretical or eventual reimbursement. This may of course mitigate a theoretical perverse incentive for a District to treat only patients from outside its District: for example Districts well above their target in London with an imputed low average cost per patient treated in order to live within their budget, such as the West Lambeth District in London, may be thought to benefit from importing patients—but only if they are reimbursed adequately quickly, and/or their target is affected in a benign manner with regard to future calculations of allocation.

The complexity is illustrated by the following considerations. A District which sees itself set a much lower target than its historic record of allocation (whether justly or unjustly, in that District's view) has a number of choices. It can attempt to cut spending in order to reach its lower target, presumably in practice over a number of years. Quite apart from the fact that targets are constantly shifting, however this is a dangerous policy. For how does it cut spending? It can say, do not treat patients from outside the District—in which case its target is lowered further as it loses 'cross-boundary' flow money for imported patients. It may therefore be locked into a vicious circle of decline. Or it can say it will try to treat only or mostly patients from *outside* the District. This may boost its target by boosting cross-boundary flow adjustment. But it will lose its own patients if other Districts do the same, in a 'beggar my neighbour' policy (Bevan and Beech, 1987). In other words, the essence of the problem is a low target for its resident population. This cannot be altered by such manipulations.

Rationing

The District, pre-White Paper, had no control over the behaviour of its own residents. The London Districts for example have traditionally had more services and more usage of services per population—even after adjusting for need—than other areas of the country. This may or may not be just. Those who argue that the health service is underfunded generally say that even in the London Districts there are many cases of unmet need. Epidemiological work and case load monitoring has suggested this.

However, even if it were hypothesised that consumption per capita in these Districts ought to be reduced to the national average level, achieving this would be very difficult. Prior to the recommendations of the 1989 White Paper at any rate, if a District sought to cut services to its own population, people could merely seek services elsewhere, in other Districts. 'Rationing' was done informally, if at all, by providers—clinicians in the main rather than managers. Post-White Paper, rationing is to be institutionalised, and conducted 'rationally' by managers.

It is not difficult to see, given this morass of complexity, that abolishing the cross-boundary flow discrepancy and seeking to move to either a model of direct trading or a model of Regional Strategic Movement was attractive. The question in practice has been: which is more attractive, and by what criteria? Such criteria are political, managerial and ethical (given the significance of equity as the motor of resource allocation based on need in public health care systems).

The White Paper

Considering competition first, it is as well to start with the Prime Minister's Review of the Health Service conducted throughout 1988 and the resulting White Paper in February 1989. This embraces the concept of the internal market as advocated by Enthoven and indeed goes further in advocating a competitive strategy for the provision of health care, with Districts as purchasing agents.

Firstly, the financing of health care (still to be funded from general taxation and subsequent distribution of resources to Regions and Districts) is to be separated from the provision of health care. In the past Districts have, in an *ad hoc* manner, received monies and provided services. They are now to purchase and contract for services, from themselves amongst others. In some cases this may merely be an accounting exercise.

A hospital, whether or not opted out of health authority control, has to price its services in order to achieve contracts with its local Districts, other Districts, the private sector or with GPs holding practice budgets for hospital care. To furnish a realistic price—and to prevent the private sector being squeezed out of business—capital accounting has to be undertaken and incorporated into the price of any particular service in any particular specialty the hospital offers. The purchaser has to pay a price which includes a capital charge. The development of practice budgets for hospital care by qualifying GP practices fragments the system of financing of health care. For the qualifying practices receive their budgets direct from the Region, and the resulting deficit from the funds available for allocation to Districts thus has to be spread over the Districts.

Therefore the tidy textbook advantages of the market (the rationale for the White Paper's objectives) may be in severe doubt in practice. If a District has to decide what care is necessary for different groups within its resident population, make contracts with a range of providers and allocate monies for contracts with opted-out hospitals as well as with the other range of District and GP services, a significant element of flexibility in the provision of services necessitated by temporary or unforeseen need will be lost. The language of contracts may not after all be useful in the management of flexible public health services. One of the great international advantages of the NHS has been its capacity for cost control at the aggregate level with flexibility in distributing care at the local level by Regions and Districts.

There is, for example, in the United States a considerable problem with Health Maintenance Organisations whose catchment populations are not large enough to allow them to distribute risk and 'cross-subsidise' the needy from less needy patients' premiums. Importing the disadvantages of a less global, less publicly planned service, as well as the advantages of the market place, may be one consequence of the White Paper.

Strategic Planning by the Backdoor?

NHS Regions are to be slimmed down considerably, losing much of their 'direct labour' function. Many of their functional tasks will disappear. The intention is to make them leaner, fitter and more strategic corporations. What is meant by 'more strategic' must be clarified. There is a possible need for Regions to advise—if not more—on the best Region-wide mix and distribution of services; to 'rent' capital to providers within Districts; and therefore to combine elements of Regional Strategic Planning/Management with competition (competition in that, once the location and type of service is advocated, there can be tendering for its provision). The alternative is to abdicate such a role and leave it wholly up to Districts whether to provide services themselves, seek them elsewhere and so on.

If the former, more active Regional role occurs, then the internal market will be reduced in practice either to a system of competitive tendering for a stipulated delivery of services in a stipulated location or to a paper exercise which merely continues, (albeit in the language of District contracts!), regionally-mandated cross-boundary flows or Regionally-mandated core services for District catchment populations. If the latter passive role by Regions is chosen, a considerable amount of duplication of services may occur as Districts develop services in order to try and compete in the long term: there may indeed be an unintended boost to District self-sufficiency as Districts contract with providers within their boundaries. The alternative is widespread closures as services are concentrated according to the laws of specialisation and comparative advantage in different Districts.

In practice, an internal market is likely to mean most care contracted for locally by Districts, with referrals afar only occurring at the margin. Worries that the internal market will mean long travel to care are legitimate. However, Alain Enthoven interprets the new system as implying localised care by contract—not as compelling travelling on a large scale. The big question is always the long term effect upon such options of politics and NHS management priorities formed in line with political priorities of the day. Guidelines should be laid down as much as possible from the centre as to overall criteria: how much redistribution and closure is to be permitted; what local services must be available to a population (that is, how precisely should core services be defined, and who within the District ought to provide them); and how the ground rules for fair competition are to be developed, to prevent, for example, opted out hospitals with special development monies from the Department of Health competing unfairly with other providers.

Turning to the allegedly superseded planning-based approach, what are the characteristics of the Regional Strategic Management/Planning model which give rise to both advantages and disadvantages? Firstly, some (not all) of the complexities in sub-Regional resource allocation formulae, especially in the reimbursement of Authorities for cross-boundary flows, are abolished if one replaces a resource allocation-led model with a planning-led model. However the question still must be resolved as to whether it is a capital planning-led model or a revenue planning-led model. Given Treasury and general government restrictions hitherto on flexible use of capital in the National Health Service, most radical-sounding planning models have in fact been only revenue-based models. After the effects of the 1989 White Paper policy are registered, a greater flexibility in the use of capital may be possible; but it is unlikely that an overtly regional activist role in planning, even an advisory or indicative one, will exist. In consequence, more ambitious Regional Strategic Planning, overcoming some of the restrictions of pre-1989 versions, is unlikely to see the light of day. The next section reviews such approaches, so that disadvantages and advantages of different options may be learned for the future—when planning and competition will have to co-exist, with neither exclusively chosen.

SECTION III

Specific Approaches

In this section, actual policy in Regions (which are kept anonymous) is described. The main emphasis is on 'First' Regional Health Authority so that the complications of a planning strategy can be highlighted. Other approaches are then briefly reviewed for comparative purposes, on the assumption that the first analysis has set the scene and also provided some detail on the thorny issues confronting management in such a strategy.

Regional Planning in 'First' Regional Health Authority

From the evolution of the Resource Allocation Working Party in 1976 until the Financial Year 1980/81, First Regional Health Authority used RAWP in order to make allocations to its Districts with only a few differences from the national formula. The planning of mental handicap was treated outside the RAWP framework; a different formula was used for acute mental illness services; and catchment populations were gauged using a 'treatment intensity' model. There had for some time been controversy as to whether the geographical population of Districts ought to be used for allocation purposes, or whether catchment populations different from District boundaries ought to be used. Where cross-boundary flows are common or even endemic the latter course seems sensible.

It is really a question of whether cross-boundary flows are considered as temporary aberrations from District populations (implicitly to be treated within Districts) or whether they are to be treated as permanent and therefore the building blocks of catchment populations. In any one year the difference is immaterial. However, when applying growth or contraction to budgets for the future, it makes a difference to the District allocation how the District's catchment population is calculated. The four models generally discussed in NHS debates are the net flow model; the 'ebb and flow' model; the proportionate flow model; and the treatment intensity model (Beech and Bevan, 1987). For those interested in technical differences, the reference is useful. The importance of which version is chosen is related to the assumptions made in each version. If these assumptions are not realised, then the aim of RAWP—distributing resources to populations according to need—is not realised, and existing differential use of service unrelated to need may be built in or reinforced, in the formula. The actual technical details are not developed here. It should briefly be pointed out however that the treatment intensity model has been claimed to be more realistic in that its primary assumption is that clinical behaviour is not affected by whether or not the patient comes from within or without the District.

Nevertheless, give or take a few divergences and technical differences, First was using RAWP directly translated from the national formula as justified in the 1976 RAWP report. Between 1981 and 1984, there was increasing dissatisfaction with the RAWP formula merely being translated mechanistically down from national to sub-Regional level.

In 1983/84, a new team of Regional officers wanted to diminish the import of what they called 'untargeted growth'—the provision of funds without specific service plans in mind. In other words they wanted to establish a rationale for a *planning-led model.*

The first task therefore was to develop the rationale for an alternative system. The guiding assumption was that, in an era of resource constraint, specific service plans had to be justified in terms of their utility to Regional (and by implication national) objectives for the health service. Strengthening the review process, whereby the Department of Health reviews a Region's progress by reference to its objectives and Regions do the same for Districts, created an atmosphere in which Region wanted to be sure about its Districts' objectives, in order to justify them nationally, and also created a framework within which the Region could have more leverage over its Districts: that is, they could be in trouble in the Review process.

The difficulty unforeseen at this stage however—applying nationally but in First Region in particular—was the difficulty of implementing an ambitious planning strategy when new development monies were unavailable.

Some of the guiding assumptions behind the new approach stemmed from a belief in the importance of maintaining and developing a policy of RCCS—financing the 'revenue consequences of capital spending'—in other words ensuring that revenue was distributed to allow the fruits of capital spending to be realised. The Region wanted to learn from mistakes elsewhere in the service, which had seen capital and revenue policy treated separately and often new capital developments coming on stream with no revenue to support them. Thus it supported and sponsored:

(1) the development of bridging funds, to help in a transitional period, and the development of a specific budget for Regional specialties known as the 'Regional Specialties Reserve', in order to meet national targets and to encourage certain specialties to develop faster than others

in line with Regional priorities. This meant that only a selected number of Districts, five out of the Region, were in receipt of these monies:

(2) the development of a bidding approach in the District for other than major capital developments. It is interesting to note that, prior to RAWP, bidding for funds on the basis of plans existed both at national and Regional level. A major challenge at this stage therefore was the development of a new objective system rather than a return to the old subjective, 'political' and *ad hoc* criteria for assessing bids and guiding Districts in the creation of bids.

The development of criteria for a District bidding process took four years. In 1984/85, there was very little guidance to Districts, who were told 'good work would be rewarded' in the allocation of revenue budgets. In 1985/86 some guidelines were developed as to how to identify service deficiencies in each District Health Authority—these were generally defined in terms of inputs such as number of beds or numbers of staff in different categories. (That is, outputs or outcomes from health services were not the main building block in the planning process.) Identification, for example, of bed gaps or staffing gaps led to priorities being assembled for each DHA. In 1986/87, this approach was extended in translating service gaps to District Health Authorities into how they might make good their gaps in provision.

Influences on the Development of the Model

A new team of officers had taken over; and in October 1983 the Griffiths Inquiry recommended the implementation of general management in the National Health Service. The former Regional Treasurer became Regional General Manager in First. This guaranteed a strong financial input into the rationale for the model. Next, the DHSS had strengthened the planning process in October 1984 with the imposition of annual programmes to accompany longer term plans. This provided an opportunity for the Region to make its Districts specify the services they required and how they planned to deliver them. Next, as referred to above, the DHSS/RHA/DHA review process gave the RHAs leverage with the District as well as an obligation to the Department of Health. A new Regional General Manager was strongly committed to the model, and one of his key colleagues had experience of the service planning approach at unit level in a London District and was keen to develop it further.

Responses of Districts

As might be expected, Districts were fairly cynical as well as slow to respond. There was considerable lack of understanding of the process. Had the main change been a clearly identifiable change in the RAWP formula, Districts might have been able to see the 'nitty gritty' financial implications of each change in the formula for each District (as for example, Regions were able to see the implications of the Review of RAWP recommendations in 1988).

However they generally failed to look at the fine print and understanding of the statistical basis of the new model was not high. Thus a cynical attitude did not translate into strong argument against the model. Responses nevertheless fell generally into three categories:

(1) The gainers tended to be the currently deprived Districts, and these Districts naturally gave a (cautious) welcome to the model while mistrusting its ability to move resources quickly enough or definitively enough;

(2) The losers tended to be Districts currently with heavy acute provision, who interestingly argued that their responsibility for other Districts' patients (cross-boundary flows) were insufficiently recognised by the model. (It is interesting that a planning-led model, intended to address RAWP's problems including this particular one, was attracting the same criticism.);

(3) Districts unsure whether they would gain or lose were even more apathetic than the others.

It was pointed out quite perceptively by a number of Districts that implementation of the model called for a big cultural change in the service in a very short period of time. There was a move from a resource based model of untargeted growth to a service planning model, which is a more radical change than many recognised.

The DHAs were generally consulted through technical workshops and presentations, but consultation and discussion was considered inadequate by some Districts.

Problems in Implementation

With the departure of the Regional General Manager and a key colleague, the model lost its two greatest 'product champions'. Next, changing political circumstances and their policy implications affected the development of the model. The Regional Strategy as a whole had envisaged a move of emphasis from acute services to development of the 'priority services', in line with govenment priorities from the mid-1970s onwards.

However, by the late 1980s these assumptions were proving unrealistic, as national priorities led to a re-emphasis of acute 'headline' medicine in response to a perception of 'NHS crisis' filtered through the media. This led to waiting list initiatives, involving priorities such as a 'blitz' on hip replacements; and the need to secure funding for major teaching hospitals in response to media highlighting of ward closures (especially in London in 1985 and Birmingham in 1987) interfered with earlier (or, it could be argued, longer term) priorities.

This converted the Region's planning model in practice into very much an *ad hoc* approach which had to respond to political pressures. The danger with a planning model based on bids is that there will not be enough of an 'objective' basis (on the lines of the RAWP formula, for example) to withstand political pressures.

The changing financial climate also meant that there was not enough money to fund new developments unless closures and reorientations of service were achieved at least as early, fully and efficiently as predicted by the model. This was far from the case, and in the absence of new monies, the development side of the model fell by the wayside. One component of the model planned to claw back resources from inefficient District Health Authorities in order to fund new service developments. This became unrealistic, as to continue with the approach would have meant significant ward closures at a time when such were considered to be both nationally and Regionally politically unacceptable. Complications resulting from the national failure to fund fully annual pay rounds led to further pressure on the Region's finances. Crucially the fact that the model concerned the distribution of revenue monies meant that the link to capital planning was tenuous. Capital planning was a much slower process, and changing revenue priorities were unable to be reflected in changing capital priorities. Finally, it is important to note that the data on which the more optimistic predictions of success were based may not have been adequate.

Advantages of the Approach

The Region believed that a service planning-led approach would prevent monies being distributed to the Districts for vague or unmonitored purposes. It allowed a dialogue between the Regions and Districts which was clear as to what the RHA was trying to achieve, and at least in theory allowed the rendering compatible of national, Regional and District priorities. With an activist role for the Region, Districts have to 'deliver' on their bids, and Regional monitoring of Districts is easier than in more diffuse systems.

Disadvantages of the Approach

Undoubtedly a Regional planning-led model diminishes District autonomy and reduces options and choices in certain circumstances for Districts. There is a potential for involvement by the Region in District decision-making without necessarily an adequate intellectual, or analytical or managerial capacity at Region to do so on a continuing basis. District Health Authorities may feel a lack of 'ownership' of their plans. There may also be a lack of flexibility in allowing Districts to come to terms with new needs. Power relations within District Health Authorities may be affected, as for example, the District Treasurer or Director of Finance sees a decline in his influence and autonomy as a result of a Regional-led plan with a strong financial basis.

More detail on the Model's Rationale

Known as a service provision model, the aim was to use Regional funds to produce specific service plans and goals throughout the Region. An initial decision was taken as to priorities for allocating resources to different client groups (for example, the mentally ill; the mentally handicapped) and then various planning criteria (ranging from norms to expected uptake of services by populations of certain characteristics) were used to set targets for service provision in different specialties in different Districts.

In particular, a population's likely need for services was predicted *given* average or 'reasonable' use, in a population of such demographic and epidemiological characteristics, of specific services, broken down by care group and specialty and incorporating weightings for morbidity. Such planning models may be similar to resource allocation models, with the addition in planning models of assumptions as to location of services irrespective of District boundaries—whereas resource allocation models tend to think in terms of allocation to Districts, or at least Districts' catchment populations. But the two may converge.

Also built into the model were assumptions about efficiency and the 'expected cost' of delivering certain types of services. This led to a costed strategy, which translated assumed case load in different Districts into financial targets. Aside from this, Regional priorities—such as the Regional specialties already referred to, and for example, a boost to health visiting—were accounted before the residue of money was available for direct distribution to Districts.Cross-boundary flows were accounted for by continuing the principle of catchment populations.

Some assumptions were made as to the ability of Districts to provide services within stipulated budgets, i.e. as to relative levels of efficiency among Districts, in deciding where services were to be provided. The approach did not generally differ from sub-Regional RAWP in assuming a fair degree of District self sufficiency. The main financial imperative lay in the need for Districts to fulfil Regional expectations about cost and efficiency in different specialties and hospitals.

If these assumptions were not met, continuing with Regional plans priorities would mean closures. But it was not merely a question of efficiency. The assumptions of the model as to patient flows and changing patient flows over time were not realised. In consequence services which it was anticipated could be run down and closed often could not be.

Outcome

As a result of the difficulties identified, the model foundered and was abandoned in 1987/88. In the absence of a return to straightforward use of sub-Regional RAWP (by now generally abandoned or amended throughout the NHS), the Region was in something of a quandary regarding the future, prior to the White Paper. The need to concentrate services in line with Regional strategic objectives may be achieved by taking a multi-District approach, involving federations of Districts, to the provision of certain specialties. However, with the advent of the 1989 White Paper, it is more likely that concentration to reap the benefits of economies of scale may be stimulated by a market mechanism rather than a planning approach. That is, supra-District specialties (whether or not specifically earmarked Regional specialties) will be expected to evolve as a result of Districts' rational decision-making and resultant contracts for services, placed by consortia of Districts rather than mandated by Regional planning. It is interesting to note here that the strategic objectives to which it is hoped the market can contribute may be the same as those which in earlier periods were sought from strategic planning. This will not be the case if the development of provider market-dominated NHS is not accompanied by overall strategic plans based on identification of patient and population need and viable strategies for meeting that need.

In Retrospect: Key Questions to consider about such a Model Are:

1. What specific planning criteria might be used in the development of such a model?

2. How might Districts be involved more effectively in the development of such a model?

3. What might be the basis for predicting different patient flows in the future by comparison with the past?

4. How might capital and revenue planning be better combined?

5. To what extent do personalities, national political pressures,

regional political pressures and other behavioural factors affect policies such as this one?

Other Strategic Planning Models

First Regional Health Authority allocated resources to Districts as a result of the planning model (the service provision model) adopted. Thus a resource allocation formula based on the national RAWP formula was abandoned, but the District was still the recipient of a global allocation of funds. The difference was that resources for each District were now calculated by reference to expected workload for the various providing facilities (hospitals and units) in that District, with assumptions about efficiency built in. Variants of the Regional Strategic Planning/Management model have been attempted in other Regions in the NHS—in two in particular.

'Second' Regional Health Authority

In one, another strategic planning approach was developed with a view to allocating resources to Districts. The strategy consisted in modelling need for health care and then (pre-White Paper) building in assumptions about the distribution of facilities, which were based on the ability or otherwise of patients to travel, reasonable catchment areas and similar concerns. Need was considered to be gauged by usage of services, defined in terms of the Standardised Discharge Ratio: the number of discharges or admissions for age and sex as in a Standardised Mortality Ratio (to prevent 'double counting' of age and sex factors in allocating resources). One problem is that the Standardised Discharge Ratio does not account for length of stay or cost of particular services. There are ways of seeking to build in such factors, as the model attempted.

However, even if one accepts at a conceptual level that usage of services is a surrogate for need of services, there is still a need to control for the supply and distribution of facilities. Otherwise greater usage of hospital services, for example, in one area may be explained simply by the greater profusion and availability of services in that area. Therefore an attempt to 'control for supply' is necessary. This can be done using various mathematical models. They vary from the simple assumption that availability of services (for example, populations living in different electoral wards) varies directly with the proximity of services or inversely with the distance from services. More complex and realistic models, such as the gravity model, can also be used. Such models attempt to trace natural flows of patients to facilities, and compute factors such as ease of travel, distance, habit and patients' assumptions.

Such models can then be used to attempt to adjust for the existing provision of facilities—in other words, the aim is to predict the usage of services that would occur based on health need without the further effect of the supply variable. Such models can be used either to 'control for' uneven supply of facilities when using admission rates to gauge need *or* to plan services equitably recognising the complex nature of people's habits and the factors which affect their uptake of services. They are two sides of the same coin—explaining usage helps to predict usage if a new service mix is planned.

Procedures used to measure need may include statistical regression analysis of usage of facilities against social factors. In most cases the electoral ward is taken as the unit of analysis, thought to be suitable because it is small enough to allow comparison between different wards with different social characteristics yet with similar access to facilities. That is, geographical distances may be small yet social characteristics may vary significantly. Need for services (gauged by the surrogate measure, usage of services) is correlated statistically with a variety of social factors, available from national census data, local authority social services data and other sources. This produces complex regression analysis which identifies need—specialty by specialty—with social characteristics. These can then be translated into predictions of need for different electoral wards and later aggregations of electoral wards. (One can go below the level of the electoral ward to the Enumeration District. Doing so may produce smaller and more homogenous populations; but a major problem arises in that the populations involved may be too small to allow meaningful statistical comparison.)

Second Region had moved through a variety of means of calculating global catchment populations to the development of a small area-based system to gauge particular needs for particular services, and to allocate accordingly to providers on behalf of catchment populations (via Districts). Such models start by defining small areas' needs for different types of health care—for example, starting with the electoral ward as a building block of population. The next stage is to model access according to the usual criteria for how to locate potential services, assumptions about distance to care and so forth.

Post-White Paper, the Region has modified the strategy to allow overt comparison of such catchment targets with Districts' resident targets, through the actual costing of cross-boundary flows from one District to another. In this way, gradual future changes in planning can be incorporated—or market competition can incrementally be developed to replace the directed flows to one provider implicit in planning.

It is in order to model appropriate provision given particular needs for particular services in particular areas, and to be able to see how changing need within a care group or for one type of service in one area, can affect allocations, that the 'small area' approach to gauging populations' needs is chosen. Furthermore the planning of services on a small area basis can be linked to a similar methodology for resource allocation in which changing targets can be specifically linked to changes in imputed services for specific care groups. Global catchment populations derived mathematically (such as the net flow, proportionate flow and treatment intensity methods) cannot be used in the same disaggregated way.

Second Region, in following such a rationale has refined its separate formulae for allocation of resources for different 'care groups', distinguishing between:

immediate in-patients
non-immediate in-patients
day cases
outpatients
casualty patients
mental illness
mental handicap
community
and other, small categories

For each group, a separate formula for resource allocation is devised, and the overall allocation to Districts incorporates the separate calculations. It is however also a planning methodology, which can be used to predict particular local needs for services. Planning and resource allocation are, after all, two sides of the same coin.

Post-White Paper, the need is to decide the District's resident population targets, *then* to decide how 'top down' the Region is to be in mandating the continuation and actual costing of inter-District flow, so that Districts' *catchment* (or provider) targets can be derived—or alternatively how *laissez-faire* the Region is to be in leaving it up to Districts to trade autonomously. The Department of Health in reality has realised that a full market model is not possible, certainly in the short and medium terms.

This is not least because certain Districts (e.g. inner-city Districts) might lose 'impossibly'

(i) due to their resident populations being less than their catchment populations; and,

(ii) due to quick movements to target, instigated by Regions or by the Department of Health.

(iii) due to gaining purchasing Districts no longer using the funds newly at their disposal as purchasers to buy services from the losing Districts, which previously were reimbursed directly by Regions as providers.

(iv) due to new formulae gauging their needs to be less within the Region overall.

In practice, therefore, movements will be gradual, by contrast with Departmental allocations to Regions, which are supposed to have occurred by 1991.

A different approach would remove the significance of the Districts altogether, and use the Region to allocate resources to particular facilities directly. Interestingly, the 1989 White Paper, albeit in very different language, also advocated that rational choice ought to be made about where within a Region's services are provided. The White Paper implied that Districts ought to make decisions as to where their resident populations could best receive care, and then to trade in the market place to contract for that care. That is, the assumption of District self-sufficiency was challenged, allegedly to be replaced by a trading model based on the internal market. However a Regional Strategic Planning model may be a way of achieving the same or similar aims: that is, the goal is to decide where patients can most realistically achieve quality, cost effective care and then to finance appropriate facilities directly by their workload. One of the major problems of sub-Regional resource allocation formulae, such as the sub-Regional RAWP formula, has been the fact that specific hospitals, units, specialties, and departments may not have been financed in proportion to their workload. In other words, relating revenue and reward to workload has not occurred. This is because Districts received sub-Regional RAWP allocations and subsequently allocated money to hospitals, specialties within them and other services on a historic basis within their allocations. If an efficiency drive for example boosted the workload of a hospital significantly, this might have had no effect on its budget unless through bureaucratic or 'political' means.

However, the Regional Strategic Planning model would seek to get round this type of perverseness by modelling the workload (and changes in workload where relevant) provided by different facilities and rewarding them accordingly. Thus both planning and the market may be geared to achieving the same ends. It has been remarked that it is only planning which can achieve the text book advantages of the market. One could equally argue that it is only the market which can achieve the textbook advantages of planning. The lesson is that they should not be seen simplistically as opposites.

'Third' Region

An alternative option to that of First Region which had sought to implement a planning-led approach compatible with revenue allocations to Districts on existing lines, is to implement a more radical planning-led approach. Third Region sought to implement a form of Regional

Strategic Planning based on equity. Its methodology consisted in the following steps (Bevan and Waring, 1984):

(a) to estimate need in each District, by specialty, to generate predictions of caseload—in other words, the needs of a District's resident populations;

(b) to model access, taking into account existing hospital distribution and capacity, to provide for closures and new developments, given reasonable assumptions about travel to care by different types of patient in different specialties—(definition of 'reasonable' involving exploration of current patterns of travel and catchment population);

(c) to cost options under (b);

(d) to identify manpower and other needs to fulfil the strategy: that is, to put flesh on the bones of the planning strategy.

The rationale for the Region doing this is that Districts cannot 'plan for equity' on their own for adequately large populations, given catchments.

Prior to the White Paper, Districts did not have control over their own residents' use of services. Therefore, District-based strategies could be undermined by patients being 'cross-boundary flows' out of the District (seeking care elsewhere) and thereby incurring costs under the RAWP formula to the District, reducing its future allocation.

Post-White Paper, Districts are supposed to have control over their residents' use of services, and this is allegedly to be 'contracted for' directly, after agreements with GPs as to referral among other complex considerations. However, this is a statement of 'pure' intent which will only be approached—at most—in reality. As a result, the rationale for a Regional role to plan services remains to some extent.

CONCLUSION

Unlike the other case studies in the book, this one primarily consists in general strategic review of policy. It incorporates comment on the broad strategic issues confronting British health policy—competition, planning, resource allocation, and their reconciliation—which clearly bear either directly or indirectly upon the particular areas examined in the earlier studies.

The challenge confronting resource allocation policy is to combine equity in gauging need through formulae for resident populations with pragmatic links to planning for the provision of services to meet need—whether or not Districts are purchasers for their residents.

Competitive strategies should be encouraged at the margin, but not as replacements for the beneficial aspects of public planning.

Nationally, in a rush to ensure the South-East of England does not lose more money, it is unfair to downgrade objective measures of morbidity such as the standardised mortality ratio, which correlates well with both morbidity and social deprivation.

Sub-Regionally, the problems of metropolitan inner-cities and other areas with special needs should not be addressed by 'over complicating' formulae but by special or 'extra' district allocations. The equally valid claims of other areas are not then irrevocably distorted.

Both nationally and sub-Regionally, strategic planning should be called in as an aid to allocating resources. The approaches to planning briefly discussed in this study derived from a pre-White Paper NHS, when 'planning' had not become a dirty word. But they contain useful pointers for the future (as well as disadvantages), even in an age of contracting and alleged competition.

As raised in the introduction, there are thus two basic issues in deriving Regional policies for resource allocation. *Firstly*, need has to be measured geographically, including differential need by different social classes and care groups. *Secondly*, assumptions have to be made about whether the provision of services to meet the need can be left to the market, with Districts as purchasers, or steered by Region, as a strategic planner of whatever degree of activism.

'First' and 'Third' Regions above sought to be, respectively, moderately and extremely activist in planning services. That is, they addressed not only the *first* but *second* issues above. Post-White Paper, therefore, they have had to amend their strategies or at least incorporate them into a competitive language. 'Third' Region, for example, has encouraged consortia of 'mega Districts' which will be the purchasers of mixes of provision along the lines intended by the former 'Regional Strategic Planning' approach—although inevitably different in some aspects.

'Second' Region might also have gone down the road of activist planning. Post-White Paper, it has concentrated on the mechanics of the formulae to measure populations' need—and has sought to balance District autonomy with a Regional Steering role. Many Regions, indeed, which have moved from the old RAWP system for measuring need to more detailed gauges based on usage are in a similar position.

PART II

POLICY PRIORITIES

CHAPTER 6

Case Study: Waiting Lists—Coventry

INTRODUCTION

In a period of unprecedented debate about the future of the National Health Service there can be few more potent symbols of the shortcomings of the NHS than the existence of waiting lists for non urgent inpatient treatment. Since its inception in 1948 there has been concern about waiting lists which have remained stubbornly above the 500,000 patient mark. Academic discussion has focused on the vexed question of interpreting waiting list statistics rather than on how they might be reduced. Recently discussions about waiting lists have been linked to the equally thorny debate about variations in GP referrals rates.

Implicit in economists' discussions about waiting lists is that they result from a mismatch between supply and demand created by the absence of the price mechanism to allocate resources in the NHS. Waiting lists are a consequence of the excess demand for health care and are used to ration health care in the absence of rationing by price. From this analysis flowed government attempts to affect the supply side of the equation by increasing capacity (beds, operating theatres) or utilising existing capacity more effectively. Furthermore there was an implicit assumption that supply side deficiencies leading to lengthy waiting lists was caused by inadequate resources for treatment. However other observers (Culyer and Cullis, 1976) had less comforting explanations for the persistence of waiting lists. They argued that Say's law operated in the NHS and an increased supply of beds would create its own demand.

This lack of consensus over remedies to reduce waiting lists did not prevent governments trying to tackle the problem. In 1975 the Labour government made £5m available in 1975/76 to fund schemes devoted to reducing waiting lists. This strategy of ear marking funds for particular purposes was developed by the Conservative government after 1979. The late 1980s have witnessed a renewed interest in the issue of tackling waiting lists. This reflects the political potency of the issue as the Conservative government's handling of the NHS has been increasingly carefully scrutinised. It has become important to reduce waiting lists as a mark of the success of their policies towards the NHS.

Complementing this central pressure to reduce waiting lists have been developments which have assisted this process. NHS managers have been encouraged to view the management of health services as analogous to management in the private sector and to adopt private sector management practices. This has encouraged greater emphasis on customer satisfaction and increased awareness that lengthy waiting lists contribute to user dissatisfaction. Increased managerial autonomy and power since the implementation of the Griffiths report has enabled managers to explore other avenues in reducing waiting lists notably cooperation with the private sector and entering into contracts with other health authorities. The scale of these types of initiative is set to expand rapidly under the Government's proposals to reform the NHS (Department of Health, 1989a). It has also been argued that as a society becomes more affluent people become less tolerant of deficiencies in service like waiting lists.

Lies, Damned Lies, and Statistics

The importance of timely and accurate information for good management decision-making is now widely recognised in the NHS. The implementation of the Körner reports has been the first national step along this route. One constant obstacle to tackling waiting lists has been the questionable accuracy of the information they contain making managers reluctant to act on the data. The most common criticism is that waiting lists are inaccurate and include people who are dead, have been operated on or include elderly patients who will not be given an operation. Waiting lists also do not give any idea of how long patients have been waiting. It is also argued that waiting lists for inpatient treatment should not be looked at in isolation from outpatient waiting times as tackling inpatient waiting lists may lengthen outpatient waiting times. Hence there is concern that relieving pressure on one area of the NHS will transfer pressure to another area. Finally critics of the Government suggest that the figures have been manipulated to reduce the waiting list figure below its true level.

Waiting list statistics in England were collected in two ways. The number of patients on the waiting list at 31 March and 30 September were collected half yearly on the SBH 203 returns. This procedure has been modified by the implementation of the Körner proposals. Less detailed data is collected annually as part of the SH3 Hospital Return. Health authorities have to breakdown the Waiting List Return by speciality and categorise patients as urgent or non-urgent. Urgent cases who have been on the waiting list for more than a year are shown separately. One difficulty inherent in the categorisation is that no central guidance is given as to how urgency is defined. This is left to clinical judgement which gives rise to variations in classification across the country and difficulties in comparing health authorities or even different specialities within the same authority. Furthermore it is unclear how patients should be categorised whose status changes from non-urgent during the course of their wait.

A number of other criticisms have been levelled at the accuracy of the figures. First, a number of surgeons use a booking system which serves to reduce the waiting list statistics. In this system when a patient is seen in an outpatient clinic and requires inpatient treatment a date is offered for that operation. This is agreed between surgeon and patient and the case is booked for that date. There is consequently no need for that patient to be placed on a waiting list and therefore booked cases do not appear on the waiting list returns.

A second source of underestimation arises because the government has altered the manner in which the waiting list statistic is compiled. In September 1979 the DHS instructed health authorities not to include people waiting for day surgery on the Waiting List Returns. This was an idiosyncratic decision as day surgery has been expanded rapidly precisely to reduce waiting lists. Circular HSC (IS) 181 on 'Reduction of Waiting Times for Inpatient Admission: Management Arrangements' specifically advised that: 'The provision of facilities for day surgery can help reduce the routine element of a waiting list'. A further change in March 1980 related to the description of the degree of urgency of treatment. Authorities who used intermediate degrees of urgency between urgent and non-urgent were instructed to classify these intermediate categories of patients as non-urgent.

Although critics have focused on the under-estimation of waiting lists governments have been more concerned with perceived inflation in waiting lists. Several studies have indicated that routine returns on the number of patients on waiting lists over estimate the number of patients eventually admitted to hospital (Lourie, 1978; Donaldson *et al.* 1984; Porter, 1985). Recent work in Oxford Regional Health Authority compared Waiting List Returns and Hospital Activity Analysis for the major surgical specialities between 1974 and 1983. This comparison revealed that twenty-eight per cent of the waiting list comprised patients who were not eventually admitted to hospital within the Region (Lee, Don, Goldacre, 1987). One perennial problem with these type of studies is if the data being compared is comparable.

In December 1984 the DHSS asked all health authorities to review their inpatient waiting lists and remove patients who had been treated or who no longer required treatment. The DHSS suggested that at least ten per cent of all patients on waiting lists would not eventually require treatment. The review had to be completed by March 1985. The government was disappointed with the results of the review which did not precipitate a rapid fall in waiting lists. Government figures indicate that numbers on the waiting lists fell from 682,599 in September 1984 to 674,453 in March 1985 and to 661,249 in September 1985.

Yates (1987) has demonstrated that a rushed central review was doomed to failure. A proper review of waiting lists is a complicated and time consuming exercise which requires the patient to be written to and in the absence of a reply the general practitioner concerned needs to be consulted. Additionally clerical time and cooperation from consultants is necessary to check the information gained and agreement obtained for removing individuals from the waiting list. Consequently Yates discovered that in many cases waiting list reviews had been conducted in an inadequate manner.

The debate about the validity of waiting lists has proved inconclusive. Yates draws a rather lame conclusion:

> There is no way of knowing whether the over estimates balance the under estimates. The evidence clearly shows that waiting list data is imperfect but there is no convincing evidence which suggests that it is completely false. (Yates 1987, p. 13)

Consequently interest in waiting times—the length of time it takes for a patient to be admitted for treatment—has increased. One potential advantage is that it would more accurately gauge how long patients have to wait and remove the misleading division between inpatients and outpatients. Inpatient waiting lists ignore the possibility that an individual may have been waiting a long time for an outpatient appointment. Consultants preferences vary, some prefer to give immediate outpatient appointments and then allow patients to wait a considerable time on an inpatient waiting list, conversely other consultants prefer to allow patients to wait for an outpatient appointment but then bring patients in quickly for inpatient treatment. These variations in practice distort waiting list figures but would be revealed if the focus was on the total waiting time. Unfortunately no data is collected by the DHSS on outpatient waiting times.

An additional complication is the effect of an inpatient waiting list on clinical practice (Sanderson, 1982). The knowledge that a waiting list exists may encourage surgeons to place patients on a waiting list prior to when an operation is actually required. This is to enable patients to advance up the waiting list so that when they are admitted they are ready for their procedure. This type of behaviour clearly has the potential to exacerbate a waiting list problem.

To summarise, inadequacies clearly exist in the waiting list data available. Claims about inflation in lists need to be treated cautiously as it is not clear that individual examples of where lists are inflated can be applied universally. There is a strong political imperative for government to reduce the waiting list figures as the change in the way the figures are compiled demonstrates. Although data on waiting times would be a better gauge of the experience for consumers, as this data is not collected by government there is less political pressure to rectify long waiting times. Consequently the Conservative government has concentrated its attention on the potentially perilous statistic of waiting lists.

The Causes of Waiting Lists

Waiting lists are frequently viewed as inherent to a publicly funded health service where the price of health care is set too low to prevent excess demand. This arises in the NHS as although users pay for health care from general taxation there is no financial cost in terms of payment for service at the point of entry to the system. Indeed one of the guiding principles of the NHS was that health care should be available at the point of delivery regardless of the ability to pay. Health economists have argued that the absence of a price mechanism results in consumers treating health care as free thus creating excess demand.

This position has been modified in recent years as the existence of barriers to health care have been identified. It has become a common place to note that it is not individuals which directly demand hospital care but that this demand is filtered through professionals who have to translate this demand into a request for treatment. In this process there is scope to filter out demand. Similarly commentators have drawn attention to the barriers to health care faced by individuals from lower occupational classes (Townsend, Davidson, 1982). Sharp increases in prescription charges since 1979 have also eroded the concept of free health care at the point of delivery. Consequently excess demand may exist but it is not self evident that this is due to the lack of a price mechanism as price barriers and professional barriers also may prevent demand being expressed.

The nature of the demand for health care can alter and should not be viewed as static. The demographic changes which the UK is experiencing with an ageing population who make greater demands on the health service is one reason often cited for an increase in demand. Advances in new technology which increases the scope for medical intervention and raise people's expectations of what the NHS can remedy is a further potential source of increased demand and therefore increased waiting lists. This reasoning has been criticised by Yates (1987). He argued that the NHS was in danger of trying to resolve its waiting list problem without sufficient knowledge of those waiting lists. Assumptions about waiting lists containing large numbers of elderly patients waiting for highly sophisticated medicine were found to be erroneous.

Yates in a 1986 survey of 31,224 patients on thirty-three of the largest inpatient surgical waiting lists in Wales and the West Midlands found that waiting lists were not dominated by elderly patients except in ophthalmology. Furthermore waiting lists were not made up of patients who require difficult or advanced surgical treatment, in general surgery of 7,476 patients recorded on the list, 3,353 patients (45%) were waiting for varicose veins or hernia operations. A similar picture emerged in the other specialities. A question mark over the evidence on the numbers of elderly patients waiting is the possibility that elderly people are filtered out of the system before they reach the waiting list. However, managers and clinicians will in the main focus their attention on existing waiting lists not invisible demand.

In the absence of a straightforward relationship between supply, demand and waiting lists, as shown by wide variations in waiting lists across Districts, forensic analysis has been carried out on individual Authorities examining particular causes of long waiting lists. The focus in this type of analysis is to shift from the macro level to the micro level and examine how efficiently resources are being used. The concentration is on how effectively operating theatres and beds are being used.

A report by the Public Accounts Committee (1988) on the use of operating theatres in the NHS was highly critical of consultants who cancelled operations at short notice. The report found that cancellations varied in 1987 between eight and eighteen per cent in each month. This report followed an earlier National Audit Office (1987) report which found under utilisation of operating theatres in a number of health authorities. However this information itself is not necessarily an indication of inefficiency. Operating theatres can not be viewed in isolation but need to be placed in the context of the workload of the whole hospital.

For example, an operation can only proceed if the theatres are adequately staffed but shortages of theatre staff are well documented. Similarly operations can only proceed if full post operative care is available on the wards of which the availability of beds is central. Consequently although poorly managed use of operating theatres may exacerbate a waiting list problem the underlying pathology of the problem needs to be addressed first. Similar issues need to be tackled in utilising beds efficiently.

To summarise, no clear picture emerges of the causes of waiting lists. The cosy explanation which viewed waiting lists as an inevitable adjunct of a publicly provided service where demand will outstrip supply is viewed as unsatisfactory. Changes in the nature of demand due to demographic changes and government policy have to be incorporated. Furthermore health economists acknowledge that the market for health care is distinct from the theoretical models of neoclassical economics but largely ignore this in postulating that waiting lists are caused by excess demand. This is essentially a fatalistic diagnosis which severely limits managerial action. However health authorities such as Coventry documented below have tackled their waiting list difficulties in innovative and imaginative ways. This seems to suggest that efforts need to be focused at local level where in Yates's terms the anatomy of waiting lists can be examined and action targeted at the problems revealed. It may emerge that for example, theatres are being under utilised but the diversity of waiting list problems seems to preclude the adoption of national panaceas.

Waiting List Initiatives to Date: An Overview

A number of initiatives have been taken to improve the waiting lists situation at national and local level. The initiative which has gained the most publicity in the last couple of years has been the government's national waiting list initiative which was launched in October 1986. The allocation of specific monies to alleviate waiting list difficulties had a precedent in the 1970s when the Labour government allocated £5m in 1975/76 to schemes aimed at reducing waiting lists. A follow up scheme was planned in 1976/77. The scheme was not monitored to the same extent as the 1980's initiatives and industrial action in the winter of 1978 in the NHS contributed to a rise in waiting lists at the end of the 1970s.

The Labour government in 1979 established a Working Party to examine waiting times in outpatient appointments and inpatient treatment for the orthopaedic speciality. Orthopaedics were chosen because their existed long waiting lists in this speciality and the situation was deteriorating. The Working Party was under the Chairmanship of Mr Robert Duthie who was an orthopaedic surgeon and the group reported in 1981. The report concluded that there were enormous variations in size of waiting list which were caused by many factors, not simply a shortage of resources. Consequently local action was necessary to remedy the situation and the starting point needed to be Districts undertaking their own internal reviews with the aim of alleviating bottle necks in the system. However in the absence of health authorities and government action to initiate the proposals, the potential of the report remained unfulfilled.

In the absence of a sustained impetus to remedy the situation from government or the NHS, consumer groups have begun to apply pressure by highlighting lengthy waiting lists and encouraging consumers to obtain a better service through referrals to Districts with shorter waiting lists. The College of Health has been in the vanguard of this movement, publishing an annual guide to hospital waiting lists. The College of Health believes that in the short-term government action will not ease the situation and that a more immediate solution for patients who face a long wait is to seek referral to another hospital. The College of Health has made accessible to consumers information that was previously not released by health authorities. However consumers need to be prepared to travel to other hospitals and obtaining the initial referral is not always straightforward. Finally despite considerable publicity the annual guide is not widely known about.

In the absence of marked progress the govenment was becoming increasingly concerned about waiting lists in the run up to the last general election at a time when their record on the NHS looked fragile to the electorate. On 21 July 1986 Norman Fowler the Secretary of State for Health wrote to Regional Chairmen in the following terms:

> I know you agree we must respond to the continuing problem of patients having to wait too long for consultation and treatment. Despite the efforts which have already been made in many Districts, waiting lists and times for inpatient treatment are still a cause for concern . . . The problem deserves priority attention and I should be grateful if you would ensure that this is achieved.
>
> Because waiting times and their causes vary greatly from place to place, there is no universal solution. I am therefore asking you to arrange for the position on waiting lists and times to be reviewed in every District in your Region in order to establish the extent of the problem, its nature and cause.

Regional Chairmen were asked to report back by the end of October 1986. This proved to be the first sounding for a specific national initiative on waiting lists. Waiting lists had been on the NHS Management Board's management agenda which set out priorities for NHS management since its birth. Additionally in December 1984 health authorities had been asked to carry out a validation exercise on their waiting lists and remove patients no longer requiring treatment.

In October 1986 the govenment unveiled a national waiting list initiative to tackle the waiting list problem. The government was concerned that the national waiting list was set to rise from the 31 March 1986 position of 673,000. The government allocated an extra £25m in 1987/88 (Table 10) to help health authorities to reduce their waiting lists. It was envisaged this would fund 350 projects throughout England and treat an extra 100,000 patients. This worked out at a modest £250 per case. Sir Roy Griffiths, Deputy Chairman of the NHS Management Board led the team which assessed health authority projects to reduce waiting lists. The initiative was repeated in 1988/89 when a further £30m was allocated.

TABLE 10. *Allocations of Waiting List Fund Monies to Regional Health Authorities.*

	Allocation (£m)	
REGION	*1987/88*	*1988/89*
Northern	1·700	1·925
Yorkshire	1·757	2·072
Trent	2·410	2·845
East Anglia	1·018	1·046
North West Thames	1·590	2·316
North East Thames	2·070	2·637
South East Thames	2·040	2·350
South West Thames	1·330	2·013
Wessex	1·400	1·609
Oxford	1·010	1·163
South Western	1·650	1·915
West Midlands	2·880	3·304
Mersey	1·350	1·633
North Western	2·295	2·531

SOURCE. *BMJ*: 28 February 1987, 1988

The waiting list initiative has been viewed as a political gimmick to demonstrate the government's commitment to the NHS. This was undoubtedly an aspect of the initiative. However the methods adopted were in keeping with other aspects of government policy towards the NHS. It was an attempt to move away from central directives by government via Health Circular and instead in line with the Griffiths philosophy of management devolution health authorities were to be given incentives to tackle waiting lists. In this approach health authorities were allowed to reduce waiting lists in any manner they thought fit and were judged on the basis of performance.

This flexibility has helped to spawn varied local initiatives. Since 1983 when the government made competitive tendering for ancillary services mandatory in the NHS contracting out has gained favour as an option in providing services. A number of health authorities have contracted with private hospitals to reduce waiting lists. In 1985 Bath Health Authority paid the private Bath clinic to undertake over 120 children's Ear, Nose, and Throat operations (Yates, 1987). An expanding variant of this approach is to contract with other health authorities to carry out procedures. In Bolton analysis of their orthopaedic waiting lists showed the existence of blockages, namely a shortage of beds and theatre time. This focused attention on contracting with another authority and agreement was reached with North Manchester Health Authority for their consultants to assess patients at Bolton's outpatient clinics followed by admission to North Manchester's Ancoats Hospital where spare capacity existed (Brunt and Peel, 1989).

A related approach seeks to use existing capacity and staff at unorthodox times of the week. In Chichester the acute services Unit Management Team undertook an initiative to reduce orthopaedic waiting lists. An evening session from 6pm to 10pm was held every week day for six weeks and 129 cases were completed (Heppenstall, 1985). An initiative in Bristol where 102 patients were admitted for Ear, Nose and Throat operations was undertaken at the weekend (Griffits *et al.*, 1988). The aim of these types of schemes was to harness existing capacity at unpopular times allowing cose effective surgery. At Worthing the problems of bed shortage was eliminated by the use of a local hotel as a residential base with nursing cover provided on site (James, 1989).

Day surgery, where patients are admitted and undergo a minor surgical, medical, diagnostic or therapeutic procedure and are discharged that day, has increased in popularity in the last two decades. In the 1970s day surgery became fashionable and more district general hospitals developed their own units. Day surgery had a number of advantages. It avoids having to admit patients requiring surgery to an inpatient bed allowing these beds to be reserved for patients requiring major surgery or emergency admissions. Conversely the existence of a separate day surgery unit prevents minor cases being cancelled due to pressure on acute hospital beds. Day surgery can create savings in three main areas.

1. The ability to close the ward at night and at weekends economising on salaries of nursing and ancillary staff. Furthermore by enabling staff to work normal working hours staff who leave the NHS because of having to work unsocial hours can be retained.

2. Hotel services for example, meals which would be necessary for inpatients, are not required.

3. The shorter time spent by each patient in hospital permits more patients to be treated in the same hospital.

Finally patients often prefer to minimise the time they spend in hospital. As long waiting lists frequently contain large numbers of minor cases the increased use of day surgery has become a popular remedy to tackle waiting list problems. In 1985 the Royal College of Surgeons gave its support to the expansion of day surgery and thus helped to set the seal on an increase in day cases from 449,600 cases in 1979 to 962,800 cases in 1985.

The Coventry Initiative

Coventry Health Authority is situated in the West Midlands Regional Health Authority and provides health care for a population of 312,000 in Coventry. The District had a revenue budget of £61m in 1988/89 and is split into three management units. This case study focuses on the City Unit which has a £14m revenue budget per annum. The Unit contains the Coventry and Warwickshire Hospital a 205 bed hospital where orthopaedic services for the District are concentrated. In addition theatre sessions are used at St Gerrards, Coleshill, a small hospital run by nuns, for minor and intermediary cases. Opthalmology services are the responsibility of the Unit and are provided at the forty-two bedded Paybody Hospital. The Coventry and Warwickshire Hospital also provides outpatient clinics and Accident and Emergency services.

Towards the end of 1985 as a result of the implementation of General Management a new District General Manager was appointed. He inherited a number of lengthy waiting lists particularly in orthopaedics, ophthalmology, and general surgery. In 1984 a District Health Authority Members' Working Group had been set up to examine the waiting list problem. It had suggested that the use of beds and operating theatre sessions needed to be better coordinated and had recommended the appointment of a bed coordinator to fulfil this role. However this appointment had not been successful as the person concerned had not known the hospital well and had not been sufficiently assertive to coax the consultants into new ways of managing their lists. The other recommendations of the member Working Party also had a limited effect.

The new District General Manager viewed the reduction of waiting lists as one of his central objectives. This concern was strengthened by the appointment of a new Chairman in Spring 1986 who shared his interest in reducing waiting lists. The District General Manager believed that there was a poor use of resources in the District with an imbalance between the required numbers of surgeons and anaesthetists. A related problem was the difficulty of attracting junior medical staff for the Accident and Emergency department and in orthopaedics. The information systems were poor, preventing adequate analysis of the waiting list problem. Finally there was very little day surgery being carried out although as two day theatres existed in the Accident and Emergency department they were in poor condition and scarcely used. This created frustration as work which could have been carried out on a day case basis was clogging up lists in the main theatres.

A number of methods were employed to bring about a climate of change. Performance indicators were one means of bringing about a change in perception of the problem and therefore facilitated subsequent management action. In December 1985 the Inter-Authority Comparisons and Consultancy (IAAC) standard profile and exceptions were sent to all Chairmen of divisions, for circulation to consultants. When further information was requested follow up meetings were held with management and the District Information Officer. Information derived from the performance indicators was incorporated into the planning guidelines and circulated to units. Targets began to be set for reduction in the inpatient waiting list per thousand catchment population and other similar performance related objectives.

John Yates at Birmingham University, a specialist in the reduction of waiting lists, was approached to examine the anatomy of the long waiting lists in the District. This was prior to the West Midlands Regional Health Authority request to John Yates to undertake the same task for the worst Districts in the Region, and a subsequent request to repeat the exercise for the twenty-two districts with the longest lists nationally.

Yates first examined the general surgery list and during the summer of 1986 made a study of orthopaedics. The results showed that orthopaedics was suffering from a lack of capacity. Beds and theatres were being used well when available with bed occupancy close to eighty per cent and an average turnover interval. However levels of day surgery were very low and there was a high percentage of trauma work which had a disruptive effect on the ability of the District to carry out cold elective orthopaedic work. The orthopaedic inpatient waiting list covered 1,034 patients of which 547 non-urgent patients had been on the list over a year (Table 11).

Discussion with the orthopaedic division highlighted the difficulties in the Accident and Emergency department which was having an adverse effect on cold orthopaedic surgery. The Accident and Emergency department did not have a consultant in charge and this was coupled with the shortage of junior orthopaedic staff. Consequently inexperienced junior staff in casualty tended to admit a lot of patients who subsequently did not require an operation. This situation was partially remedied by the appointment of an additional orthopaedic consultant on

TABLE 11. *Orthopaedic Inpatient Waiting List 1984–1989*

		Total	Non-Urgent (waiting over one year)	
March	1984	1,671	1,015	
September	1984	1,564	944	
March	1985	1,286	697	Effect of review
September	1985	1,207	689	of waiting List in
March	1986	1,045	506	January 1985
September	1986	1,034	547	
March	1987	1,093	432	
September	1987	910	344	
March	1988	518	175	
September	1988	429	72	
March	1989	336	16	

1985 % Rank position: waiting list per CP 72
waiting list per bed 44
% Urgent wait >1 month 70
% Urgent wait >1 year 95

SOURCE: Coventry Health Authority, 1989.

the understanding that the division would assign a high priority to the reduction of waiting lists. Consequently the consultant appointed had a special responsibility for overseeing junior staff in the Accident & Emergency department.

In September 1986 the Unit General Manager for the City Unit took up his post and began to pursue the reduction of waiting lists as a top priority. It was during this period that the government indicated its intent to publish a specific fund for the reduction of waiting lists. This was to be targeted at the five major surgical specialities—orthopaedics, general surgery, ENT, gynaecology, and ophthalmology. The initiative was also to concentrate on the Districts with the longest waiting lists. Coventry fell into this category, for example in ophthalmology in September 1986 1,535 patients were on the waiting list with 521 waiting for over one year. Only eleven Districts in the United Kingdom had a worse position (Table 12).

The Unit General Manager examined the situation in orthopaedics and ophthalmology, the specialities that were his responsibility. The difficulties in orthopaedics had been identified as a capacity problem. In ophthalmology the situation was different. Performance indicators and discussions with clinicians revealed a poor use of resources with low occupancy rates and theatre usage. This was partially a problem of a

TABLE 12. *Ophthalmology Inpatient Waiting List 1985–1989*

		Total	Non-Urgent Waiting Over One Year
March	1985	1,115	457
September	1985	1,121	477
March	1986	1,120	432
September	1986	1,428	524
March	1987	1,087	275
September	1987	851	133
March	1988	763	53
September	1988	639	30
March	1989	513	0

1985 % Rank position: Waiting list per CP 88
Waiting List per bed 88
% Urgent wait >1 month 70
% Non-urgent wait >1 year 94

SOURCE: Coventry Health Authority, 1989.

lack of anaesthetic cover which inhibited surgical activity, but also a poorly managed use of beds and theatres.

It was clear that although orthopaedics and ophthalmology both had long waiting lists the problems they faced were very different requiring different solutions. In orthopaedics management had to find extra capacity. Potential solutions included the use of private hospital facilities, other NHS facilities in the District or building capacity particularly a day surgery unit. The high admission rates through the Accident and Emergency department also warranted attention. In ophthalmology there was a need for additional anaesthetic sessions to enable further operating sessions to take place and better planning of lists to enable an increased throughput. For both specialities additional funding had to be found as the Unit faced a £·5m overspend for the year 1986/87.

The Unit began to prepare bids for the waiting list initiative at the end of 1986. The preparations were made easier by the discussions already in progress. In orthopaedics the lack of capacity was planned to be alleviated by using an extra session at Coleshill, building a new day surgery unit at Coventry and Warwickshire Hospital and carrying out extra work at Coventry and Warwickshire Hospital. The Unit General Manager began negotiations with the Administrator at St Gerrards Hospital, Coleshill, which had a vacant session which was available for the City Unit. The aim was to use the additional operating session at

St Gerrards for minor cases releasing resources to enable an additional 100 joint replacement operations at the Coventry and Warwickshire Hospital.

Negotiations between the hospitals resulted in an agreement that the City Unit would pay £50,000 per annum for the session but this left a number of issues to be resolved:

1. The anticipated case load in a session. This covered not only the number of cases in a session but also the case mix.

2. The number of sessions to be held per year.

3. The rules about stand-in surgeons when the desired surgeon was not available.

4. The method of payment and the situation if either party cancelled a session.

A target of 250 cases admitted from the waiting list over 50 sessions was agreed. Penalty clauses were to be used flexibly and would only apply if more than two sessions per annum were cancelled. In this event if the session was cancelled due to an oversight on Coleshills part they would pay the City Unit £1,000 (the cost of one session). Conversely if the cancellation arose due to a problem on the Coventry and Warwickshire side they would pay Coleshill fifty per cent of the cost of a session, i.e. £500. The full costed proposal which was submitted to Region for the waiting list initiative monies is detailed in Table 13

The City Unit also wanted to increase the low levels of day surgery being carried out. During the 1970s it became accepted that day surgery

TABLE 13. *Resource Consequences of Coleshill Session and Additional Joint Replacement Work at Coventry and Warwickshire—Waiting List Initiative 1987/88.*

Item	£
Coleshill session (includes nursing, hotel, drugs, dressings)	60,000
Surgical time (additional GP session to cover surgeon's visits to Coleshill)	2,000
Anaesthetic time (one GPCA session)	2,000
Prostheses, Coventry and Warwickshire (assumes use of most popular leg and knee prostheses)	31,000
Prostheses, Coleshill (minimal)	—
Total	95,000

SOURCE: Coventry Health Authority, 1986.

was best accommodated in autonomous units. This meant that day beds were additional to the inpatient one's which could be utilised for more major surgery and that the unit could close at night and at weekends saving on hotel costs.

Furthermore the autonomy of the unit prevented the cancellation of day surgery due to emergency work. In Coventry the lack of theatre capacity further strengthened the case for building a new designated day surgery unit. The Unit bid for £190,000 for the capital cost of building the Unit and planned to raise a further £60,000 to equip the Unit through charitable donations from the Coventry and Warwickshire Hospital 150th Anniversary Appeal. It was planned that the Day Surgery Unit would allow an additional 1,250 minor orthopaedic operations per annum and enable an additional 250 major joint replacement operations to be carried out.

The financial compilation of the bids was carried out without recourse to detailed financial information. Coventry was not a resource management pilot site and consequently had little information on the link between workload and costs. Consequently bids had to be compiled by asking staff what they would require to fulfil the targets in terms of staff and equipment. The costing of consumable items like syringes and drugs was particularly difficult and informed guesses had to be made of how many swabs might be used in a typical operation. For management the objective was to ensure that the bids were successful and priced at a level which at worst would not incur losses and at best would produce a small surplus for the Unit. The City Unit ensured that their bids were competitive when the Region compared cost per case across Districts by not asking for increased consultant time and by using GP anaesthetists for operations.

The Director of Finance from the Regional Health Authority assisted by John Yates met a team from Coventry to discuss the bids. The aim was to establish that a clear realistic target and cost had been set by the District. The Region ranked all the bids it received as follows:

1. High priority bids which would have a significant effect on waiting lists times, are fully validated and can be implemented by 1 April, 1987.

2. Bids which would have a significant effect on waiting lists/times, but some details of which required final clarification and agreement.

3. Bids which appeared likely to have a significant effect on waiting list/times, were often imaginative and innovative but often required more investigation.

4. Bids which required further investigation before a decision could be made.

The City Unit's bids predominantly fell into category one and all the bids were successful. On 2 March 1987 the District was informed that £506,300 out of a total Regional allocation of £2·88m had been allocated to Coventry and over £320,000 had been allocated to the City Unit to tackle orthopaedic and ophthalmology waiting lists. The acceptance of the money was conditional on acceptance of a number of rules set down by the Region:

1. Waiting list funding represented an earmarked allocation for the financial year 1987/88 and was only to be spent on the specific project for which it was provided. No guaranteed commitment was given for funding of the scheme in 1988/89.

2. Districts were required to submit forms KHMO6A and KHMO7A detailing quarterly the number of admissions, waiting list and waiting times information.

3. Failure to achieve targets would result in the reduction or withdrawal of the allocation. This would only be carried out after discussion with the District General Manager.

4. The success of the contract was measured in terms of an increase in cold admissions and not by changes in the size of the waiting list. Although it was expected that waiting time would decrease, Districts were not penalised if waiting list figures went up nor would they necessarily fail to receive funding in the second year if they had managed to substantially decrease their waiting lists.

5. Progress was to be monitored regularly at Performance Review Meetings.

The Initiative Underway

Coventry made a prompt start in April 1987 and this was underpinned by complementary measures including the appointment of a new bed/theatre coordinator, use of pre-operative assessments and a new admissions policy. The Unit also gave detailed attention to its information needs. This coincided with the implementation of the Körner minimum data sets but extended beyond Körner. Special data collection of monthly admissions and operations ensured management had an up to the minute picture of progress in the waiting list initiatives. Particular attention was paid to information on cancelled admissions and sessions and reasons had to be provided for these cancellations.

By July the initiative was proceeding well and the City Unit was ahead of its targets. The bid for 100 joint replacements at the Coventry and Warwickshire Hospital was enhanced and the Region provided an extra £75,000 for 200 extra operations. In addition a further £24,000 was made available to perform an extra 100 operations at Paybody Hospital of which fifty were cataract operations. By the end of November 1987 in orthopaedics to have been on course 1,600 out of the target figure of 2,400 would need to have been performed while the actual figure was 1,814 a gain of 214 operations. Similarly in ophthalmology the annual target was 1,700 operations resulting in a target of 1,133 for the end of November. The actual position was 1,187 a gain of 52. This led the Director of Performance Review and Administration at the Region to comment:

> Coventry and East Birmingham had severe financial difficulties but their achievements on the waiting lists has been nothing short of magnificent.

The Regional picture was more mixed. A resumé of the position in October 1987 across the Region showed that many schemes had started late. This was often due to the inability to win the cooperation of clinical staff and at the end of the year several Districts had to refund money to the Region for not fulfilling their targets. This proved to be a serious set back for Districts which had employed new staff to fulfil their targets and then were saddled with the additional cost as Region clawed back money for work not completed.

The Region also outlined its approach for the second year of the waiting list initiative. The first slice of money had been targeted at the Districts with the worst record. In the second round although the priority remained to improve the longest waiting lists in the Region, this was only to be done where schemes had been successfully implemented in 1987/88. The Region therefore took into account previous performance in its attempt to reward success.

Coventry began to prepare its bids for the second year with considerable confidence given the reduction in waiting lists (Tables 11/12). Throughput had also risen strongly with a fifteen per cent increase in orthopaedic throughput at the Coventry and Warwickshire (Table 14), a forty-seven per cent increase at Coleshill and a thirty-three per cent rise at Paybody. The City Unit's priority for 1988/89 was to obtain the revenue funding for the Day Surgery Unit to match the capital injected by the Region the previous year. A bid for £248,000 was submitted for six orthopaedic sessions which would have a target of 1,250 day cases. It would have been difficult for the Region to refuse this bid having provided the capital to build the Unit. The session at Coleshill was planned to continue and the workload at Coventry and Warwickshire Hospital was to increase to allow an additional 300 cases to be performed. £196,400 was requested for these activities. In ophthalmology further work was to be carried out at Paybody Hospital. The Region accepted the bids and the City Unit in 1988 continued to fulfil its targets.

TABLE 14. *Throughput in Orthopaedics and Ophthalmology 1987/88*

Hospital	*Orthopaedics* March 1987	March 1988	*Ophthalmology* March 1987	March 1988
Coventry and Warwickshire	1,200	1,380	—	—
Coleshill	850	*1,250*	—	—
Total		2,630		
Target		2,400		
Paybody	—	—	1,300	1,730
Target				1,700

SOURCE: Coventry Health Authority, 1988.

Measures to Complement the Waiting List Initiative: From Validation to Pre-operative Assessment Clinics

The success of the waiting list initiative in the City Unit was achieved by a range of management actions not immediately visible from the waiting list bids. One adjunct to the waiting list initiative were the reviews of activity in each speciality in the acute sector. They were prepared once a year and compared activity levels over time with other places using performance indicator information. These were then discussed with the consultants concerned. A bi-annual waiting list report was prepared for Health Authority members to keep them abreast of developments. In addition to the validation exercise carried out by all Health Authorities in early 1985 an annual review of all patients waiting more than six months for treatment was instituted. A separate study in orthopaedics during 1986 was made of all patients waiting over five years for treatment. Details of the patient's name, unit number, length of time on the list and condition were sent to each consultant.

A potential consequence of a long waiting list is that when patients are called for admission after a period of months or years since their previous outpatient appointment the patient may not be ready for surgery. A further possibility is that due to lengthy waiting lists a consultant will place a patient on the waiting list in anticipation that by the time the patient reaches the point for admission their condition will have advanced sufficiently to require surgery. In the case of cataract operations this phenomenon has been demonstrated (Sanderson, 1982). This type of behaviour which amounts to an informed guess of future medical need raises the possibility that patients could be admitted at the

TABLE 15. *Evaluation of the Ophthalmic Pre-Operative Assessment Clinic for Waiting List Patients: 1988*

A	Patients sent for to attend clinic		402
B	Patient attending clinic		335
C	Patients who cancelled their operation		34
D	Patients who did not attend the clinic		33
E	Patients admitted for operation		269
REASONS FOR NOT ADMITTING PATIENTS AFTER ASSESSMENT AT PRE-OPERATIVE CLINIC (B–E)			
1.	Vision improved		12
2.	Chest condition		4
3.	Hypertension		11
4.	Diabetic		5
5.	Anaemia		3
6.	Others		
	6·1 did not want operation	5	
	6·2 on holiday at admission date	3	
	6·3 other general illness	6	
	6·4 other ophthalmic condition	10	
	6·5 no benefit from operation	7	
		31	31
		Total	66

SOURCE: Ophthalmic Department, Coventry Health Authority, 1989

wrong time leading to cancellation of the operation. To prevent these type of difficulties the ophthalmology department at the Coventry and Warwickshire Hospital instigated a pre-operative assessment clinic for waiting list patients.

The clinic had two aims. First, to detect physical, physiological and social needs prior to surgery. Second, to educate the patient and his/her family about forthcoming hospitalisation. Patients were called up four-to-six weeks prior to their operation and were checked to see that appropriate medical investigations had been completed. The patient's general health and fitness for the operation were tested and their home circumstances assessed. If all the criteria were fulfilled the patient was informed of their date of admission. The results of an evaluation carried out in 1988 (Table 15) shows that only sixty-seven per cent of patients sent for were eventually admitted for surgery. In the absence of the assessment clinic this would have resulted in wasted admissions.

The Role of the Bed Coordinator

The increased activity levels planned under the waiting list initiative assumed improved management of theatre time and beds. A bed coordinator was appointed in 1985 but proved not to be a success as the post holder failed to gain the confidence of the clinical staff and was not sufficiently knowledgeable to alter clinicial management of theatre time. In the autumn of 1987 the Theatre Nursing Officer was appointed as the new Bed Coordinator. She proceeded to change the manner in which lists were chosen.

Formerly surgeons had come to the hospital to compile their own operating lists. This created a situation in which surgeons assigned priority to urgent cases and procedures which they found challenging. The length of time the patient had been on the list was not necessarily the over-riding criteria for compiling lists. The bed coordinator wanted to compile the lists herself in order to achieve a good mix of patients on a list ranging from major cases to minor procedures. Furthermore length of wait would be an important consideration and less importance would be attached to the preferences of individual consultants.

A further responsibility of the bed coordinator was the management of inpatient beds in conjunction with the rehabilitation team. The team which included paramedical staff, nursing staff, a social worker, and the responsible consultant discussed each patient on the surgical and orthopaedic wards once a week. Recommendations were made based on the needs and outlook for individual patients. This active monitoring of patients ensured that patients were kept in hospital for an appropriate length of time and facilitated an equitable use of beds between different consultants. The rehabilitation team were also able to arrange the social needs of patients ready for their discharge at an early stage. This prevented patients staying in hospital unnecessarily because, for example, an essential adaptation of the patients home had not been carried out.

The drive to reduce waiting lists encouraged the view that the problem was remedial and not insoluble. This helped to foster an innovative culture where other ideas were adopted to tackle waiting lists. In ophthalmology a short notice list was assembled in which patients who were ready for admission having had the necessary tests could be admitted at short notice to ensure the maximum use of a list if another patient cancelled at short notice.

In order to increase the throughput of minor operations, general practitioners were written to and asked to refer patients who although already referred could be re-referred to a special extra clinic where they could be quickly assessed for day surgery. The establishment of the clinic reflected the fact that the inpatient to outpatient workload was becoming imbalanced with the level of day surgery outstripping the supply from outpatients, there was a danger that the Day Surgery Unit would be hoist with its own petard as the supply of day cases dried up. The clinic proved initially not to be a success as general practitioners did not respond very well probably reflecting the administrative task involved in targeting particular patients from their case load for more rapid admission. However during 1989 the message had begun to filter through to GP's and the number of referrals has increased. Nonetheless the City Unit began to examine other options for maintaining the flow of patients and funding the increased capital.

Extending the Initiative: The Use of the Internal Market

The Region has always provided the waiting list monies to the participating Districts on the clear understanding that there was no guarantee that work funded in one year would necessarily be funded in the future. This was a source of anxiety to the City Unit who were receiving in some years in excess of £$\frac{1}{2}$m out of a basic budget of £14m. This money had helped to ease the financial difficulties the unit faced. Consequently senior management began to investigate the possibility of carrying out operations for other Districts on a contract basis and making available facilities to the private sector.

Coventry had gained a reputation in the Region for being very successful in tackling its waiting lists. The Region was supportive of the idea of an internal market where health authorities could purchase clinical services from each other at an agreed price and a defined workload. The Region's primary objective was the reduction of waiting lists and it was not concerned where the work was performed as long as it was carried out cost effectively and to a satisfactory standard. The City Unit therefore entered into a contract with South Birmingham Health Authority to take 100 minor and intermediary orthopaedic cases from their waiting list and the City Unit was paid £30,000. In a similar venture Worcester Health Authority had 300 minor orthopaedic cases taken on by Coventry for £100,000. Clearly this entailed an addition to the workload of the Coventry staff. To give an incentive to the medical staff half of the surplus on the £30,000 contract was paid into the orthopaedic division Trust Fund to assist their research. Clearly in the light of the government White Paper *Working for Patients* (Department of Health, 1989a), this type of internal market arrangement is set to expand rapidly and Coventry are in a good position to capitalise on these developments.

The internal market was only one strategy used by the City Unit. A further option was to cooperate with the private sector. The Day Surgery Unit could accommodate ten sessions per week of which six were funded through the waiting list initiative. A further 1⅔ sessions were funded by the District for plastic surgery and dental work this left 2⅓ sessions vacant. Bioplan Holdings were looking for day surgery facilities in the West Midlands and had approached Coventry Health Authority with a view to building a new unit. The Unit General Manager of the City Unit approached Bioplan and offered them facilities which were already being built thereby reducing the lead time necessary.

Agreement was reached that Bioplan would rent a session at the Day Surgery Unit for the use of their private patients. This session was to be staffed by NHS personnel and this led to opposition from District trade union representatives. In order to win trade union acceptance for the scheme Bioplan agreed to contribute approximately £28,000 for improving the facilities in the nurses changing rooms. Bioplan also agreed to pay for non-orthopaedic instruments needed in the Day Surgery Unit as these instruments had not been purchased as the Unit had been predominantly used for orthopaedic work.

A Day Surgery Management Board was established to advise on operational matters that arose between Bioplan and Coventry Health Authority. Further cooperation is envisaged, with the building of a new inpatient unit, endoscopy facilities, and additional day surgery facilities at another acute hospital in the District. The City Unit has found the venture beneficial. They have managed to secure funding for improvements to staff facilities and by negotiating a commercial price with Bioplan for their session been able to build in a surplus which can be used for other activities.

Impact on the Unit

The waiting list initiatives and cooperation with other Districts and the private sector has changed the perception of the hospital in the District and the City itself. The Coventry and Warwickshire Hospital tended to be overshadowed by the larger District General Hospital and there was a feeling that resources tended to flow to that hospital. This position has altered with beneficial effects on the morale of staff. A tangible sign of this raised profile has been the good publicity in the local paper for the hospital where previously it was seldom mentioned except in a critical light.

The increased workload falls on staff which may lead to other activities being squeezed out of the hospital routine. High levels of day surgery require a large input from consultant staff if the lists are to be completed on time. This may make it difficult for clinical staff to devote much time to teaching. Conversely better planning of theatre time with a realistic number of cases on the list can ensure that lists do not over run enabling staff to leave promptly.

Performing work for other Health Authorities can also draw a mixed response from staff. They wish to safeguard the needs of local people first and would be reluctant to be carrying out work from further afield if they were not satisfied that local patients needs were being met. This situation should not arise as contracts with other Health Authorities are pursued after local needs have been catered for and where spare capacity still exists. Nonetheless if work for other Authorities is seen as lucrative the suspicion might arise that this work is being taken on in preference to the needs of local patients. Nursing staff are less likely to be aware of these circumstances unless they looked at the patients details. Clinical staff may take a less sanguine view of the internal market as clinical issues of good practice may arise. A surgeon may not wish other consultants to follow up his work in outpatients but it may prove difficult for patients to travel long distances for follow up consultations.

CONCLUSION

Waiting lists have become the Achilles Heel of the NHS. A central justification for the proposed reform of the NHS is to increase the amount of choice available to patients. Implicit in the proposals are the notion that waiting lists represent a denial of choice and that patients consequently suffer. This theme has also been adopted by drug companies in promoting drugs to GPs which purport to make the wait more tolerant. One advert carries the caption 'Prostrate trouble: He can't jump the queue, but you can ease the waiting.'

In this atmosphere of disquiet the government launched its waiting list initiative in 1986/87. Coventry Health Authority which had a legacy of long waiting lists was targeted by the Region and this coincided with internal initiatives to tackle the problem. Coventry has continued to be successful in ameliorating waiting lists and in winning money from the Region. In the third year of the initiative for activity in 1989/90 the City Unit has been allocated funding to continue the orthopaedic work at Coleshill and at the Coventry and Warwickshire Hospital Day Surgery Unit. The waiting list position has improved particularly in terms of reducing the number of patients waiting over a year for their treatment. In June 1986 only 14·1 per cent of all patients had waited over a year for treatment, compared with 26·7 per cent a year before. The proportion of cases performed as day cases also rose with 132 per cent more day cases performed in April-September 1988 compared with the same period in 1987.

The success of the initiative in the City Unit contrasts with the position in certain other Health Authorities where the initiative has been marked by late starts and non-fulfilment of targets. An advantage the City Unit had was the Coventry and Warwickshire Hospital is dominated by the orthopaedic speciality. Consequently there was limited scope for disagreements between specialities over allocations of beds, etc, which has complicated this type of initiative in other authorities.

Medical–Managerial Cooperation

The cooperation of medical staff was essential to the success of the initiative. This was achieved by senior management drawing out the potential benefits for the Unit in terms of the welcome injection of resource the initiative would bring. Furthermore as the initiative widened to encompass work from other Health Authorities specific funds for research were made available to groups of clinicians as an additional incentive. Management also built upon the latent frustration in the Unit, that day case work was clogging up operating lists. The use of contracts with the Region which set clear targets, helped to establish a clear dialogue with clinicians facilitating negotiation over what was possible.

The negative feature of this clarity is the inflexibility it can bring in its wake. The penalties for not fulfilling the targets are severe and if a large amount of emergency work jeopardises fulfilment of the target this may lead to Authorities having to carry out surgical blitzes on minor cases to achieve their targets. This type of action and the waiting list initiative more generally can therefore distort priorities as Health Authorities scramble for earmarked funds. The likelihood of this occurring was evident in Coventry where an imbalance existed between inpatient and outpatient waiting lists and times. Management were aware of the difficulties but it was proving difficult to obtain the same commitment from Region to tackle outpatient problems. However as outpatients and inpatients waiting times became imbalanced an insufficient flow of patients for surgery from outpatients was becoming evident.

The availability of earmarked central funding can also be a two edged sword with the danger existing of activity levels being ratcheted up by special funding leaving Health Authorities with a difficult situation if that funding then evaporates. This was emphasised by the City Unit

General Manager in his introduction to his 1989/90 bid for waiting list funds:

> Progress in the second year of the waiting lists initiative remains good, but it must be emphasised that current workload can only be maintained through the availability of specially targeted funding.

The irony is that the waiting list initiative emphasised the need for local management to tackle the waiting list problem as they saw fit and not through central prescription. However local management's greatest constraint is the uncertainty surrounding future funding. There is a temptation for Regions to respond by allocating money to the same Authorities each year. However this may simply accentuate the gap between good and poor performers leading to a vicious circle developing where good performers are allocated additional funds while poor performers languish and are penalised. This reduction of equity is one likely consequence of an internal market where resources flow to hospitals that perform well.

The experience of the City Unit at Coventry demonstrates the effect that a committed onslaught by management and clinicians can have on a waiting list problem despite the familiar shortcomings of information systems which makes the preparation of bids an uncertain proposition. However the national picture is less comforting with the latest figures for March 1989 showing a rise in the national inpatient waiting list to 704,700 up 2·0 per cent on September 1988 and up 3·8 per cent on the corresponding period for 1988. The figures are the highest since March 1983 when the number was inflated by the effects of the 1982 health workers pay dispute. Government ministers' described this situation as disappointing. The suspicion remains that the waiting list initiative although being usefully harnassed by Districts like Coventry is a political gimmick in which money is returned to Health Authorities which they were deprived of from other sources of funding. The lack of interest shown in tackling outpatient waiting times or lists for which statistics are not collected is a major oversight as the inpatient and outpatient waiting list problem needs to be tackled jointly and the artificial division between the two broken. As long as the division is maintained and current government policy is sustained the impact of the national waiting list initiative is likely to remain modest.

CHAPTER 7

Case study: Community Care—Macclesfield

THEORETICAL INTRODUCTION: MANY SOURCES OF FINANCE AND MANY ADMINISTERING AGENCIES

Prior to the implementation of the National Health Service and Community Care Bill of 1989-90, there were many sources of finance for care for priority groups. The NHS vote from the Department of Health is administered by health authorities for the purposes of providing and running hospitals, community health services (and to a much lesser extent) a few NHS nursing homes. The Department of Social Security organises transfer payments, pensions, income support or supplementary benefits, and various other allowances, which are administered through Social Security Offices for various purposes such as support at home, contributions to local authority services and payment for care in private residential homes and private nursing homes. Personal social services, also paid for from the central Department of Social Security in part, go to help local authorities fulfil various purposes such as the running of homes.

This latter category of central expenditure goes to support local expenditure by local authorities, using revenue firstly from Rates and later from the Community Charge. Such authorities used also to be supported by the *Department of Environment*, which through the former Rate Support Grant helped to provide the finance for residential homes and sheltered housing. Support to local authorities under the community charge arrangements are more piecemeal. The Department of the Environment also provides housing subsidies which are administered through the agency of housing associations for the purpose of providing housing for priority groups such as the elderly and mentally handicapped. Local Rates, replaced by the Community Charge in 1990 (1988 in Scotland), are the local source of finance relevant to our argument.

Furthermore there is finance from personal resources and charitable sources which go to provide various services in the private, voluntary as well as public sectors. At the outset one can notice a vast scope for complication. Let us consider the case of one individual requiring care. Should he be in a long-stay NHS hospital, an NHS nursing home, a residential home, sheltered housing, a private nursing home, a home in the community, or living at home with his family if he has one? All these options have different medical and social purposes as well as different costs (Maynard and Smith, 1983).

(i). *Long-stay NHS hospitals*

Almost all of their cost is borne by the NHS (the Department of Health), although a tiny increment of the retirement pension is used as a transfer payment to pay for long-stay care in NHS hospitals within certain limits.

(ii). *NHS nursing homes*

NHS nursing homes are too few and far between, and costing figures are not reliable. However it is clear that their cost also is borne substantially by the NHS.

When considering the next options, it is important to distinguish between public and private finance for care. Unlike in the case of NHS institutions which are paid for from the public purse, local authority homes and, of course, private nursing homes receive income from private sources, from individuals and their families. The following discussion, in attributing proportions of *public expenditure*, ignores this private component—not because it is not important, but because the discussion attempts to analyse the different contributions from different government departments and public agencies. The proportions are percentages of the public expenditure.

(iii). *Residential Homes (local authority or private)*

In the aggregate, three quarters of their costs, approximately, is borne by local authorities (broadly the cost of the home including capital, plus the cost of nursing in the home) and almost one quarter is borne by the Department of Social Security, which provides funds for supplementary retirement pensions to be used in such homes.

(iv). *Sheltered Housing (local authority or private)*

In this case two thirds of the aggregate cost is borne by the Department of Health, approximately, and the rest by local authorities.

(v). *Private Nursing Homes*

Almost all of the public financing cost is borne by the Department of Social Security, through its paying for places in such homes for those who qualify. This category provides a good example of the problems of 'sudden cut-off points'. Below a certain income threshold one is eligible for public funds for staying in such a home; but above that threshold, and below another threshold, much of the entitlement is lost; and above the second threshold, all entitlement is lost. (Exact figures are not inserted as they naturally change from year to year).

(vi). *Living at Home*

While difficult to cost, the public finance to support living at home breaks-down approximately with two thirds of the cost borne by the Department of Social Security and the rest by local authorities.

Consequences for Policy

There are therefore financial barriers to guaranteeing the most effective care for the individual. A poor family may be forced to see a relative go into an NHS hospital, because eligibility for public finance for nursing homes is just missed and this is the only option truly available. Naturally a required level of medical and/or nursing care is necessary for admission. Otherwise the poor family which just misses eligibility for certain public benefits may be forced to care for the individual at home, under all sorts of pressure.

In other words, the institution or form of care which one receives may in the end be determined by what amount of money is available and what budget can be used at the time one registers the need. This does not guarantee that it is the cheapest, let alone the most cost-effective, or the most socially effective form of care, which will be chosen. The point of contact with the system, whether it is a general practitioner, the social worker, or the bureaucrat, the district nurse or the health visitor, may also determine somewhat arbitrarily what type of care one receives.

Naturally health authorities and local authorities' social services departments have sought joint planning and cooperation to get round these barriers. However, they are generally forced to play at the margins, given the variety of the financial and structural barriers they face.

It is characteristic of government that it will face one variable at a time. In trying to prevent inefficiency in the NHS and 'bed blocking' through the use of expensive care by people perhaps with the minimal medical need, the social security regulations were liberalised in 1983 (without the requirement of legislation, through merely the interpretation of existing legislation) to allow access to private nursing homes. However, although still cheaper than 'bed blocking', in the main, the soaring cost of these institutions—and the mushrooming provision in response to the newly determined demand from the government—led to restrictions and ceilings placed on the amount of reimbursement available for different categories of patient, in May 1985. People who could no longer afford the top-up fee in many cases returned to block beds in hospitals, which are at least free at the point of use.

Thus in tackling one variable at a time, the government finds itself punching a balloon; punching down one blown up budget may merely lead the balloon to swell in another area.

It is in this context that the Audit Commission Report, *Making a Reality of Community Care* (Audit Commission, 1986) and the subsequent report by Sir Roy Griffiths, *Community Care: Agenda For Action* (Griffiths, 1988) emerged.

Overall their objectives are to rationalise funding for community care, to provide short-term bridging funding to allow versions of community care to develop, and to coordinate the spending of social security money and various monies available for community care through the Department of Health and Personal Social Services, to promote organisational unity, to stimulate new staffing and other demarcations, to stimulate further voluntary agencies, and to give ministerial responsibility for community care to a Minister of State.

It should be pointed out at the outset however that such rationalisation was only to apply to community care. The barriers to effective decision-making, discussed already, occur at a more basic point in decision-making by the potential client and the professionals involved: before the form of community care is decided upon, it is necessary to decide whether community care *is* either the best *or* the most cost effective option for that individual. Greater rationalisation of funding, not just within the boundaries of community care, is necessary. This has led some to advocate a variety of solutions to the financial fragmentation and frequent perverse incentives which arise. One proposed solution is an equal ability to recover costs by all providing agencies. This could lead to the abolition of charging by non-NHS agencies, or the introduction of charging by NHS agencies for specified categories of patient. Secondly, this suggests that the joint finance is increased. This would allow local authorities to have more access to health authority money. However, joint finance was always just intended to be a 'marginal' policy to grease the wheels of the existing system. Expanding it significantly would make it one more inflexible wedge in a still fragmented arena.

More promisingly the role of the 'board' or the 'gate-keeping manager' to manage care has been proposed, both prior to Sir Roy Griffith's report and subsequent to it. This would provide one gatekeeper who would at least take a global decision for the individual based on a global assessment of that individual's needs and the potential funds available. The Griffiths report has taken further the idea of inter-agency charging: in recommending one purchasing agent (the local authority's social services department), the aim is to stimulate a provider market of provision—within which the NHS might or might not compete, depending upon government priorities as to the overall role of the NHS in chronic care (is that after all the NHS's core business, it is argued).

Problems in Making and Implementing Policy

Major problems have therefore been:

the separation of hospital and community health service and local authority spending;

financial control over local authorities by the Treasury which has prevented innovative schemes often being able to get off the ground (with innovative authorities often ironically being penalised for financial overspending);

the difficulty in monitoring and mandating expenditure through the Rate Support Grant (or Community Charge 'Revenue Support Grant', following the establishment of some distribution from the centre to prevent inequity being too stark);

consequent limitations on joint finance as a bridge builder;

and overall, the different financial implications of different policies to different agencies.

It should be stressed that there is no UK-wide model for either community care or for the coordination of care for priority groups in general. There are naturally behavioural and organisational impediments to effective planning, which have been analysed in the case of the Department of Health, the Scottish Home and Health Department and the Welsh Office respectively (Hunter and Wistow, 1987). Finally, a failure to appreciate the likely cost of effective community care led to the alleged 'new priority for the 1980s appearing less attractive as the 1980s progressed; and greater uncertainty as to overall policy.

It is by no means clear that community care is desired by many 'priority' individuals. The continuing challenge is naturally to cost different types of care for different types of group to help decision makers, hopefully in charge of global budgets in the future, to help individuals.

The Policy of Community Care

The policy of community care has been central to the development of health and personal social services for over a quarter of a century. Yet its evolution has been slow with limited tangible results beyond the ubiquitous references in official government documents. In the late 1980's the pace of change has quickened and community care has become synonymous with the closure of the long-stay institutions. This has acted as a catalyst to those opposed to the policy who have pointed to the lack of community provision available as proof of the failure of the policy. A series of critical reports (Social Services Committee, 1985, Audit Commission, 1986) fuelled these debates and the gravity of the situation led the government to ask Sir Roy Griffiths to undertake a full scale review of community care. The Report was published in March 1988 (Griffiths, 1988) and the government finally responded in July 1989, with a White Paper following in November (Department of Health, 1989c). This ended the silence which had prevailed since the government's publication of the White Paper on the future of the NHS (Department of Health, 1989a) which focused exclusively on the acute services and neglected future options for community care. This lengthy delay was attributed to Griffiths' advocacy of a greater role for local authorities, which was unpalatable to a government pursuing a deliberate strategy of weakening local authorities.

The Evolution of Community Care

The ebb and flow of the debate about the effectiveness of community care has been muddied by the lack of a clear definition of community care. The extent to which communities exist and can be supportive of clients leaving long-stay hospitals has been questioned. The pressure group SANE has been lobbying against the closure of long-stay hospitals.

The demise of community was one of the central themes of early sociological writers such as deTonnies and Durkheim who attributed this decline to the removal of the need to live in a highly localised world. The development of the welfare state has further loosened the need for community. The perception that individuals had become too dependent on the State was central to the post 1979 Conservative Government appeal. The Conservatives have tried to revitalise the idea of community but this has sat uncomfortably with their more recent 'market liberal' emphasis on individualism. This has spawned essentially negative community action against perceived threats, a recent example being the lobbying in Kent against the Channel Tunnel railway link. Paradoxically this new self-interested sense of community may pose a threat to the success of community care, as communities may organise against the placement of people with learning difficulties in the community. Consequently policy-makers have not always been sufficiently clear about what role they expected the community to play in establishing successful community care.

Critics have frequently failed to distinguish between the philosophy of community care and the outcomes of that policy. As Jones (Jones,

1976) demonstrates community care can be interpreted in very different ways which serve different purposes. For politicians it may be a useful piece of rhetoric or endorsed as a cheap option. Health authorities view it as an opportunity to increase the quality of care and move away from an institutional model of care while friends and relatives may be conscious about the increased responsibilities they may have to bear.

The Social Services Committee (HMSO, 1985) was unable to offer an absolute definition of community care. They argued community care rested on a number of general principles which suggested a preference for home life over institutional care and emphasised the pursuit of an ordinary lifestyle for people with learning difficulties or mental health problems rather than a model of service premised on their separation from the rest of society. There has been an increasing acceptance of these principles to provide services, but the elaboration of principles, has not necessarily resulted in services which have remained true to these principles. The difficulty for health authorities and other agencies has been that these principles give little guidance to the nature of services to be provided. Consequently financial and other imperatives have blown this fragile basis for services planning off course.

The decision to close Mary Dendy and other long-stay hospitals stems from the gradual drift to community care which commenced after the second world war. The policy encompassed not only people with learning difficulties and those who were mentally ill but included the elderly and children. The 1946 Curtis Report implicitly acknowledged community care by suggesting that children should be cared for in private homes or small group homes rather than in large institutional establishments. However it was the establishment of the Royal Commission on Mental Illness and Deficiency in 1954 whose recommendations laid the basis for the 1959 Mental Health Act which first recommended a shift to community care (Martin, 1984).

Health policy is rarely the product simply of high level recommendations but mirrors changing professional and public perceptions. This was true for the adoption of community care which was stimulated by changing professional practice and the low esteem in which long-stay institutions were held following a series of scandals in the 1960s.

The advent of psychotropic drugs in the 1950s heralded a new era of unbridled optimisim for psychiatry, in which it was believed that the attributes of the new drugs would enable people with mental health problems to live in the community. They also served to challenge the traditional custodial role of long-stay institutions and move towards a more active therapeutic role for hospitals. This process was accelerated by the incorporation of the mental hospitals into the administrative framework of the NHS which broke down the isolation of the long-stay hospitals.

It was this degree of insularity which had contributed to the low standards which surfaced dramatically in the 1960s. Emergent anxieties about over crowded hospitals providing low standards of care had prompted the formation of Aid for the Elderly in Government Institutions (AEGIS). This generated a debate in the pages of *The Times* which led Robb of AEGIS to document the conditions in particular long-stay institutions; drawing on the experience of nursing and social work staff. The book *Sans Everything: A case to Answer* was a savage indictment of conditions in long-stay institutions. Although the committees' of Inquiry established by the Minister of Health, K Robinson, to investigate the allegations concluded that the book contained gross exaggerations the finger of suspicion remained pointed at the long-stay hospitals and public opinion had been galvanised against the long-stay institutions. A series of fires highlighted other short-comings in the management of long-stay institutions.

It was not long before further allegations appeared concerning the Ely Hospital in Cardiff which catered for people with a mental handicap and the mentally ill. On this occasion the Committee of Inquiry was uncompromising in its criticism of staff and management at the Hospital. The glare of publicity that now focused on long-stay hospitals revealed further ill treatment at Farleigh Hospital near Bristol and Whittingham Hospital, Lancashire. The scandals placed the defenders of long-stay institutions on the defensive and injected a new urgency into the search for alternative models of care.

The scandals in the long-stay institutions appeared to vindicate writers such as Goffman (1968) who had argued in *Asylums* that the institution became of greater importance than the individuals it was meant to serve, creating an environment in which the quality of life for their inmates was diminished. Consequently the growing hostility to the long-stay institutions in the 1960s coupled with the development of new drugs spurred on the belief that community care would be both more humane and cheaper than long-stay provision. This powerful combination led to the first unequivocal adoption of community care policy in *Better services for the Mentally Handicapped* published in 1971.

This proposed a major shift of emphasis from hospitals to community care advocating a run down of hospital beds to half the 1971 level of 52,000 and recommended that no new large hospitals were built. In their place local authority funded care was to expand but while there were promises of improving the existing hospitals the document had scant detail on how the new model of community care was to be provided and financed.

This strategy was reiterated in the 1976 *Priorities for Health and Personal Social Services* document which emphasised a preventative and community care approach and highlighted current need in mental handicap, mental illness, elderly and childrens' services which were designated as priority areas. The degree to which community care was becoming the accepted orthodoxy was illustrated by the recommendations of the Jay Committee in 1979. The report examined mental handicap nursing and questioned the need for specialised hospital provision arguing that mental handicap was a disability not an illness making hospitalisation inappropriate. This was a significant extension of the community care philosophy as even though the 1971 document had envisaged a reduction in beds for people with a mental handicap it had never fundamentally questioned the need for some form of hospital provision. The acceptance of the Jay philosophy opened the way for the complete closure of long-stay hospitals. The question was no longer, should the hospitals close rather it was the pace of change which was to dominate debate in the 1980s.

The 1980s witnessed the concept of community care becoming tarnished since the heady days of the 1960s and 1970s. Community care has at worst become an evocative slogan which gives little indication of how services should be provided and monitored. Community care has not been immune from the climate of financial stringency that has buffeted the NHS. Indeed the pressure on acute services has often been difficult to resist leading to a diversion of resources away from priority areas such as community care to acute provision. The dominance of the acute sector in government thinking was reiterated in the 1989 White Paper *Working for Patients* (Department of Health, 1989a) which focused exclusively on the future of the acute sector.

The rupturing of the cross-party consensus that marked the earlier years of the NHS led to a questioning of the degree to which the state should be involved in social care provision. The Conservative government since 1979 has encouraged the private sector and voluntary sector to be more involved in areas where traditionally the state has taken the lead. The prominence in Conservative ideology of the role of the family in the provision of services has seen a subtle shift from care in the community which implied statutory support for people living in private homes to a policy of care by the community which implies a reduced role for statutory provision and an increased role for informal provision. The clearest statement of this shift of policy came in the White Paper *Growing Older*.

> Whatever level of public expenditure proves practicable, and however it is distributed, the primary sources of support and care for the elderly people are informal and voluntary. These spring from the personal ties of friendship and neighbourhood. They are irreplaceable. It is a role of public authorities to sustain and where necessary, develop—but never, displace—such support and care. Care in the community must increasingly mean care by the community. (DHSS, 1981)

The anxieties about community care which have surfaced in the 1980s reflect not only reservations about the shifting definition of what constitutes community care but the maturity of the policy itself. In the 1960s and 1970s the debate about community care was couched in theoretical terms due to the lack of evidence about the effects of the policy. In the 1980s there has been a number of surveys and reports on the consequences of community care. There has also been international evidence about the Italian and American experiences of closure of long-stay hospitals.

Community Care: Problems in Policy and Practice

Advocates of community care commence from a critique of long-stay institutions which curtail an individuals ability to fulfil their potential. It is argued that individuals can lead more ordinary lives in the community where social networks of family and friends can be more easily sustained. In this way services can be tailored to meet individual needs and enhance the quality of life. Critics believe that the principle of community care is not proven and combine this attack on community care in practice with criticism of the underlying philosophy it embodies.

The first strand is philosophical, this questions the assumption that people with learning difficulties can live ordinary lives in the community. The concept of normalisation is viewed as hopelessly idealistic and misinterpreted as placing an obligation on individuals to conform to an artificially imposed definition of normality. Consequently striving for normalisation does not 'enhance' choice but restricts choice.

The second strand is operational and suggests that it is more difficult for people with learning difficulties to take advantage of opportunities in the community. At a hospital, leisure facilities are available on site and economies of scale ensure a wider choice. In the community even if facilities are available they are not as accessible. Furthermore community facilities often are not developed and community care is viewed as simply an exercise in closing hospitals. As the pace of change has accelerated in the 1980s both sides have lobbied increasingly strongly in support of their position.

The most influential and critical report on the state of community care was a survey carried out by the Audit Commission in 1986. (Audit Commission, 1986). This expressed grave concern at

> the lack of progress in shifting the balance towards community care: and identified structured impediments to the implementation of community care.

The report estimated that £6 billion was spent on community care for the elderly, mentally ill, mentally handicapped, and physically disabled but the money is inappropriately targeted leading to poor value for money. The NHS accounts for half the £6b spent while personal social services spends nearly £26m on community care and the remainder is social security payments. The Commissions criticism extended beyond their formal remit of ensuring value for money in the public sector. They were critical of the fact that although there were 37,000 fewer mentally ill and mentally handicapped patients in hospital in 1986 than 10 years earlier there was no record of what had happened to those who had been discharged. But this is not to suggest that the Commission felt health authorities were meeting their targets in reducing the population of mental handicap hospitals as outlined in 1971. Community care for people with learning difficulties should use up 33·4 per cent of total expenditure, according to *Better Services for the Mentally Handicapped* but only 21 per cent of the resource is being used in this manner. Therefore the report made it clear that extensive weaknesses existed in the framework, it is to these we now turn in more detail.

The strategies on community care point to the tremendous variations in provision and expenditure across the country. For adults with a mental handicap local authority expenditure varies by a factor of six. In 1984/85 gross expenditure per head of population ranged from £11·65 in Camden to £1·04 in Sutton. It is the financial mechanism which contribute to these variations which have been heavily criticised.

The Audit Commission highlighted the peculiar lack of incentives to the implementation of community care. The financial arrangements do not reflect the changing balance of responsibility envisaged with the shift to community care, given that the bulk of resource is distributed through the NHS. However there is no mechanism to reward or penalise the health service. The RAWP formula is primarily concerned with global distribution to individual regions rather than the distribution of that resource within a region between different client groups.

For local authorities the shift to community care has frequently been experienced as an attempt by the NHS to disengage itself from a complex and expensive area of care and place this responsibility on local authorities. For local authorities who have been attempting to maintain levels of services in an environment of reduced Rate Support Grants and increased statutory responsibilities the prospect of having to fund and manage new areas of care was viewed with trepidation.

Joint finance is the best known mechanism for switching resources from health to local authorities and was envisaged as a way of facilitating the cumbersome joint planning machinery. The expectations for joint finance outweigh the resources assigned to the programme, with only approximately £110m available annually a fraction of the £6b spent on community care. Consequently the impact of joint finance is likely to be modest. Joint finance also tends to support existing projects and is tapered so that after eight years the local authority will be financing the project in full. There has been a marked reluctance by local authorities to take on these new responsibilities. There is also a suspicion amongst health authorities that joint finance money has not been targeted appropriately and been used to maintain services that would have been provided by local authorities even in the absence of joint finance arrangements. Furthermore Hunter (1987) argues that as joint finance monies are included in the 1% of revenue that health authorities are allowed to carry forward there are limited incentives to use the money effectively because of the threat to their carry over arrangements.

There has been no shortage of suggested remedies to improve the workings of the joint finance machinery. Glennerster (1984) believed that in view of the shortcomings of the joint planning machinery tinkering with the machinery by increased individual responsibility as suggested in *Progress For Partnership* (1984) would have limited results. The emphasis on improving joint planning structures does not appear to address the financial disincentives to joint planning, consequently a more fundamental shift which changed the statutory responsibilities for the provision of services with resources flowing to that agency has gained support.

The other central mechanism for shifting resources to fund community care initiatives has been the dowries which are attached to individuals entering the community from long-stay institutions as pump priming money to help establish community provision. However these dowries which are usually about £10,000 neither reflect the true cost of keeping individuals in the community and fail to acknowledge that individuals who would have entered long-stay hospitals will no longer have this facility available, increasing the pool of need in the community. Health authorities are also reluctant to release funds until the savings from bed reductions have been realised militating against their effectiveness. This situation is made more difficult by the lack of adequate bridging funds which might have been used to cover the double running costs as services are run down and new services provided to take their place.

The difficulties in finding adequate financial mechanisms reflect greater uncertainties about the ability of local authorities and health authorities to work together cooperatively. They are very different types of organisation with diverse control and accountability mechanisms. NHS managers tend to have greater autonomy in making decisions about community care initiatives while social services managers need to refer back to their elected members. Conversely health authorities have been required to plan ten years in advance while social services managers may not view community care as a priority area compared to their legal responsibilities in connection with child abuse and the homeless. Conversely health authority managers are constrained by powerful professional groups who have lobbied to maintain acute services and divert resources intended for community care initiatives. The different philosophy of the two organisations complicates joint working with the NHS being geared to a medical model based on a curative approach as opposed to the social services ethos which focuses on the social needs of individuals and is less orientated to capital projects.

In recent years new concerns have emerged which go beyond the perennial criticism of joint planning machinery. Due to the unfavourable economic climate health and local authorities are making increasing use of social security benefits to fund community care. This is not cost effective as it leads to a bias towards the provision of residential care which may be inappropriate but is reinforced as residential care attracts the largest benefit payments. This runs counter to the thrust of the community care initiative. Consequently the steep rise in social security benefit payments has distorted the priorities of community care and may not reflect need.

To summarise the administrative and financial arrangements which are the framework for provision of community care have proved to be an uncertain foundation for community care. The collaborative mechanisms established to facilitate inter-organisational cooperation have not always been sufficient to bridge the essential lack of incentives to enable community care to become a reality. Consequently there have been a series of reports on changing the system of community care.

Griffiths II: Agenda for Action?

Following this trenchant criticism from the Audit Commission, in December 1986, Norman Fowler the former DHSS Secretary of State asked Sir Roy Griffiths, the Prime Minister's health adviser to undertake a review of community care policy. He was set the following terms of reference:

> To review the way in which public funds are used to support community care policy and to advise me on the options that would improve the use of these funds as a contribution to more effective community care

The remit for Griffiths made it clear that the review was not to comment on the adequacy of existing funding nor to focus on the shortcomings of the system rather it was to make recommendations on improvements to the existing financing and management of community care. Consequently Griffiths outlined a broad agenda for change.

The thrust of Griffith's proposals was philosophically in tune with the governments desire to inject market forces into areas previously devoid of these considerations. Similarly it addresses the governments dislike of having services funded and provided by the same agency.

The Griffiths report was, in a more modest form, a precursor for the White Paper *Working for Patients* (Department of Health, 1989a) in its advocacy of separating the funding of services from their provision.

The proposals emphasise the need for a strengthened management function in the provision of community care. At the centre a clearer strategic role for central government is envisaged with a designated minister responsible for community care. The Minister should establish clear objectives; ensure local plans fulfil these objectives and should monitor the development of local plans. Funding for these plans was to be provided by specific community care grants approved by central government.

At local level a leading role was to be played by social services departments who were to prepare local plans in collaboration with health authorities and other agencies. The basis for these plans was to be the objectives established by central government and the assessment of need. Social services departments were not necessarily to provide services but rather

> Social Services Authorities should see themselves as the arrangers and purchasers of care services—not as monopolistic providers. (Griffiths, 1988, Paragraph 3.4)

health authorities were left with a residual role, they were to concern themselves with provision of services for clients who had unambiguously health needs.

The response to Griffiths was generally a positive one. A survey by the Kings Fund Institute (1988) found not surprisingly that 91 per cent of social services directors supported the proposals as opposed to 40 per cent of health service managers. Supporters were encouraged by a vision of increased flexibility and clearer lines of accountability which the proposals seemed to offer. However a number of difficulties remain. The governments preference for market lead solutions tends to ignore even neoclassical economic notions of market failure. In the provision of community care where services are often being provided for vulnerable individuals consumer sovereignty is not applicable and consequently reliance on the market may open up the possibility of abuse. Griffiths seems to implictly acknowledge this possibility when stressing the need for monitoring. However the difficulties local authorities already experience in trying to monitor services effectively is testimony to the problems involved.

Another dimension of the philosophical thrust in Griffiths concerns the assumptions about the role of the family in the provision of community care. Griffiths adopts the government view outlined above that care in the community should in the first instance be care by the community. This effectively means care by families and a large body of research indicates that women largely carry this burden. Yet women's increased participation in the labour market and higher rates of divorce raise doubts about women's capacity or willingness to provide this informal care. (Allen, 1987). It also cannot be assumed that people have a preference for informal care over formal/statutory care (Phillipson, 1988). Consequently a market orientation may be inappropriate for providing community care and the assumption that informal care is preferable and readily available is not proven.

The ability of the centre to effectively monitor local plans and act as a focus to disseminate good practice has been questioned. (Hunter, Judge, 1988). The paradox is that the Griffiths report emphasises local accountability and decentralisation yet advocates a complex centralised monitoring system.

By the end of 1989, the government had published its White Paper on community care, which accepted the thrust of the Griffiths proposals. Local authorities were to be the new 'purchasers' of care, yet—or rather, because of this—their providing role was to be diminished. Private providers, along with voluntary agencies, were to be further encouraged.

The overall problem, however, of deciding *where* a client ought to receive care was not necessarily to be addressed. To allow choice (within a budget) of the best care for clients, and best care-mix or client-mix, requires the global purchaser to make a choice from not just *within* alternative 'community care' providers but *between* community care and other variants of care. After all, getting 'bed-blockers' out of hospital and needy individuals *into* hospital may be the dominant need. Yet political, financial, and managerial fragmentation of overall budgets —coupled with the NHS being 'free' unlike other forms of care— prevents overall coordination.

Community Care: Existing Models of Good Practice

Although the spotlight in the debate about community care has increasingly focused on the shortcomings of community provision, despite difficulties good practice has developed. In the field of services for people with learning difficulties the core and cluster model has come to prominence. This model is closely associated with the Kings Fund Working Party on *An Ordinary Life* (1980) which established the concept of a 'local' residential service which would be 'comprehensive' in that it would not exclude individuals because they were defined by society as too handicapped.

At a fundamental level the Kings Fund proposals were underpinned by the philosophy of normalisation. This term is associated with the work of W. Wolfensberger (1972). The central tenet of this philosophy is that people with learning difficulties have the same needs and rights as ordinary people but may need assistance to meet these needs. Wolfensberger argues that people with learning difficulties are devalued in society by being primarily labelled as handicapped. This gives rise to low expectations about individuals potential leading to a vicious circle of low achievements and lower expectations. The challenge Wolfensberger argues is to break this cycle of devalued roles.

A number of principles for the planning of services flow from this philosophy. People have a right to live in ordinary housing in which they are able to make choices and take decisions for themselves enabling people with learning difficulties to grow and develop into valued members of the community and not be stigmatised and confined to long-stay institutions. Health authorities have tried to enable people with learning difficulties to mix with other groups in the community and develop relationships with people who do not necessarily have learning difficulties.

The normalisation philosophy also embodied a powerful critique of the traditional work experience and training provided by Adult Training Centres. The Kings Fund in *An Ordinary Working Life* (Kings Fund Centre, 1984) argued for real work experience to be made available to people with learning difficulties to enable greater integration into the community. The Adult Training Centres didn't fulfil this purpose. They were often unclear about their goals and not geared to development needs in which ultimately people would gain ordinary employment. This situation of devaluing individuals was reinforced by Adult Training Centres coming under the social services rubric and by the low wages paid to individuals.

One consequence of the normalisation philosophy has been the development of the self advocacy movement which began in the USA in the 1970s. The aim is to let people with learning difficulties speak up for themselves so as to have more control over their own lives by taking decisions for themselves. 'People First' the umbrella organisation of self advocacy groups has seen a rapid growth since 1980 from 40 to 300 groups enabling people who have traditionally been seen as passive recipients of services to be viewed as equals—as people first. This movement is also flowing with the tide. The need to incorporate the views of consumers in the provision of services is rapidly gaining acceptance. Consequently the self advocacy movement is growing more confident in challenging the views of professional providers.

Implications for Policy: The Core and Cluster Model

The core and cluster model consists of a network of supported homes referred to as the cluster which are administratively linked to a core. The aim is to provide flexible services in the community which meet the needs of individuals as these change over time. The model is based on two assumptions. First individuals can learn to be more independent however severe their degree of handicap. Second the service can be designed to meet individual rather than group needs.

The core acts as a focal point and a resource centre which indirectly supports the various parts of the cluster provision through professional support to families and relatives of people with learning difficulties living in the community. Units typically provide residential care for up to six people for planned rotational or emergency stays for specified periods usually up to four weeks. This respite care helps families to sustain community care. Day care facilities may also be provided and aims to cater for activities which are not easily available in other day care provision, widening the choice for people with learning difficulties and encouraging increased skill levels.

The network of cluster homes provides a range of options offering the choice of living alone or with a small number of other people in ordinary houses with varying degrees of support from full-time, part-time or visiting staff. One of the goals of the core and cluster model is to limit the number of disruptive moves that people have to make. Support and help is provided according to individual needs and it is the service and the staff which adapt rather than shifting people to more specialised units. An important corollary is that the core is not a place where the most depdendant individuals live. If intensive support is needed it should be provided in the cluster.

Central to the establishment of comprehensive local services for people with learning difficulties is the Community Mental Handicap Team. The idea was devised by the National Development Group in the mid-1970s and was developed by the National Development Team (1978) under its first director, Dr Simon. The focus was on the contribution Community Mental Handicap Teams could make to the provision of NHS services rather than encompassing social services as well. In more recent years the scope of the teams had been extended reflecting the shift to community care. A consequence has been an increase in the diversity of form the teams take.

This diversity of structure is reflected in the differing functions performed. Broadly, there is a division between teams which directly provide services to people with learning difficulties and those whose primary concern is the planning and development of new services (Mansell, 1986). Team membership is multiprofessional and consists of social workers, community nurses, clinical psychologists, a consultant psychiatrist and administrative support. Community teams have evolved from working in partnership with individuals and families providing information, advice and counselling services. Increasingly new demands are being placed on them to help in the establishment of new services as well as contributing to current provision.

Operational Implications

The core and cluster model represents a clear break with institutional forms of provision to a flexible, locally based, model of care. This presents a challenge to management and staff who have to adapt to a new philosophy of care changing roles and new methods of working.

The emphasis on a dynamic model of care which encourages increasing independence necessitates flexible staffing patterns as support levels are varied according to individual needs. The contrast for staff used to working to set routines in large institutions will be marked. In the first instance there will be the uncertainty that large scale change brings in its wake, accentuated by the lack of a clear understanding of what community care entails.

Working in a community services environment raises the level of responsibility for staff who will have less immediate access to senior staff, being geographically dispersed compared to the centralised nature of a long-stay hospital. The working environment will also differ, breaking down the hierarchal authority structures which are, in Goffman's terms, a feature of the total institution and staff will need to develop new ways of working with clients. There is also the possibility that staff may feel isolated in cluster units without the support mechanisms that were present in the hospital. Consequently, in places where community provision has been developed effectively, there has been commitment to; developing support structures for staff, regular review meetings, encouragement of team-building and a detailed training package to enable staff make the change from hospital to community.

Training and team-building activities enable anxieties to be expressed and overcome in a positive manner. Staff may be uncertain about the community care model and may be unclear about how residents will spend their day. Team-building activities help staff to be involved in the establishment of the new service. They may also feel resentful that residents are being placed in homes which are more comfortable than their own. It can be detrimental to the service if these types of doubts are allowed to fester unanswered and will be apparent to the people who live in the homes.

The potential isolation of the homes also raises important issues about how quality will be monitored. The normalisation principle assumes that transfer to a community setting will enhance individuals ability to live an ordinary life through developing new skills. Assessment is therefore important to validate the model and maintain an innovative and questioning culture. Monitoring frequently is carried out by outsiders on an irregular basis lending a punitive flavour to the process. Evaluation therefore should involve staff working in the house and be geared to the principles the service was founded upon. Consequently the degree to which residents were unable to make choices about their lifestyle and the development of competences would be an important gauge of the effectiveness of the service.

THE CLOSURE OF MARY DENDY

This case study traces the manner in which Macclesfield Health Authority grappled with the policy of community care to fulfil the Mersey Regional Health Authority's policy of closing the long-stay Mental Handicap Hospital in their district and move to a community based model of care. Mary Dendy Hospital (in Macclesfield Health Authority) planned to close in 1989 making it one of the first long-stay hospitals to completely close. Macclesfield has had to move quickly to reprovide their services. The task has not been an easy one due to the complexity of the task involved, the paucity of information about the development of community care at that time and the short time scale.

The 1982 reorganisation changed the boundaries of Crewe Health Authority. Mary Dendy Hospital which had been managed by Crewe became the responsibility of Macclesfield Health Authority. Prior to 1982 Macclesfield had a limited service for people with learning difficulties. A Community Mental Handicap Team servicing the Macclesfield area of population had been established and was fully operational from the beginning of 1980. This was a modest initiative, based at Moss Lane Hospital with a small membership of a social worker, community nurse and a secretary.

The boundary changes were the initial impetus for change in Macclesfield as not only did Mary Dendy become Macclesfield's responsibility but this change was accompanied by a seemingly more favourable resource situation and individuals committed to change. The previous chapter has documented the changing national agenda with public enquiries and government reports in the 1960s signalling a change to a new philosophy of community care.

Macclesfield Health Authority was aware of these developments and recognised that hospital care was not the most appropriate type of care for many people with learning difficulties. Members of the Mary Dendy Hospital Management Team were influenced by the *Report of the Committee of Enquiry into Mental Handicap Nusing and Care* chaired by Peggy Jay (The Jay Committee, 1979, Vol. 1) which suggested that people with learning difficulties have the right to enjoy normal patterns of life in the community. This philosophy was to significantly influence the model of care proposed in the 1982 strategy.

The District Management Team asked the Mary Dendy Hospital Management Team to prepare a strategy for Mental Handicap Services for the period 1982–91. A number of individuals were involved in preparing the strategy. The Director of Nursing Services had previously been involved in initiatives to develop community care in the West Country and had misgivings about the nature of the service developed which had concentrated exclusively on residential relocation and not sufficiently on the day care and other support service needs of those discharged to the community. He also believed that there needed to be specialised support units for those individuals who could not be or did not wish to be supported in the community.

The Consultant Psychiatrist on the Management Team was also very committed to the development of community care and supported the model of care suggested by the Jay Committee. This gave an impetus to the community care initiative at a period when medical staff in other districts were less sympathetic towards this model of care and were expressing reservations about the move to a community based service. The Unit Administrator on the Management Team supported his colleagues thinking.

The 1982 Strategy

In November 1982 the development plan for the decade 1982–91 was published. Mersey Regional policy was based on advice from the National Development Group and covered four major areas:

(i) The development of community teams

(ii) The development of community units

(iii) The reduction in size of large mental handicap hospitals

(iv) Redevelopment of the mental handicap hospital

The District acknowledged this advice and broadly endorsed the Regional policy as a basis for planning future needs. However, the Management Team was opposed to the development of community units. This was expressed in a July 1982 discussion document which was the precursor to the November strategy:

> It is within this area that we should wish to amend the policy since we feel the use of the term community unit can be misleading, as it is derived from earlier developments in community care. Community units tend to care for larger numbers than is desirable in one living unit, and the units are not always directly located within the community they are to serve, nor do they cater for the immediate community needs.
>
> *Strategic Plan For Mental Handicap Services in Macclesfield Health District.*

Community Teams

The District Strategy endorsed the first element of Regional policy the establishment of Community Mental Handicap Teams. In line with National Development advice they were to serve a catchment area of between 60,000—80,000 population and aimed to enable people with learning difficulties and their families to have the necesssary support and advice to sustain individuals in the Community. Members of the Team would counsel parents enabling them to cope with the initial trauma experienced by the family, the necessary adjustments to be made and their anxieties about the progress of their child.

The Team would also provide advice on day-to-day management which would include: methods to help achievement of developmental and self-help skills such as walking, feeding, dressing, and other advice to enable individuals to fulfil their potential and have a better quality of life. Finally members would help to arrange day care and respite care needs as appropriate. Macclesfield planned to extend their Community Mental Handicap Team network by strengthening the Macclesfield team with the addition of extra community nurses and by providing a service to the Knutsford/Wilmslow area to the north and Congleton to the south. The core membership consisted of a community mental handicap nurse and a social worker supported by the team leader and consultant psychiatrist. The team drew in other specialists as required.

Community Units

The second element in the Regional Strategy envisaged the development of community units of between twenty to twenty-four places, which the District did not support. Consequently a core and cluster model was advocated (outlined in previous section) which would provide a range of ordinary houses (the cluster) for usually three or four people to live in supported by a core unit which acts as a resource centre for the cluster units. The services the core units would provide, included being the central point for referrals and planning individuals need, as well as providing respite and emergency care for those residents in the community. The core units were designed to be flexible to accommodate all eventualities.

The Management Team believed a core and cluster model was preferable to community units primarily because of their commitment to the normalisation philosophy. They believed that people with learning difficulties have the same rights to an ordinary life as other individuals in the community. Consequently accommodation for people with learning difficulties should not be identified as different from other accommodation in the community and needs to be integrated into the community, having access to normal community facilities such as shops, public transport, etc. The houses themselves should contain facilities which the rest of society have grown accustomed to and should respect individuals needs for privacy.

The Management Team also advocated that the service needed to be local, flexible, and comprehensive. There were doubts about the ability of community units to fulfil these criteria. The larger size of these units results in them not always being located within the community they serve nor being fully integrated into the community. The community units built for a specific purpose would be difficult to change their use while ordinary houses if no longer required could simply be sold if not needed. Finally the core and cluster model offered greater flexibility in both the mix of clients possible and the use to which the accommodation could be put. The decision to adopt a core and cluster model and reject the community units model was to generate a tension between the District and the Region which was not easily remedied.

Reducing the Size of Mary Dendy Hospital

The third strand to the Regional Strategy was the reduction in size of large mental handicap hospitals and this complemented the fourth strand—the redevelopment of mental handicap hospital facilities for the core of the minority of people with learning difficulties who would need special support. Macclesfield saw the run-down of Mary Dendy Hospital as a gradual process which would result from the death of elderly residents at the hospital, a more selective admission policy locally and reducing admissions from other District Health Authorities, particularly in the North Western Regional Health Authority which had historically sent clients to Mary Dendy.

This process would be coupled with the development of community provision and the associated discharge of patients. The rationalisation of the Mary Dendy site was to proceed primarily on the basis of the needs of residents but would also take into account the condition of buildings and if expensive maintenance was required. The third criteria was to be the capital return possible. If one site could be easily sold then their might be a need to decant residents to other parts of the Mary Dendy site.

The fourth element of the strategy was the redevelopment of the Mary Dendy Hospital site to provide specialised hospital facilities for the care of people with learning difficulties who suffered from:

(i) the most profound forms of mental handicap
(ii) mental handicap and gross physical and sensory handicaps
(iii) severe behaviour disorders

The Management Team believed that there was a need for specialised provision and that the facilities should be enhanced to avoid those remaining in hospital being viewed as a residuum and not entitled to the same quality of life as individuals who were to live in the community.

The action plan based on the four elements outlined planned the reduction of beds from 350 beds in 1982/83 to 100 beds in 1990/91 (Table 16). It was planned that the strategy would be financed by bridging money from the Regional Health Authority which would be paid back by money released from the estate sales and by the gradual internal development of revenue and capital. The strategy was endorsed by the District Health Authority and was passed to the Regional Health Authority for their comments.

TABLE 16. *Planned Bed Reduction at Mary Dendy Hospital*

Year	*Bed Numbers*	*Year*	*Bed Numbers*
1982/83	350	1987/88	158
1983/84	319	1988/89	140
1984/85	268	1989/90	120
1985/86	237	1990/91	100
1986/87	187		

SOURCE: Macclesfield District Health Authority Development Plan for Mental Handicap Services 1982–91.

The Regional Health Authority Response

The Mersey Regional Health Authority had been examining its policy towards the closure of long-stay hospitals under the auspices of the

Steering Group for the Development of a Regional Policy for Services for the Mentally Ill and Mentally Handicapped. However the impetus to quicken the pace of change came when Mersey's community care strategy was raised at their Ministerial review meeting on 4 August 1983. This was at a time when government policy which advocated a shift to community care and stemming the flow of resources to the acute sector was reaching its zenith.

On 31 August 1983 Mr John Patten the Health Minister wrote to the Mersey Regional Chairman, Mr Donald Wilson, outlining the Region's task following their annual review:

> You felt that you were now in a better position to manage the rundown of large institutions now that you have completed full physical and environment surveys. On the subject of rundown, whilst I appreciate that the closure of whole hospitals is not an end in itself but the result of providing more appropriate services in other settings, targets for closure can help to provide a stimulus to other developments . . . you agreed to consider whether any faster progress could be made in this area.

Consequently the Regional Health Authority began to examine the possibility of closing a long-stay Mental Handicap Hospital in the Region in the near future.

There seemed to have been a number of factors that brought Mary Dendy Hospital to the attention of the Region as a candidate for closure. First Macclesfield had already started planning for the closure of Mary Dendy and in this process revealed a high level of commitment to the philosophy of community care and had prepared an action plan to close Mary Dendy.

Second, Mary Dendy's situation in the heart of the affluent Manchester commuter belt of Knutsford/Wilmslow and its division into four separate sites, each site comprising between twelve to forty-seven acres of land, made it a very marketable and valuable asset for the Regional Health Authority. The area is notable for its high quality housing which serves the multinational companies and professional firms located in Manchester and the southern suburbs of Altrincham, Sale, Wilmslow and Stockport. The four sites which could be disposed of separately, gave the Regional Health Authority greater flexibility and more security about its ability to dispose of the site than a single site hospital would have done.

Third, the level of dependency of the residents of Mary Dendy was by national standards relatively low. This had been revealed by the Hospital Census of 1980/81 of all long-stay hospitals using National Development Team categories and was endorsed by a visit from the National Development Group in 1980/81 which made recommendations on the Cheshire Area Health Authority which highlighted the potential for change at Mary Dendy. The higher levels of ability amongst Mary Dendy's residents can be accounted for by; the hospital's function as an annexe to Cranage Hospital which took individuals of higher dependence, and the historical legacy of Mary Dendy which had originally been a school run by one of the leading figures in the Eugenics movement. Consequently Mary Dendy had admitted 'moral defectives' who were only mildly mentally handicapped. Additional factors included that Mary Dendy is relatively small compared to some of the other mental handicap hospitals in the Region and there were no vociferous lobby groups of parents who might oppose the closure. This had been a factor in the neighbouring District of Crewe, focused on the organisation Rescare.

Consequently in August and September 1983 at meetings of the Regional Mental Illness and Mental Handicap Review Group the Regional Nursing Officer began to explore with Macclesfield District Health Authority the possibility of earlier closure of Mary Dendy Hospital excluding Soss Moss Hospital. It was agreed that no upgrading work should be carried out on wards which were expected to close in under two years. This alerted Macclesfield to the possibility of closure before 1991, but at this stage the Mersey Regional Health Authority had not given Macclesfield clear intentions about closure before 1991.

At the Mersey Regional Health Authority meeting of October 1983 it was agreed a Joint Working Party with Macclesfield District Health Authority should be established to identify the necessary pre-requisites to closure, to suggest alternative solutions and to decide on a strategy. The Regional Health Authority acknowledged Ministerial pressure to close Mary Dendy prior to 1991 siting their belief that this would help the development of community care by setting an example to other districts which would act as a catalyst for change. The proposal was endorsed and it was agreed that the idea of a joint review should be broached with Macclesfield at their annual review meeting with the Region on 17 October 1983.

At the district review meeting the Regional Administrator stressed the need to speed up the closure of Mary Dendy and the necessity of establishing a joint working party with Macclesfield to include social services representatives as necessary. The Regional Administrator reiterated the urgency of the task with a report required in six months time so that the Region had time to consider its response before the 1984 ministerial review. Macclesfield management had serious reservations about a quicker closure of the hospital.

First, the plans outlined in the strategy were advocating a model of care which was more radical than the community unit model which was the accepted model of care at that time, consequently the magnitude of the change planned both philosophically and physically made Macclesfield's managers wary of moving too quickly and jeopardising their ability to carry their staff with them. This feeling was heightened by the knowledge that Mary Dendy Hospital had not been immune from the spate of inquiries into allegations of insensitive treatment of residents in long-stay hospitals in the 1960s and 1970s.

A further concern was the major financial implications of a compressed closure programme. The District anticipated that this would increase the need for bridging finance as provision would have to be identified before capital and revenue could be released from the rundown of Mary Dendy. In order to address these issues and the feasibility of earlier closure of Mary Dendy, Macclesfield agreed to the Region's suggestion that a working party should be established.

The Mary Dendy Hospital Working Party

At the Regional Health Authority meeting in October 1983 the Regional Administrator had proposed that four regional officers should sit on the Working Party. They included the Regional Nursing Officer, the Regional Service Planning Officer, the Senior Assistant Regional Treasurer and a Specialist in Community Medicine. In Macclesfield there was uncertainty about who should be represented on the Working Party. The District Administrator was pressurised by the Regional Administrator to keep the membership of the Working Party small in order to make rapid progress. For example, on 2 December 1983 the Regional Administrator had written to the District Administrator vetoing an increase in the membership of the Macclesfield District Health Authority Working Party.

However the Mary Dendy Unit Management Team all wished to participate in the Working Party as they had drawn up the strategy. This request was granted and helped to reassure the Unit Management Team that the Working Party would not be biased too greatly to Regional and District needs. Social services representation on the Working Party constituted the District Officer for Social Services (Macclesfield) and the District Officer for Social Services (Congelton).

The first meeting of the Working Party was convened on 12 December 1983 and the formal terms of reference were agreed as follows:

> In the light of the ministerial review tasks and district review meeting
>
> (i) To identify the necessary prerequisites to the closure of Mary Dendy Hospital.

(ii) To identify alternative solutions together with their financial and other costs with a view to accelerating the transfer of services from the hospital.

(iii) To prepare a recommended strategy (for the Regional/District review meeting in April/May 1984).

(iv) That Soss Moss would continue as a long-term facility within the District, as part of the overall pattern of service.

The Working Party met approximately monthly and discussions were dominated by a number of issues.

The strategy document that Macclesfield had prepared in 1982 had amended Regional policy by not endorsing the concept of community units. This difference in perspective was to surface forcibly in the Working Party meetings. The Regional officers were proposing a model of care based on developments in Wessex Regional Health Authority which at the time involved the establishment of twenty to twenty-four community units as the alternative provision to the closure of long-stay hospitals.

A group of Regional officers had visited Wessex Regional Health Authority in the previous year and spent a couple of days being shown their service. It was clear to these officers that the Wessex model of twenty to twenty-four place units were significantly cheaper than a group home accommodating four to six residents. However they had reservations about the size of the units and felt that twelve to sixteen place unit might be a better size to create a community environment.

Regional officers believed that within the financial constraints they faced it would be better to plan for a model of care which could be provided comprehensively for all those in need than to plan a service based on four to six place homes which would be very expensive and risked not being completed. This would leave a situation where service provision would be patchy, with excellent provision in some areas matched by a paucity of services in other areas.

Macclesfield's managers were opposed to the Wessex model of care and reiterated the arguments they had outlined in the 1982 strategy. They regarded the community units of twenty to twenty-four places as being too large. The Region was prepared to reduce the size of the units to twelve to sixteen places, but this failed to placate Macclesfield as their critique was broader than solely a concern for the number of residents in each unit. They felt that the concept of community units possibly based in vacant NHS accommodation did not embody the philosophy of an ordinary life which underpinned their strategy. Macclesfield argued that the Region's proposals were little advance on the existing provision at Mary Dendy because the site was already split into separate units. Consequently if twenty to twenty-four bed community units were going to be provided this was already available in a nascent form on the Mary Dendy site and therefore no changes were needed.

The discussions on philosophy underpinned the deliberations of the Working Party and were bound up with the financing of the project. Macclesfield Health Authority were concerned that the Region should not view community care as a cheap option. Conversely the Region had a suspicion that as the closure of Mary Dendy was a pilot project to be funded centrally by the Region, the District would try and maximise the resources they obtained from the Region.

The differences in philosophy were resolved by the Region ceding to the Districts proposed model of care. The Region's prime concern was to fulfil the Minsterial deadline on the closure of Mary Dendy and this could not be achieved without the full cooperation of Macclesfield Health Authority. Furthermore the Region's advocacy of the Wessex model was based on pragmatic considerations of cost and knowledge of existing services elsewhere rather than a model grounded in particular principles. Therefore the Region was more ready to compromise than Macclesfield Health Authority and the core and cluster model was adopted as the basis for planning the new provision.

Social Services Perspectives

Social service representatives were more sympathetic to the position being endorsed by Macclesfield Health Authority than Mersey Regional Health Authority. Nonetheless although Congelton and Macclesfield Social Services are accountable to Cheshire County Council the District officers had sufficient autonomy to enable different approaches to emerge. Congelton Social Services had carried out a review of its Mental Handicap Strategy published as the Lifetime Report which endorsed a similar model of care to the core and cluster philosophy. Consequently Congelton Social Services were supportive of the Macclesfield Health Authority approach. Macclesfield Social Services were less committed to a particular model of care and accepted funding for community unit style provision with the proviso that adaptations were made to enable the hostels to provide a community style environment.

Social services representatives recognised the magnitude of the change being proposed. Services for people with learning difficulties had been the responsibility of the NHS and community initiatives had been ad hoc and uncoordinated. The closure of a long-stay hospital like Mary Dendy was an implicit acknowledgement that a mental handicap was not an illness and therefore not an NHS responsibility. It followed that providing services for people with learning difficulties was a social responsibility for the local authority and this in turn raised the question of future funding and organisational arrangements.

Cheshire Social Services were not prepared to adopt new responsibilities at the expense of existing services. Consequently Cheshire were anxious that the community care initiatives allowed new funding to be made available to them to match their new responsibilities. They were unwilling to enter into arrangements that attached a sum of money to each patient leaving hospital. This is intended to help local authorities fund new developments. However this type of dowry system is geared to providing services for individuals leaving long-stay hospitals rather than providing a comprehensive service for the community.

Social services regarded dowry systems as flawed for four reasons. First the level of dowries set at between £12–£16,000 is used by health authorities as an encouragement to social services to provide services for individuals leaving hospital, but does not reflect the true costs of providing those services. Second, dowries only cover individuals leaving hospital but ignore the needs of those already in the community. Third, dowries are unable to accommodate the costs of keeping individuals in the community who would formerly have entered long-stay hospitals. Social services therefore insisted that funding was provided for services for the whole community in perpetuity.

Finally social services were not prepared to provide services at the levels of expenditure which prevailed in the NHS. They regarded health authority services for people with learning difficulties as seriously underfunded and were not prepared to emulate this level of funding in providing new services. The funding arrangements agreed between Mersey Regional Health Authority and Cheshire County Council was contained in a legal document known as the Heads of Agreement.

The Assessment Process

At the first meeting of the Mary Dendy Hospital Working Party it had been agreed to establish a number of working groups to examine various topics which included evaluation of the existing building fabric at Mary Dendy, staff training needs, and the preparation of patient profiles. The Regional Administrator continued to cajole the District Administrator to enable the process to be completed by the Regional/District Review in May 1984 and increasingly stressed the need to complete the joint assessments of patients. On 23 February 1984 the Regional Administrator wrote to the District Administrator expressing concern that at the previous Working Party meeting 'not as much information was available as had been hoped' and requested that eighty of the assessments be available at the next meeting on 5 March. The Regional Administrator reiterated that 'a steady momentum must be maintained'.

The patient profiles were the central process used to establish the needs of individual clients and provided the information to plan the types of provision required. It was envisaged as a planning exercise which would establish the type of services needed rather than as an assessment process designed to specify each individuals total needs. The Director of Nursing Services was charged with convening this group with assistance from the Consultant Psychiatrist and a Social Services representative. Although assessments of patients had taken place before, notably in the 1983 Census of Mental Handicap patients this assessment had not been carried out jointly with Social Services nor had the previous assessments been drawn up with a view to provide proposals for placements in the community.

An assessment panel was convened which included the nursing officer, pre-discharge Sister from Mary Dendy Hospital, Consultant Psychiatrist, Clinical Psychologist and Social Work representatives from the Social Services. The panel had four to five months to carry out 274 assessments leaving approximately thirty patients unassessed as these patients were regarded as having meaningful links with Authorities outside the Macclesfield catchment area.

There was considerable reluctance by clinical staff to become involved in the assessment process as they felt that the short time available was insufficient to assess clients needs adequately. It was unacceptable to decide individuals futures on the basis of a rough assessment process. The Nursing Officer who chaired the assessment panel argued that the assessments were only to be used as a guide to the range of facilities required and that individual placements would be decided in more detail at a later stage. He emphasised that if the assessment panel failed to carry out their task the strategy would be drawn up without the clinical input the assessment could provide.

The first task of the assessment panel was to decide the assessment process to be used. Due to the time-scale involved the panel used the National Development Team categories to assess patients as this system was quick, efficient and easy to use. This system was a modification of the Wessex Social and Physical Incapacity/Speech, Self Help and Literacy Scale (SPI/SSL) (Table 17). The assessment panel used the existing data from the 1983 Hospital Census and discussed residents abilities with their current carers. In this manner 274 residents were assessed into four groups.

Members of the assessment panel expressed reservations about the manner in which the assessments were carried out. There were potential advantages in using the assessment for planning purposes rather than as a blueprint for individual placements because the latter process causes difficulties. As needs change fairly rapidly the individual placements

TABLE 17. *Details of Mental Handicap Assessment Form Specification used in the Grouping of Patients*

The Development Team classifies people with learning difficulties in long-term care over the age of five into one of four main groups to indicate the degree of handicap, and the type of care required.

GROUP I

Criteria: Competent in all areas of self-help, ambulant, continent, no behaviour problems, not disruptive in any way.

Opinion: Could be discharged home or to hostel immediately without any special facilities necessary for management, apart from those normally provided in a local authority hostel. Some may be appropriately placed in group homes.

GROUP II

Criteria: Continent, ambulant, almost completely self-sufficient with mild problems of behaviour which could be corrected with a short period of treatment and self-help training. A number could be considered for self-care training units.

Opinion: Should be suitable immediately for discharge home or to a hostel, where, after a short period of pre-discharge training they would be suitable for discharge to a group home or other form of independent living in the community.

GROUP III

Criteria: Continent with lapses at night. Some are mildly over-active with occasional mild behaviour problems. All are said to be easily managed and would benefit from specific training. If discharged to a hostel, staff ratios would need to be higher than for those in Groups I and II.

Opinion: Considered suitable for care in the community after intensive training, and with greater supervision than is usually required by those in Groups I and II.

GROUP IV

Criteria: Severe double incontinence, multiple physical handicaps, severe epilepsy, extreme hyperkinetic behaviour, aggression to self and others.

Opinion: The majority require some form of long-term residential care with a higher staff ratio than is required by those in Groups I, II and III.

SOURCE: National Development Team for Mentally Handicapped People, *4th Report* 1981–4.

will need to change and consequently the system degenerates into a constant assessment and reassessment process without any action resulting. Using the assessments as a rough planning guide should have prevented these types of difficulties because if seventy residents were classified as Group 1 even though some assessments would change there would be sufficient flexibility to allow individuals to be placed in the appropriate accommodation. This process would be facilitated because a resident's need would be decided immediately prior to entering the community and not at the planning stage.

Members of the assessment panel having been reassured that the assessments were only for rough planning purposes believed individual placements would be decided at a later date. Although this was the intention and a clinical subgroup was established for this purpose the effectiveness of this group was premised on the assumption that the initial assessments had been reasonably accurate. This proved to be unfounded. The assessment panel members had not worked together as a group before and it took time to establish a consensus on the way in which the assessment criteria were to be used and the priority to be given to certain attributes. There were few members of the assessment panel who knew the residents well and this increased the panels dependence on ward staff to complete the assessments.

This had a number of implications. First, staff who helped with the process may not have been very clear about the purpose of the assessments and may not have filled in the forms very carefully. Second, by drawing on a wide range of staff without a benchmark to check the assessment against there was more likelihood of inaccuracies and differing criteria entering the assessments undetected. Third, in some services poor staffing levels could affect the ability of residents to fulfil the criteria. For example, continence is a key criteria in the assessment yet if staff levels are low and staff become disinterested, staff may allow residents to become incontinent and remain soiled by failing to encourage residents to go to the toilet. Consequently the environment itself influences the assessments and the assessments may end up assessing the environment as much as the residents. Finally the staff also became anxious about the assessment process as it was a clear indication that change was being envisaged. The process contributed to the organisational turbulence and may have encouraged staff to assess patients in a manner which safeguarded their own futures. The vagueness of the categories would have made this type of response easier.

Despite these potential difficulties the panel continued to proceed with the assessments and by mid-1984 all the assessments had been completed. The nature of provision planned for residents reflected the results of the assessments.

Criteria for Different Types of Accommodation

The different types of accommodation planned represented a spectrum of care with staffed hostels and elderly persons homes having a high staff ratio in contrast to ordinary elderly persons homes, staffed group homes and dependent living at the other end of the spectrum. A wide range of factors were used in planning individual placements and the criteria used are summarised below:

---

1. Staffed hostels

Some or all of the following likely to apply:

- limited self-help skills
- no experience of cooking
- unable to handle or budget money
- unable to go out into the community unaccompanied
- limited communication skills
- physical or behavioural problems requiring twenty-four hour staffing
- considerable institutionalisation

This group needed twenty-four hour waking staff.

2. Staffed group homes

Some or all of the following likely to apply:

- some self-help skills and potential to further develop self-help and domestic skills
- able to handle and understand at least small amounts of money
- able to go out into community unaccompanied
- reasonable communication skills
- likely to benefit from training

This group needed twenty-four hour staffing but for some individuals sleeping-in staff would be adequate.

3. Unstaffed group homes

Some or all of the following likely to apply:

- able to cook for self without supervision
- able to dress appropriately and attend to own personal hygiene
- able to understand money and budget it unaided or with limited supervision
- no behavioural problems
- able to use community facilities
- good communication skills

Individuals in this group needed some regular daily supervision.

4. Staffed bedsits

These represented the borderline area between staffed and unstaffed group homes and individuals in them reflected this having reasonable self-care skills but still needing regular supervision.

5. Ordinary elderly persons homes

Met the usual criteria for elderly persons homes except a little more active than usual in elderly persons homes.

6. Elderly persons homes with high staff ratio

Met criteria for ordinary elderly persons homes, except presented physical or behavioural problems which made them unacceptable in an ordinary elderly persons home.

7. Small elderly persons homes

Met criteria for ordinary elderly persons homes but felt would benefit from the greater independence and intimacy of smaller elderly persons homes.

8. Staffed group home for elderly

Met criteria for staffed group homes, as above.

SOURCE: Criteria for Different Types of Accommodation: Macclesfield Health Authority, July 1984.

The patient assessments were matched with the accommodation required leading to recommendations for 274 placements (which excluded the patients thought to have meaningful links).

The Working Party Report

The core task of the Working Party had been the patient assessments and the matching of these assessments to provision. Consequently the completion of the assessments led to the publication of the feasibility study and enabled the deadline to be met. Members of the Working Party viewed the report as a broad statement of intent rather than a blueprint for the future. They believed that further work would be necessary on financial estimates.

The bulk of the report concerned the type of provision necessary and recommended placements (Table 18). The Working Party believed that ninety-three patients needed to remain in hospital accommodation which although a high figure was attributed to the elderly nature of the Mary Dendy population. It was proposed that future hospital provision should be based at Soss Moss Hospital which was part of Mary Dendy but this would require substantial capital investment. The Working Party embraced the core and cluster model of care advocated by Macclesfield but in considering the feasibility of closing Mary Dendy Hospital within five years identified a number of potential difficulties. First, the long lead times in converting or building properties.

Second, the capital costs involved which due to the compression of the scheme would be greatly increased. Third, a consequence of the greater capital costs would be increased revenue expenditure in addition to the double running costs which community care schemes spawn. Fourth, the acquisition of properties themselves could prove difficult

TABLE 18. *Placements Recommended for Mary Dendy Residents*

Placements Recommended	Groups 1	2	3	4	Total All Groups	
Hospital Accommodation Necessary	6	24	27	36	93	
Core and Cluster: 24 hr staff	4	28	10	8	50	62
Core and Cluster: staff am, pm, w/e	6	4	0	0	10	
Core and Cluster: staff am, pm, 7 days	1	0	0	0	1	
Core and Cluster: Staff evenings	1	0	0	0	1	
Group Homes for the Elderly (24 hr staff)	5	0	1	0	6	
Group Homes for the Physically handicapped (24 hr staff)	1	1	0	0	2	
Elderly Persons Homes: ordinary	10	7	5	1	23	44
Elderly Persons Homes: small	4	2	0	0	6	
Elderly Persons Homes: High Staff Ratio	9	1	2	3	15	
Fully Staffed Residential Centres	15	14	21	11	61	
Warden Supervised Accommodation	2	0	0	0	2	
Staffed Hostel for Mentally Ill	1	0	0	0	1	
Independent Living	3	0	0	0	3	
Total placements recommended	68	81	66	59	274	

SOURCE: Joint Working Party Report, July 1984

due to local opposition to Health Authority plans and the lengthy procedures followed for the acquisition of property in the NHS. The report concluded that if adequate resources were made available the closure of Mary Dendy Hospital was possible within three to four years. However this would be dependent on considerable capital investment and commitment from all the agencies involved. The required action plan envisaged:

(i) A full option appraisal of suggested schemes for the provision within three years of suitable hospital accommodation for the remaining ninety-three residents with a view to upgrading Soss Moss Hospital.

(ii) The sale of Mary Dendy Hospital to release capital and revenue resources, using the planning and expertise of the estate agents to gain maximum values.

(iii) The acquisition of several large units of property to provide day care and work experience units at a capital cost of between £46,000 and £1,600,000.

(iv) The provision of sufficient revenue resources from transferred or new funds to run all day units.

(v) The acquisition of fifteen to twenty units within three years for core and cluster accommodation for sixty-two patients in local neighbourhoods.

(vi) The acquisition of group homes within three years at a cost of £1,125,000 for sixty-one elderly patients together with the necessary revenue provision.

(vii) The introduction of a major staff training programme to cope with the change and different approach to care.

(viii) A study into a coordinated approach to the role of housing corporations in providing some accommodation.

(ix) The establishment of a Steering Group drawn from health and social services to implement the action plan.

The Report was accepted by Mersey Regional Health Authority with certain minor comments concerning the financial costs of the strategy. As a result the Mary Dendy Hospital Working Party's role was downgraded and the emphasis increasingly shifted to District level and the forums established to implement the strategy.

Implementing the Strategy

The multi-disciplinary nature of those involved in the closure of Mary Dendy required the establishment of several specific groups drawn from health and social services to enable closure to proceed smoothly and for alternative provision to be established. The Mary Dendy Hospital Working Party had been established specifically to examine the feasibility of earlier closure. It had completed this task and consequently became largely redundant as the initial planning stage was complete. The Working Party lumbered on until May 1986 due to the desire of the Region to monitor closely developments in Macclesfield. However the Working Party was increasingly usurped by the Implementation Group.

The Implementation Group emerged out of the Working Party and consisted of senior officers predominantly from Macclesfield Health Authority although there were officers from the Regional Health Authority and social services. The group was given overall responsibility for the implementation of the community care strategy. They were responsible for keeping within the financial target established. This had been delegated to the group by the Regional Health Authority and they approved all developments and monitored progress. The Implementation Group met monthly and was for some time chaired by the Administrator, other members of the Unit Management Team were also represented including; The Director of Nursing Services and the Consultant Psychiatrist. The Implementation Group did not involve itself with the minutiae of implementation but confined itself to a strategic role.

The Steering Group was established to take on the operational tasks delegated by the Implementation Group. It was established in September 1984 to look initially at commissioning cluster accommodation in Wilmslow and thereafter other such developments. There was some duplication in membership between the two groups as the three members of the Unit Management Team were on the Steering Committee, chaired by the Unit Administrator initially. However the other members were individuals specifically concerned with aspects of commissioning and discharge from the hospital. This included a Works Officer, Clinical Psychologist, Social Worker and a Community Nursing Officer.

The Steering Group prepared the properties for residents. It examined properties and ensured any necessary adaptations were made as well as choosing the necessary equipment for the houses. This was to meet DHSS requirements on fire regulations and floor space but in a manner that was in keeping with the normalisation philosophy. The Steering Group discussed staffing levels for the houses and arranged other community services which included day care and GP support. Finally specific issues such as the need for a public relations initiative or requirements for voluntary support were raised.

The final group established was known as the Sub-Group which was a purely clinical group. Its initiation was stimulated by the knowledge that the assessment process was only a rough planning guide and to establish individuals placements would require detailed discussions of individual cases. Consequently the Sub-Group was responsible for identifying residents for all health and social services developments. This was on the basis of criteria from the Steering Group which helped the Sub-Group to select possible clients. The Sub-Group's membership consisted of the Community Nursing Officer, Consultant Psychiatrist, Clinical Psychologist, Director of Nursing Services and the leader of the Community Mental Handicap Team.

Identifying Groups of Houses

The process of identifying residents for houses ran into difficulties during 1985. A problem existed that the movement of residents into the community by the Sub-Group did not correlate with the joint assessment results on which most of the plans had been based. The greatest concern came from social services who were worried that more dependent individuals were being sent to social services elderly persons homes than originally envisaged. This had clear implications for social services in terms of higher staffing levels, etc. There was some suspicion that Macclesfield District was trying to place responsibility for a number of more dependent residents on social services.

The reality was that the mismatch was likely given the nature of the initial assessments as a rough guide. The difficulty was that the initial assessments were converted into a planning blueprint but this action did not have the support of the Sub-Group members who wished to place residents on a more comprehensive set of criteria than had been possible during the initial assessments which had been geared to meeting the Region's deadline. For example, the Sub-Group members many of whom had been on the assessment panel took account of friendship between individuals in deciding placements which may have overridden a crude categorisation into a particular National Development Team category.

This hiatus led to a special meeting between health and social services managers in June 1985 and the procedure for identifying residents for developments, which had been largely left to the Sub-Group, was changed. The Sub-Group was to be given more information from the Steering Group on which to base its initial selection of clients. This information included:

(a) location of the development
(b) size and room distribution
(c) advice on aids and adaptations
(d) projected staffing levels
(e) special criteria

These criteria were to be matched to the joint assessment information and in this manner a list of names would be selected. The Sub-Group had to highlight any discrepancies from the joint assessment information to the Steering Group.

This adjustment to the identification of groups still led to variations from the original assessments which created friction with Social Services. The Implementation Group decided in July 1986 to undertake a full-scale review of the assessments carried out in 1984. This was termed the Mid-Term Review.

The Mid-Term Review

The immediate stimulus for the Review were the difficulties with the elderly persons homes placements. The criteria for admission and philosophy in local authority elderly persons homes did not match the needs of the Mary Dendy residents. They tended to be very active for their age whereas elderly persons homes clients were less active and required less in terms of day activities. This led to some clients being returned to hospital and others refusing to move to community places because they feared not gaining from the experience.

This was not the sole reason, for the Mid-Term Review. Individuals had begun to be discharged and this was providing valuable information on how residents were coping in the community which could be used to make future assessments more accurate. It was also half way into the project and therefore an appropriate time to take stock of developments. The assessment panel was also eager to use a different assessment method.

The Implementation Group established the Mid-Term Review Group in July 1986. The Group consisted of a clinical psychologist, community nursing officer, social worker and project officer from the Social Services. They used the STAR (Social Training Achievement Record) profile assessment system instead of National Development Team categories. The STAR profile scoring sheet is designed as a criterion-based record of social competence and is called STAR because of the resemblance of the summary sheet to a star (Appendix 1).

This system was considered superior to the use of National Development Team categories for three reasons. First, the system had a higher degree of objectivity due to its concentration on specific measurable skills, for example, the ablity to wash and dry dishes. Second, STAR had previously been used in a clinical setting and therefore a benchmark was available against which to check the outcomes of the assessments. Finally the system was easily understood.

The Review Group carried out their task in a different manner from the original assessments. The Group worked as two separate sub-groups during each session to enable a final recommendation to be made. The Clinical Psychologist and the Social Services projects officer spoke to ward staff and completed the STAR profile. The Community Nursing Officer and the Social Worker found out other information on residents by looking at records and speaking to staff involved in clients day time activities. The Social Services Day Services Officer participated in this process by gathering background information about day activities when available. The Group took note of other appropriate factors, for example, the ward environment and its effect on individual development. Friendships with other residents and the expressed wishes of residents were also taken into account in preparing supporting notes for the profiles.

The assessments of 206 residents were carried out during the period August 1986 to November 1986 and ninety-three recommendations (45 per cent of the total) at the Mid-Term Review were different from those in the joint Assessments. Of these ninety-three, fifty-one (55 per cent) were 'increased' recommendations at the Mid-Term Review (i.e. individuals were recommended for a more independent type of living than previously). The detailed changes are summarised below (Table 19).

TABLE 19. *Changed Recommendations Resulting from the Mid-Term Review.*

	Number	*Percentage*
Increased Recommendations		
Remain in Hospital: Staffed Hostel	25	49
Elderly Persons Home: Staffed Hostel	1	2
Staffed Hostel: Staffed Group Home	12	24
Elderly Persons Homes: Staffed Group Home	5	10
Remain in Hospital: Staffed Group Home	5	10
Hostel: Mentally Ill: Staffed Group Home	1	2
Staffed Group Home: Independent Living	1	2
Remain in Hospital: Therapeutic Unit	1	2
	51	
Reduced Recommendations		
Staffed Group Home: Staffed Hostel	14	33
Independent Living: Staffed Hostel	1	2
Staffed Hostel: Remain in Hospital	10	24
Staffed Group Home: Remain in Hospital	7	17
Eldely Person Home: Remain in Hospital	9	21
Behavioural Unit: Remain in Hospital	1	2
	42	

SOURCE: Final Report of Mid-Term Review Group, Macclesfield District Health Authority, 1986.

The Review Group cited three main reasons for the changes, from the original joint assessments. First, changes in residents themselves particularly physical deterioration which featured as a significant factor in the reduced recommendations. Second, when the original assessments were carried out there were no specific resource assumptions. The Mid-Term Review Group knew the services were being developed which made it easier to match individuals to resources available. Finally, the joint assessments made a number of inconclusive recommendations where there were some doubts about individuals suitability or the availability of resources. The Review Group were able to resolve these uncertainties with more precise recommendations. The main implication of the changed recommendations was the need for twenty-six more residential unit places than had been planned. In addition to this, eight staffed group home places were specifically needed for physically handicapped people. The reduced need for places in elderly persons homes led to no new placements for this type of accommodation being made.

The Mid-Term Review therefore took stock of how well implementation was proceeding and gathered information which was of assistance in planning and in determining the exact type of cluster homes which were to match residents needs. The information was also useful in the detailed planning of the day centres. The review had confirmed the centrality of the assessment process to the implementation of the community care strategy. The accuracy of some of the first joint assessments had not been sufficient for detailed planning of placements and in addition to this residents needs had changed exacerbating the difficulties of planning correctly. The Mid-Term Review Group had been able to make adjustments to the planning process at a stage when adjustments could still be made and this was an important aspect in the strategy succeeding.

The Review Group had faced a difficult task in completing the assessments. The wards were given up to a month's notice of the reviews and asked to arrange for staff that knew the residents well to be available. Despite this, the Review Team found wards often unprepared for the Team's visits and some staff were unhelpful about having their staff interiewed by the Review Group. The problems, the Review Team felt, were a manifestation of the opposition some staff felt towards the care in the community plans. This was a central challenge for management because the success of plans for discharging residents largely depended on the cooperation and commitment of staff.

The Staff Response

The core and cluster model envisaged by Macclesfield Health Authority represented a clear break with institutional forms of provision to a flexible locally based model of care. This involved fundamental changes in the way services were delivered and staffed. The Director of Nursing Services explained the changing situation in the following terms:

> As with all new conceptual and practical developments it is inevitable that numerous changes will take place. In this situation the fundamental principles of recognising individual needs and matching the provision of services to meet those identified needs are paramount and will require changes in the delivery of service. Current working practices, patterns of duty and attitudes towards care have evolved over a number of years to meet the needs of a custodial and institutional environment. The future care pattern is based on the needs of individuals and recognising individual rights. This will require us to adjust our working practices in a way that best meets the individual needs of the mentally handicapped population.

It was clear that there was considerable anxiety about the closure of Mary Dendy and potential for opposition to the Authority's plan. Management made two early decisions which helped to engender support for their proposals. First the Authority gave a promise that there would be no compulsory redundancies. This was given after a manpower planning exercise revealed that staffing levels of direct care staff would remain broadly unchanged.

The nursing establishment was 193·81 WTE at Mary Dendy Hospital and the community care proposals envisaged a total requirement of 185·66 WTE, although there was a marked reduction in the number of state enrolled nurses required, (Appendix 2). The situation was more problematic for ancillary staff. The nature of the change of philosophy and the flexibility inherent in community developments meant that large numbers of support staff were not required. A reduction from 47·48 WTE to 8·40 WTE was planned. The majority of this reduction being composed of domestic and catering staff. The mandatory introduction of competitive tendering which the community unit tried to have deferred, prevented the no compulsory redundancy strategy being achieved in this particular instance. However, apart from this exception the commitment was adhered to and this proved to be important in eroding opposition to the community care strategy.

The second decision was to involve staff as early as possible concerning the future shape of the service and to be open about the strategy being proposed. A series of meetings were held with staff side representatives in early 1985 and a guarantee given that there would be no compulsory redundancies providing staff were flexible in terms of where they would be moved in the future. Furthermore no staff would have to move to social services provision. Macclesfield management were beginning to meet not only with COHSE, NUPE, and the RCN who represented staff at Mary Dendy but also representatives of social services management and staff organisations which included NUPE and NALGO.

A central set of issues concerned the case of transfer by Health Authority staff to social services terms and conditions of employment and the impact of such change for both agencies.

Discussions between the agencies in mid-1985 revealed large areas of common ground in relation to conditions of service. For salaried staff the availability of jobs in the Health Service was stable. Posts available in the social services were primarily managerial and offered attractive terms and conditions of service. For manual staff pay and conditions were comparable with local authority conditions offering marginally better enhancements. Consequently transfer to local authority employment was not a contentious issue as conditions were favourable.

Recognition of service presented difficulties as Health Authority length of service was not recognised by local authority employees in consideration of leave or maternity leave. The implication was that staff transferring were faced with a fairly significant reduction in their leave entitlement and were also disadvantaged in respect of maternity leave based on qualifying service. It proved impossible to resolve this issue as it impinged on national agreements and employment law.

The third issue initially appeared the most intractable but was satisfactorily resolved. It concerned the transfer of superannuation payments. There were different retirement ages which affected the rate at which service was counted, but by changing the rate at which service was counted, pension entitlements were not affected by the transfer of employment. Finally nursing staff were anxious about recognition of their qualifications in social services provision. Although this stimulated attempts to bring about a joint qualification which did not come to fruition, the likely increase in pay on transfer reassured nursing staff. Macclesfield management also succeeded in getting agreement that Health Authority applicants for social services posts would be treated as internal applications by social services. There was uneasiness from NALGO which represented social services staff about the potential increase in competition for posts but their agreement was given. This was a major achievement for Macclesfield's management and gave a fillip to Health Authority staff.

Internally management were seeking adjustments to working practices. The philosophy of community care with the emphasis on treating people with learning difficulties as individuals and continuity of care sought to break the compartmentalisation of care prevalent in long-stay institutions. This specifically involved a shift away from the idea of having separate night staff. Managers wanted shifts to be of a rotational nature to enable staff to be fully involved both in the development and execution of individual care plans. It was hoped this would foster an awareness of the total needs of the individuals and enable residents to meet their full potential.

There was considerable opposition to the abolition of the long day (which ran from 7 am to 7 pm) and the proposal to abolish the separate night shift. There were a lot of women who worked this shift to link with their husbands shifts and they were vociferous in their opposition to change. This opposition had a resonance with deeper anxieties about the closure of Mary Dendy, which concerned the shift from a predictable job in a known environment to the uncertainty of new surroundings and a changed philosophy of care. Management sought to facilitate change in a number of ways. The assurances on job security have already been mentioned. This was part of a major effort to involve and inform staff of what exactly was happening. Management were generally not prescriptive about the changes required and did not have a blueprint for working arrangements in the houses. Management harnessed the considerable level of staff support particularly amongst the younger staff.

A team building approach was adopted to establish new working patterns. Initially the Director of Nursing Services had intended to allow suitable patterns to develop. However at a meeting with staff organisations in March 1986 fears were expressed that this was creating too much uncertainty for staff. Consequently in May 1986 broad criteria for working patterns were suggested which built on answers staff had given on previous training courses. The key parameters are summarised in Table 20.

TABLE 20. *Working Patterns for Staff Employed by Macclesfield Health Authority in Establishments Providing Care in Community Settings*

Criteria	*Hours*
Working Day	No staff would be required to work in excess of $8\frac{1}{2}$ hours in any one period of duty.
Working Week	75 hours per fortnight with a maximum of 8 consecutive working days.
Meal Breaks	$\frac{1}{2}$ hour per working shift.
Night Duty	All staff to be available for at least 8 weeks during the course of a year.
'Sleep in' Duties	A maximum of one shift per week.
Core Time	To be identified by the individual manager.
Split Shift	Abolished.

SOURCE: Macclesfield Health Authority, Mental Handicap Unit, July 1986.

The guidelines enabled senior staff to take away staff on team building exercises and to formulate, in conjunction with staff, the most appropriate working patterns for the new service. This had a major impact on enabling change to be brought about as staff felt they were having an impact shaping the new service. It also enabled COHSE who represented many of the staff at Mary Dendy to accept the changes as they were following the lead of sections of their membership.

Management tried to win over reluctant staff by taking them to the new developments and giving them a chance to work there for a couple of weeks to ease their anxieties. The transition was eased by the retention of the hospital resource at Soss Moss which enabled a more gradual change and allowed some staff who felt more comfortable in a hospital environment to remain there. Although ultimately this has postponed changes concerning the role of night staff which management still wish to resolve.

Ultimately resistance failed for four main reasons. First, management adopted a sophisticated industrial relations strategy which allayed staff anxiety by letting them participate in the change while safeguarding job security. Second, the nature of the Mary Dendy site which is split into separate units imposed divisions on the workforce which prevented orchestrated resistance and allowed committed staff to distance themselves from the opposition. Third, as new developments came on stream and staff began to move a momentum of change was created which was impossible to resist. Finally it would have been difficult for the trade unions to oppose a progressive policy and as the closure was being properly funded by the Regional Health Authority they were anxious to use it as an example to other Health Authorities of the terms and conditions they expected in other community care developments.

Training Strategy

At the first meeting of the Mary Dendy Hospital Working Party in December 1983 the need for training and retraining for staff was raised as important in helping to achieve the changed philosophy of care. A training sub-group was established with Regional, District and Social Services representatives present. At certain times representatives of the NHSTA, the CCETSW, and ENB were represented.

The feasibility study published in July 1984 included a short statement on training needs which endorsed a number of principles:

1. The training strategy had to involve both health and social services personnel.

2. While agreed on the necessity for joint planning for training, any programme subsequently implemented is dealing with staff with a range of experience and training and any programme had to meet different needs and would not necessarily be joint throughout.

3. Staff groups whose needs had to be considered included: qualified NHS staff (nurses); unqualified NHS staff; qualified Social Services staff (residential, day care and field work); unqualified Social Services staff; new recruits

4. The training programme had to include the following components: combined training in relation to general philosophy and principles of a community service; specialist skill development; team building; management and supervisory skills.

5. The need for a training analysis from which to develop and cost a package.

To take this work forward in January 1985 the Joint Training Implications sub-group was formally constituted. In July 1985 they produced a four phase strategy for the training plan they wrote. They were identified as:

Phase 1. Implications of change training for key priority target groups.

Phase 2. Intensive research study into skills analysis/training need identification.

Phase 3. Implementation of the requirements identified in the study.

Phase 4: The long-term strategy. Qualifying and post-qualifying training.

The first phase was between health and social services and was aimed at first-time managers because it was believed they were crucial to the success of the strategy. The content covered the principles involved in the care of the community strategy, financing and home budget planning, community skills and team building exercises. The courses commenced in October 1985. This programme was planned, tutored and evaluated jointly by the University of Keele, Cheshire Social Services and the Health Authority. Course membership was split evenly between Social Services and the Health Authority.

The results were very positive. There were undoubtedly times when the needs of the two agency groups appeared disparate and the appropriateness of joint training for the whole duration of the course was questioned. Nonetheless the joint courses enabled misconceptions between the two organisations to be eroded and by allowing individuals from different agencies to get to know each other informally helped to strengthen working relationships. A further benefit was the opportunity to think through how the houses should be managed and gave managers the opportunity to make an assessment of their own skills.

The second phase involved the systematic analysis of training needs to provide guidance on the most effective way of training the bulk of the staff involved. A consultant was sought for six months to carry out the training needs analysis during the first half of 1986. A university department was used and set the following brief:

1. To obtain information about the training needs of first line managers and direct care staff in the residential and domiciliary parts of the Mary Dendy Hospital Care in the Community Initiative.

2. To obtain information to permit the evaluation of the effectiveness of the training initiative which will follow from the training needs analysis.

Care in the Community Training Implications, Mary Dendy Hospital, University of Manchester, 1986.

The report recommended that there should be an induction programme for all staff, a modular in-service training programme was advocated and the need for continued staff support was emphasised. The Authority had reservations about the report believing some of the questions which asked staff to tick a box if they would like some more training would create predictable results. The author of the report also expressed reservations about the task she faced (Raynes, 1987).

Consequently a training and development officer for 'care in the community', who was employed on a Regional basis, was asked to identify what training had taken place between October 1985 and October 1987, provide a methodology for that training to be evaluated and to discuss the reactions to *Care in the Community Training Implications, Mary Dendy Hospital*. The report published in Summer 1987 summarised the training to date and prepared a questionnaire which could be used to ascertain people's beliefs about the training they had received. Finally, the recommendations of the Manchester study were examined and progress towards their achievement evaluated.

The fourth phase of the training strategy had been concerned with longer term qualifying and post qualifying training. The intention in the strategy was that in the long-term a form of shared nationally recognised training could be developed which would be a tangible sign of the commitment to a multi-disciplinary approach to care. In 1986 the English National Board (ENB) outlined a new course ENB 939 'Care of People with Mental Handicap in Community Residential and Day Services'.

A multi-disciplinary planning team, involving members from Health, Social Services, Paramedics, Stockport College, and the Universities of Keele and Manchester was established in October 1986 to formulate the course. The content of the course was designed to reflect the evolving role of the carer within mental handicap. Participants strengths and needs were identified by a questionnaire before the course. An individual contract is developed which significantly influences teaching strategies, and a major element of the course is a research project. It was again found that having participants from both agencies benefited everyone and gave a greater understanding of the two services. Macclesfield's submission to the ENB to run two courses a year for five years was accepted. (Fabrizio and Buckenham, 1988.)

The emphasis on training complemented the industrial relations initiatives to enable change to be brought about earlier. The use of extensive training during a period of great change has risks attached to it. Training may be used as a substitute for good management or as a gesture to overcome resistance, which may raise expectations about a new service which cannot then be fulfilled. In Macclesfield a large amount of money was spent on training and some significant breakthroughs were achieved in terms of inter-agency collaboration but a more comprehensive evaluation of the training strategy remains to be carried out.

The Community Reaction

The 1980s has witnessed an increasing number of assaults on the concept of community care to the extent that the Government felt forced to establish its own review of the community care initiative (Griffiths, 1988). The whole community care initiative rests on the twin assumptions that residents of long-stay institutions would prefer to return to the community and that the community will allow individuals to take their place back in society.

Macclesfield found resentment and a general lack of acceptance by sections of the general public to the notion that people with learning difficulties could live an ordinary life in the community. Macclesfield's management were not unaware of the potential public response. However there were deep seated philosophical objections to the idea of a public relations strategy. The philosophy of normalisation views people with learning difficulties as having the same rights as ordinary members of society. Consequently the idea of 'selling' the strategy to the public and informing communities about their future neighbours would have been the antithesis of allowing people with learning difficulties to settle without fanfare in areas of their choice.

The Health Authority began experiencing difficulties in acquiring houses in 1984. The Authority through the relevant committees would identify a house which was thought to be appropriate for resettling a number of residents from Mary Dendy. The vendor would find out that the property was to be sold to the Health Authority and would withdraw it on their own volition or would be subject to pressure from neighbours to withdraw the property. This clearly posed a major obstacle to the Authority's ability to fulfil its plans and managers began to pursue various strategies to overcome resistance.

The first initiative involved attending a series of public meetings and explaining Macclesfield's strategy. This was not a success as the managers were not given a chance to explain their position and merely served to intensify opposition. At the same time in September 1984 the Authority organised a one-day conference in the District and invited a range of eminent speakers including Lord Glenarthor and Brian Rix from Mencap to talk about the changing perceptions of mental handicap. Members of the public were invited to attend. This one day conference in a similar manner to the latter public meetings focused unreceptive public attention on to Macclesfield's plans.

The publicity from the conference was a prelude to representations from residents of one estate in the north of the District concerning the resettlement of four Mary Dendy residents into a house on their estate. The protests were fuelled by some very emotive and inaccurate reporting by the local paper. The objectors had three principle points. First, they alleged the Authority was being secretive in its resettlement plans. Second, that the property was not sited close to amenities such as shops and third, the costs involved of the purchase of the particular house. The objectors' letters showed a lack of understanding of the difference between mental illness and mental handicap as the terms were used interchangeably and emphasised their rights as householders to maintain the value of their property.

The Health Authority pursued moving residents into the house believing that if they capitulated to public pressure an unwelcome precedent would have been established. The neighbours pursued the complaint and the Health Service Commissioner investigated the objection that the Health Authority had failed to consult the neighbours and been dismissive of residents objections. The Health Service Commissioner reported in November 1986, failed to uphold the complaint but criticised the Health Authority for not adequately informing immediate neighbours after a purchase about their future neighbours. Macclesfield felt the Commissioner had sided too greatly with the interests of neighbours against the interests of people with learning difficulties.

The Health Authority by this time was using a different strategy in the acquisition of houses. The Authority instructed the estate agent to tell the vendor the purpose for which the house was being purchased and either the vendor or the Health Authority would then inform the neighbours. Consequently Health Authority policy became the same as the recommendation of the Health Service Commissioner to tell the immediate neighbours. The Authority was also pursuing a more low key approach of trying to influence local councillors and other opinion formers to give their support to community care.

The difficulties in acquiring properties was a major cause of delay at the beginning of the implementation period. Ironically in the case of the Health Service Commissioner complaint the complainants had become so accustomed to their new neighbours that they had shed their former prejudices and were embarrassed when the complaints procedure ran its course. It would seem that the creation of the most positive images for people with learning difficulties comes about when the general public witnesses an ordinary life in practice. Ultimately this will be the manner in which the acceptance of people with learning difficulties by the community is achieved.

The Search for Properties

The delays in acquiring properties was a catalyst to endeavours to find properties through a housing association. Macclesfield management, while they wanted to gain ordinary housing in the community, did not wish to have a housing management responsibility for these properties nor did they feel it fitted in with the philosophy of normalisation if the houses were Health Authority managed. A central factor for beginning to approach housing associations was the depletion of the capital budget which would have made it difficult for the Authority to acquire all the properties they wanted. Finally a commitment from the Local Authority to provide some cluster accommodation had produced limited results and the houses were concentrated on a small number of estates.

In August 1985 the Unit Administrator first approached a Housing Association. For both agencies it was a novel situation and there were a host of issues to be resolved. The type of management the Housing Association was to provide varied from a complete package in which the Association collected the rent, maintained the grounds and carried out maintenance to situations where greater autonomy was left to the residents.

During 1986 proceedings were slow and marked by misunderstandings over how properties would be identified. The Health Authority believed that the Housing Association would be looking and buying properties for the Health Authority while the Association believed the Health Authority would be alerting them to properties they wanted. The Health Authority also detected a general lack of interest by the Association who were not very committed to a small project which required the acquisition of single houses on an occasional basis.

In 1987 the Health Authority redoubled its efforts to pursue houses through the housing association. A debate had started within management which continued into 1988 whether they were the most appropriate housing association to use. They were viewed as too slow in making bids for houses, this situation not being helped by the location of their officers away from Macclesfield. Second, the association had a poor reputation with local estate agents and was not viewed as being totally honest in the way they managed their business. Third, the association wished to retain a veto over who went into the houses which was clearly unacceptable to Macclesfield.

The Administration and Support Services Manager shared these criticisms but believed that the Association knew the needs of the Health Authority and had obtained the Halifax Building Society's agreement to grant 100 per cent mortagages. The Halifax Building Society therefore provided the capital for the houses on the basis of twenty-five year repayments and the residents paid the mortgage via the £87·50 per week benefit payments they received. Consequently it was decided to carry on with the current arrangements not least because of the difficulties of establishing the same arrangements in the near future with a different housing association.

The Administration and Support Services Manager continued to be frustrated at the lack of progress and in February 1988, with the Clinical Services Manager, paid an unannounced visit to the Association. It was during this unscheduled meeting that the Housing Association Manager finally admitted the real reasons for the delays.

First the Association was concerned about the uncertainty surrounding the future of community care and the possible outcome of the Griffiths inquiry. They were anxious about the effect on their arrangements with Macclesfield which a switch to lead responsibility for local authorities might have. Second, they were concerned about the uncertainty surrounding benefit changes and the effect reductions would have on the ability of residents to meet their mortgage repayments. Third, the Association wanted all benefit cheques to go to them so that they could ensure the mortgage repayments were the first call on residents benefits. Fourth, the rise in property prices and interest rates was raising questions about the feasibility of repaying mortgages in that manner. Finally, the Housing Association Manager admitted that their members were not convinced if the work with Macclesfield was an arena they should be entering.

The Community Unit General Manager forcibly responded to these concerns. She argued that all organisations faced uncertainties and it was not possible to predict the future. Consequently the Health Authority and the Housing Association had to address the current situation of trying to fulfil the community care strategy which necessitated a steady momentum in obtaining houses. Furthermore she argued the government would be unable to reduce benefit levels as this would jeopardise the community care policy and Macclesfield would be forced to stop discharging residents as they would not compromise the needs of those residents.

The Health Authority having cleared the air with the Association began to enjoy better relations which was facilitated by a change of local management in the Association. A number of outstanding issues were resolved. The Association had been concerned about who was responsible for maintaining a mortgage if a house became vacant or a resident left. The Health Authority in December 1988 agreed to levy a five per cent charge per resident per month to cover the eventuality of a vacancy and agreed to be ultimately responsible for covering the mortgage. In return the Housing Association had conceded that benefit cheques would be managed by individual residents who would service their own mortgages.

The degree to which benefit payments sufficiently cover mortgage repayments has involved Macclesfield's management in the search for new solutions. Macclesfield management had calculated the upper limits in property values that residents could afford on their benefit payments. This was until recently £44,000 for a three bedroomed house and £63,000 for a four bedroom house. However with interest rate rises these figures had been revised down to £37,000 and £53,000 respectively. Yet it is not possible to obtain properties for those prices in the Macclesfield area.

The Health Authority initially with the agreement of residents tried to encroach on other elements of their benefits beyond the £40·60 allocated for housing (Table 21). The Health Authority was proposing that mortgage repayments were supplemented through the £29·40 allocated to meals. The Housing Association consulted 'The Housing Association Consultancy and Advisory Service' who believed such a system raised ethical questions and was contrary to good practice as it made residents vulnerable to fluctuations in benefit levels.

TABLE 21. *Breakdown of Benefits Paid to Residents in Community Provision*

Category	*Amount*
Housing	£40·60
Meals	£29·40
Extra Care	£17·50
Personal Expenses	£10·30 or £11·50

SOURCE: Macclesfield Health Authority, 1988

In the light of these objections the Authority has been pursuing more radical solutions. Macclesfield wish to sell the properties back to the Housing Association at the market rate and use the surplus to cushion the new higher mortgages. These moves are currently being pursued but in the interim the two agencies have been able to clarify their own responsibilities:

Housing Association responsibilities:

(i) Acquire properties identified by the Health Authority.

(ii) Arrange services.

(iii) Make appointments to the Housing Corporation for consent via Section 9 of The Housing Act 1985.

(iv) Keep vendors and the Health Authority fully informed.

(v) Identify any problems and seek solutions.

(vi) Ensure mortgage is serviced.

(vii) Manage the project—ensure property is in good condition and any remedial work is carried out.

(viii) Ensure targets are met.

Health Authority responsibilities

I Liaise with Housing Association once properties have been identified in a suitable price range.

II Ensure targets are met.

III Ensure clients are identified and prepared for discharge and their relocation.

IV Provide support necessary to ensure success of individuals in the community.

V Continually monitor to identify potential problems leading to potential solutions.

VI Ensure each house is provided with carpets, furniture and curtains.

VII Endeavour to maintain optimum occupancy and reimburse the Housing Association if there is a greater than four per cent vacancy factor.

VIII Provide factual information to the Local Authority, community and medical profession to maintain good public relations.

IX Where a resident is unable to reside satisfactorily arrange more suitable alternative accommodation.

Despite the reluctance of the Housing Association to initially enter into agreements with the Health Authority the link has brought considerable benefits for the Health Authority. It is anticipated that by

March 1989, twelve cluster homes will have been provided under the auspices of the Housing Association. This represents a large capital saving to the Authority which enables management to more easily meet their plans under the community care initiative. It has also achieved the objective of removing housing management from the Authority's portfolio of activities. There has been no cost to the Authority in supporting residents in the community apart from the one off cost of furnishing and equipping the houses and Macclesfield have negotiated first call on proceeds from the houses once the mortgage has been repaid. Managerial reservations about the schemes concern the uncertainties surrounding future benefit levels and interest rate fluctuations.

Finance

The original care in the community strategy drawn up by the Unit Management Team in 1982 envisaged a long-term transfer of finance from within the institution to the community. The establishment of the Regional Working Party and the decision to compress the closure timetable to enable Mary Dendy Hospital to close by 1989 meant that a rapid transfer of finance was not possible to establish the community developments. The financial basis for the community developments therefore became a bridging exercise with additional capital and revenues injected by the Region to enable new developments to be established while maintaining existing provision.

The debates in the Mary Dendy Working Party were underpinned by financial considerations. There were disagreements between members whether community care would be a more expensive option or would create savings. The District believed the strategy would be more expensive and this has proved to be the case. The average cost of a hospital place prior to the setting up of a community facility was in the region of £8,000 per annum, the average is now closer to £13,000 per annum. In capital terms the community care exercise has involved an investment in the order of £6m, the majority of which will be recouped from the value of the hospital sale.

The most difficult financial discussions in the Working Party concerned the basis on which Macclesfield would return money to the Region as beds at Mary Dendy were vacated. Initially the Regional Health Authority were adamant that the transfer of a resident from the hospital to community provision should equate in financial terms with the loss of the cost of one bed in a hospital. The District believed that although it was theoretically possible to produce from the cost accounts a cost per bed this would be a purely theoretical cost since the marginal cost of closing one bed on a thirty bedded ward has little effect on the cost of that ward. Consequently a retraction model was adopted which tried to avoid the anomalies highlighted.

A financial model was developed based on the 1984/85 cost accounts which modelled the budgets for the service as it will appear from March 1989. This used manpower planning predictions to estimate staff numbers for the new service. A time-table for developments was agreed and retraction was based on a sliding scale which tapers the negotiated model cost on an annual basis. The difficulty with this process is that due to initial delays in obtaining houses the community provision does not match the amount of provision planned. Consequently an annual bargaining process ensues over the extent of money to be paid back to the Region for that year. This is a process which does not conform to any agreed principles and injects a degree of financial uncertainty into the District's plans.

An important aspect of the financial agreement between the Regional Health Authority and Macclesfield concerned the status of patients with links to other Health Authorities. The Regional Health Authority accepted that if a resident had been at Mary Dendy more than five years they became Macclesfield's responsibility and would be funded as such. This prevented the situation which has arisen in other parts of the country where residents are repatriated to other Authorities with dowry payments as a means to fund their provision. This type of system can create protracted negotiations between authorities which is a diversion from the establishment of community provision.

The funding for social service developments was organised in a different manner. The overall cash limit for local authority schemes was established through the 'Heads of Agreement' negotiated between Mersey Regional Health Authority and Cheshire County Council. This was a legal document in which the County Council agreed to undertake the capital projects listed in accordance with the programme agreed with the Regional Health Authority. Cheshire County Council prior to starting each project had to submit detailed costs to the Region for approval. In this manner the Regional Health Authority made available £3m for the establishment of day centres, residential centres, work experience schemes, and group homes.

There exists a widespread perception in Macclesfield Health Authority that Cheshire County Council were able to negotiate more favourable terms than the District Health Authority and were able to increase their services and estate in an area not traditionally viewed as high priority in the provision of services. This view is not shared by Regional Officers. First, it was clear that social services were not prepared to provide a service at the underfunded levels which traditionally pertained in the Health Service. Second, the nature of social services budgeting with the allocation of costs to individual cost centres involved the payment for services which in the Health Service would appear as 'a free good'. For example, if the County Surveyor carried out work for the Mary Dendy project this would be charged to the project. By contrast similar work at the Regional Health Authority would be absorbed as part of the Regional budget. Finally, the Regional Health Authority by monitoring the County Council scheme was impinging on their management prerogatives and to obtain agreement a degree of financial fluidity was needed.

In 1986 the Regional Health Authority asked the District to adopt the monitoring role for social services schemes it had been undertaking. This reflected the Regional view that the closure of Mary Dendy was proceeding well and that the remaining implementation work should be a District responsibility. It also reflected a change in management style, with the Regional General Manager keen to reduce Regional interference in District policies. Consequently the District role which had been confined to the distribution of money to social services was altered to a monitoring role.

The District had reservations about their monitoring role but began to prepare a monitoring and control system which assigned lead responsibility to the Unit General Manager with reporting through the Implementation Group. During the detailed planning stage individual scheme costs would be allowed to be varied by up to 10 per cent of the basic cost or £10,000 whichever was the smaller figure. The local authority was to provide monthly progress reports to the Steering Group and Implementation Group. At the pre-tender estimate stage the local authority was required to make a report to the Implementation Group on the capital and revenue costs.

Since the Mary Dendy exercise the Regional view of financing community care has changed dramatically. This reflects a shift in central government priorities which emphasises the centrality of acute services at the expense of the priority assigned to mental handicap and mental illness services in the 1983–85 period. The current Mersey Regional Health Authority policy is that community developments must be on a self-financing basis. The developments in the community have to be matched by the amount being released from the hospital service. This makes it difficult for other Authorities in the Region to pursue the goal of community care and to progress as rapidly as Macclesfield.

Towards March 1989: A New Service in the Making?

Despite the difficulties that the Authority experienced in obtaining housing in the community, which led to some targets and developments not being met, the picture as the target date of March 1989 approached was—of a new service in the making.

The programme for closure of Mary Dendy Hospital itself was based on the planned developments needed arising from the assessment process. This demonstrated broadly how ward numbers could be reduced over the four-year period. The decision as to which wards were to close first was made on the basis of the structural condition and suitability of the buildings involved. The site being split into four separate geographical locations enabled two of the smaller sites to be closed first, leaving the main site and Soss Moss Hospital site. The main site was closed as facilities were developed at Soss Moss and in the community.

The exercise was planned over the full four year period with the rundown of the site coinciding with the development of community provision. The management team operated on the principle that residents should be moved as little as possible. The assessment information was used to ensure that residents who were remaining in the hospital moved to the upgraded facilities at Soss Moss, allowing a spread of other residents into the remaining accommodation. There was initial overcrowding at Mary Dendy within the wards but it was agreed that wards would not close if this created overcrowding, and criteria were established for optimum ward numbers for each ward based on day and night space requirements.

Soss Moss Hospital had a total of seventy beds which included eight intensive care beds for people with learning difficulties with severe challenging behaviour needing a secure environment.

The remaining sixty-two beds are occupied by adults suffering from a degree of mental handicap in some cases with a combined physical handicap which requiring a degree of specialist medical, nursing, and paramedical input not normally coped with in the currently established community provision. The site is split between six buildings which provide fourteen place residential accommodation designed with a domestic atmosphere, to allow as much privacy as possible in the bed areas. There is a resident training and leisure centre to enable residents to enjoy a high quality of life.

The pattern of residential care has followed the broad guidelines established by the Joint Working Party and subsequently modified by the Mid-Term Review. This split provision three ways between; Soss Moss Hospital (seventy places), core and cluster accommodation (seventy-two places), and a mixture of elderly persons homes and social services residential units which provide the bulk of the remaining 120 places.

Day Care

Members of the Mary Dendy Hospital Working Party were conscious of the bad publicity that had surrounded community care in other areas due to unplanned discharges from long-stay psychiatric hospitals. The Working Party decided that to be effective residential care had to be complemented by day care and that no resident should be discharged into the community unless they had a place for day care. The strategy outlined in the Joint Working Party report in July 1984 was a two strand policy based on the provision of local day centres and the establishment of a work experience programme.

The proposals were based on the concepts outlined in the Congleton Social Services Lifetime report which suggested an integrated approach based on five guiding principles:

1. The availability of adequate day care was an essential need for every resident regardless of their residential placement.

2. There had to be a continuum of day care programmes which included the disparate elements of entertainment, training, education, and occupation commensurate with the individual's physical or mental ability and social setting.

3. There should be an avoidance of a total environment; no one was to receive all day services within one residential setting unless there were specific positive reasons for doing so.

4. The provision of services to an individual was to be managed by an individual care plan.

5. There was to be no service established in the community exclusively for Mary Dendy clients.

Three day centres have been established serving Congleton, Macclesfield and Knutsford/Wilmslow with seventy to eighty day places available. The centres are designed as access points for people with learning difficulties in the whole District whether living at home with their families or in a variety of residential units. The centres by establishing individual programme plans aim to fulfil a number of roles for clients:

(i) stimulation in which individuals can achieve personal development in areas of social skills, further education and leisure activities.

(ii) social contact through sharing social activities and making new friends.

(iii) relief for the families of clients.

The centres by providing a resource for the local community encourage self help groups, clubs, voluntary organisations, and adult education to use the facilities. This promotes a better understanding and acceptance of the needs of people with learning difficulties through community participation in the centre. Admissions are channelled by social workers to the centre manager after initial discussion at District Social Services. After admission each member is assigned a key worker who befriends, counsels and establishes with the member their programme of activities which is formally reviewed within the first six months of attendance.

Complementing the day centres has been the establishment of the work experience programme. This provides employment for people with learning difficulties in ordinary employment settings. Underpinning the programme is an attachment to the normalisation philosophy and an attempt to use ordinary resources wherever possible, only creating specialist provision where the need dictates. This implied a critique of traditional Adult Training Centres (ATCs) which did not provide opportunities to genuinely partcipate in the working life of the local community. The Congleton work scheme aims to:

> enable those clients who are sufficiently motivated to seek, gain and retain employment or work experience opportunities commensurate with their aptitude and ability.
>
> 6 January 1987: Congleton work scheme: outline description.

It provides vocational counselling on the opportunities available for clients, gives clients an understanding of the world of work and provides employment search skills. In addition to helping clients seek and retain employment the scheme operates as a catalyst for the community stimulating local employers to offer employment opportunities to clients through open employment or sheltered placement. Macclesfield operate a similar scheme through the Horizons Employment Service.

The establishment of a network of day centres and work placement schemes has prevented the negative connotations associated with community care and provided opportunities to enhance individuals potential and quality of life. In addition to this many of the facilities are suitable for use by the community and this represents a way in which community participation can be encouraged, promoting an improved image for services and reducing the isolation frequently experienced by people with learning difficulties.

Summary

There has been intense interest in community care in the 1980s heightened by speculation about the stance the government would adopt, as a series of reports have criticised government policy and inertia in this arena. This interest has spilled over into the media which has played on the publics' anxieties about the policy. Health and social services have therefore had to develop new services, and close old hospitals against a backdrop of a mistrustful community, uncertainties about the future direction of policy and the ubiquitous scramble for resources.

Macclesfield had to bring about change in this uncertain environment. In addition Mary Dendy was the first planned closure of a long-stay hospital in the Region so there was little external experience to draw on and the time-scales were compressed magnifying the scale of change. However, these circumstances although they created uncertainties also presented opportunities for bringing about changes.

The 1982 boundary changes meant that Mary Dendy became the responsibility of Macclesfield Health Authority which presented management with the opportunity to examine their policy towards community care without historical baggage fettering their thinking. The Unit Management Team therefore devised its own strategy which incorporated the closure of Mary Dendy and the development of new services in the community. Consequently, although formal impetus for closure came from the Region, Macclesfield had independently arrived at similar conclusions. This was a significant factor in achieving change demonstrating the importance that the origins of policies can have in the degree to which they are implemented.

This strong commitment to a particular model of community care, when the orthodoxy in the early 1980s was to favour the Wessex model of community care, prevailed. This example typified the importance of key individuals who possess a united vision in achieving change. In a sense this adherence to a model of community care based on normalisation principles, because it marked a departure from earlier philosophies of care, helped to sustain deep commitment to the strategy. Key individuals felt strongly it was their personal initiative in a way that went beyond notions of managerial accountability. The continuity in post of these individuals from 1983 to 1989 strengthened this involvement. This pattern of innovation corrobates Stocking's (1985) emphasis on product champions in the adoption and diffusion of new procedures. She argues that in two of her case studies, the establishment of Regional secure units and the Asian Ricketts campaign in Glasgow, the commitment of particular individuals was central to the degree of progress made.

The Region contributed to change in two main ways. Firstly, the closure of a long-stay institution had been set as a ministerial review task, at a time when the government was firmly espousing the need to reallocate resources from the acute sector towards community care. The

Regional strategy to 1994 included as a central objective, the need 'to ensure a major shift towards community care'. Although this policy was not entirely new, the tighter accountability of Regions and Districts through the review process and the emergence of general management resulted in the policy being more vigoursly pursued. The importance of the issue to the Region was seen in Duncan Nichol, the Regional General Manager being personally involved.

Secondly, it provided resources to enable the development of new services during the run down of Mary Dendy. This was particularly important as the original Unit Management Team had envisaged a gradual transfer of resources from within the hospital to the community. However, the reduction in the time-scale for closure raised costs as finance could not be released sufficiently quickly to resource the new service. Regional funding was therefore required to obtain Macclesfield's agreement to the accelerated closure of Mary Dendy.

Although the Region provided bridging finance, this left for negotiation the repayment process by the District. This created uncertainties for the District over its exact financial position but conversely allowed a degree of flexibility to ensure that money was not withdrawn too quickly before community developments were in place. However, the Regional view of financing has altered dramatically and community developments were expected to be self-financing. The publication of *Caring for People* (Department of Health, 1989c) with lead responsbility for community care passed to local authorities has further jeopardised the financial backing Regions will provide for community care.

At the District level there was limited input from District officers who devolved responsibility for the strategy to the Unit General Manager and her team of officers. The implementation of the strategy spawned a number of committees. Although there was not always sufficient clarity in the roles performed by the various committees it provided a system of checks and balances to prevent the dominance of any particular group and to increase the range of people involved.

The assessment process was central to the planning of new services. The view that the planning of new services should be based on the individual assessment of need has been prominent during the 1980s, *Working for Patients* and *Caring for People* with their emphasis on individualism and choice are both grounded in this approach. However the tools to measure need are less developed and have limitations for planning purposes. In Macclesfield the initial assessment process which was envisaged as a broad financial framework for the future pattern of provision became the plan. This reflected the desire of the Region to move as rapidly as possible and to use information that was available. However, this created disquiet at local level and stored up difficulties for the future. The Region needed to clarify the role of the assessment process and not allow the changing needs of residents to be subservient to an inflexible blueprint.

For example, this rational planning approach based on an objective needs assessment was unable to adapt to the political requirements of the strategy. As developments provoked public opposition there was a need for the Authority to place more able residents thereby helping to allay public anxieties about the strategy. Similarly flexibility was needed in finding suitable group homes and implementation should not have been constrained if a suitable house was found which could accommodate five residents rather than three or four as planned.

The closure of any hospital creates uncertainties for staff. In the case of a long-stay hospital there is the implicit assumption that hospitals are inappropriate places for people with learning difficulties to be cared for. This can be difficult for staff trained to work in hospital settings and who sometimes become institutionalised themselves, which is unsurprising when the isolation of hospitals such as Mary Dendy is considered. Hospitals also provide more predictable work and an established set of friendships. In contrast community care models by acknowledging people's rights remove the ability to use custodial practice and also change the responsibility of staff. In addition nursing staff qualifications are not recognised by many social service providers.

Industrial relations was carefully handled to allay staff anxieties, by the establishment of a no compulsory redundancy policy, and cultivating the support that existed amongst staff and trade unions. Staff were involved in the planning of new working patterns with management being open about their future intentions. There was also the need to ensure that conditions of employment were harmonised between health and social services. Social services were helpful in accommodating NHS staff and, for example, agreed that Health Authority applicants for social service posts should be treated as internal applicants.

The lack of cooperation between health and social services has frequently hindered the development of community care. In Macclesfield health and social services developed a good working relationship which prevailed even when differences occurred. Several factors were significant.

Firstly, as the closure of Mary Dendy was a Regional project with Regional funding there was less wrangling over finances than ususally occurs. The Region needed the support of social services to achieve their plan and therefore were prepared to be more generous in funding social service provision than otherwise might have been the case. It also meant that the Region was prepared to resource a strategy that included day care. This avoided the familiar social services criticism that Health Authorities are only prepared to fund residential care.

Secondly, this meant that Health Authority and social services management forged an alliance against the Region's stance on, for example, community units. This development of common interests at particular junctures of implementation helped the overall strategy and encouraged genuine joint working between both parties, as the joint training initiatives testify.

Thirdly, the experience of joint ventures between health and social services, particularly at Heather Brae in Congleton, a joint finance project which did not work satisfactorily due to the difficulties of joint management and staff integration led to the adoption of an integrated but single agency approach. This meant that although some Health Authority staff worked in social services provision, managerial responsibility and accountability were vested in one agency. This careful division of responsibilities between health and social services avoided the difficulties of joint managerial accountability across health and social service boundaries. These type of arrangements mirror the separation of purchaser from provider which the government advocates in *Caring for People.*

An additional factor that eased implementation was the decision to maintain Soss Moss Hospital. The manner in which it was retained was also important. It was not simply retained to house the remainder from Mary Dendy who needed a degree of specialist medical nursing and paramedical input not usually coped with in the existing community provision. Instead the hospital was modernised and the quality of life for residents was improved with accommodation designed to provide a domestic environment. Consequently, Soss Moss was also viewed in a postive light as providing a valued service.

Soss Moss therefore provided a safety net for people who did not adjust easily to life in the community. This was important not only for those clients but also for relatives, the wider community and staff. Some staff who found it difficult to adjust to the community care strategy were able to stay at Soss Moss and adjust more gradually to the community care policy.

Management also faced difficulties in bringing about change. The greatest obstacle proved to be the sheer difficulty of obtaining houses due to the hostility of the local community to the strategy and a similar ambivalence from the Housing Association. This led to further delays in acquiring properties. The Health Authority had difficulty in convincing the local community of the merits of their strategy. Recognition of this situation led to further attempts to promote positive images of people with learning difficulties. A joint group was established in 1988 which promoted ideas that developed positive images through, for example, the community's use of the new facilities developed as part of the Mary Dendy retraction exercise. This aimed to develop a more favourable impression of the Authority's services.

The closure of long-stay hospitals has become the most identifiable aspect of community care and become subject to increasing public scrutiny. Meanwhile during the late-1980s there was a hiatus in government policy, as it vacillated on the course it wished to adopt. For Macclesfield the luxury of inaction has not been possible as the Region, directed by the Department of Health, required the accelerated closure of Mary Dendy. For management this presented opportunities as well as risks to move more rapidly to a different pattern of provision. They have resolutely pursued this strategy supported by the Region and made few concessions to achieve their goal. Although *Caring for People* heralds fundamental changes for community care, Macclesfield have established a secure base for future service improvements.

CONCLUSION

Barriers to Appropriate Cost-Effective Care for the Elderly and Mentally Handicapped

The main barriers to coordination of care for priority groups and also for placement of individuals in the form of care most suitable to them are caused firstly, by a fragmentation in sources of finance for care, and secondly, by a resulting inadequate cooperation between the agencies responsible for the delivery of care. In a nutshell, there is no 'gatekeeper' who both holds the budget and purchases care from a suitable provider on the basis of considerations such as effectiveness of care, quality of care, happiness of the client and cost-effectiveness. There is no disputing the fact that public finance for care for priority groups, whether in the community or in some form of institution, is bound to be cash limited for the foreseeable future. The concern here is not with the overall budget going to such care but with the most effective use of that budget.

The Basic Choices and Dilemmas

Any government, organised by any political party, will be faced with the basic philosophical choice of 'choosing between variables' when giving financial subsidies to needy groups or when maintaining incomes through public expenditure. Equity, of whatever variant, may dictate that nobody's income in society is allowed to fall below a minimum norm. The dictates of efficiency and the maintenance of sensible incentives argue that 'poverty traps' and 'unemployment traps' should be avoided. That is, by doing an extra increment of work (e.g. moving from complete unemployment to a few hours work a week; or in moving from thirty hours a week to forty hours a week), one should not suffer a net loss in income; otherwise known as a more than 100 per cent rate of net taxation. In other words, if one is receiving benefit and one loses it all on gaining some income, one may be in a poverty or unemployment trap. This implies that benefit should only be lost gradually as income increases, to allow a sliding scale of diminution of benefit rather than sudden cut-off points or a sudden cut-off point, whether at the lower or higher end of the income scale.

However, determining an equity standard and what one might term an efficiency or incentive standard has implications for the overall cost of income maintenance policy. Guaranteeing a minimum income (whether through supplementary benefit, income support or any variant) *and* diminishing the perverse incentives of poverty traps, unemployment traps, or high marginal rates of taxation (whether at the lower or higher end of the scale) can be expensive. That is, the third variable, the overall cost of a policy, is determined by one's political and economic choices concerning the first two variables of equity and efficiency incentives. That is why a government committed to a social minimum income and overall cost control may be forced to institute or at least tolerate what seem like inefficient policies involving poor incentives at work.

That is, one can choose two variables: having defined equity and cost, incentive effects may be difficult to alter; having defined equity and incentives, total cost may be difficult to alter; and having defined efficiency and total cost, one's desired level of equity may not be achievable.

There may be political demands to maintain a minimum level of welfare yet also an adequate incentive to work. There may be a need to provide 'legitimation' in and of society. The argument is that, since all cannot share in the fruits of individualism, entrepreneurship and ownership of the means of production, those who do not must be guaranteed the consolation of adequate welfare. Similarly, those who have to sell their labour as opposed to owning means of production, must be guaranteed adequate reward for what are effectively jobs lacking interest or involving drudgery. Therefore, combining welfare and incentives to work may be expensive. Certain theorists of varying political perspectives have argued that this 'legitimation crisis' causes a 'fiscal crisis' as governments are forced to spend more than they can tax. This effect is accentuated when one considers that governments also need to spend to stimulate and help the accumulation of private capital.

It is thus argued that the welfare state and welfare society may involve a fiscal crisis because of inevitable discrepancies between government spending and tax revenues. The solutions proposed by market theorists, unlike their left-wing co-theorists who also share the diagnosis, is to seek to 'legitimate' a form of society with lower welfare, and yet the maintenance of adequate work incentives. Achieving this within desired cost parameters may still be difficult, and right-wing theorists may be forced to condone only minimal incentives to work in practice.

Basic changes in the social and economic structure of many 'western' countries has led to the break up of the 'old working class' (in Britain the labourist coalition; in the United States the so-called New Deal coalition) and as a result, right-wing political 'coalitions', whether temporary or not, are allowing a new normative definition of what is 'legitimate'. That is, left-wing or 'Marxist' assumptions developed in the 1960s and the 1970s about what is necessary to legitimise society may be over sanguine (from the viewpoint of reform) as to the instability of capitalism. Furthermore, it seems to be in the former non-capitalist world, such as the hitherto Eastern bloc countries, that governments have had the greatest difficulty in 'squaring the circle' between adequate revenue, adequate rewards to work and adequate levels of welfare.

It is in this context that barriers to coordination in caring for priority groups should be viewed. The aim must be to ensure that an adequate level of support (whether through income maintenance or direct provision of services) is achieved, that incentives are not perverse and that overall costs are manageable. Providing support for care, and community care in particular, may run the risk of *either* being 'too expensive' if 'incentives' to supporting families are to be maintained *or* too destructive of incentives to self-reliance *if* costs are to be constrained. Squaring the circle, or choosing which two variables of the triad (cost, equity and incentive) are most important, is the perennial political dilemma.

APPENDIX 1

The Star File

Social Training Achievement Record

SUMMARY

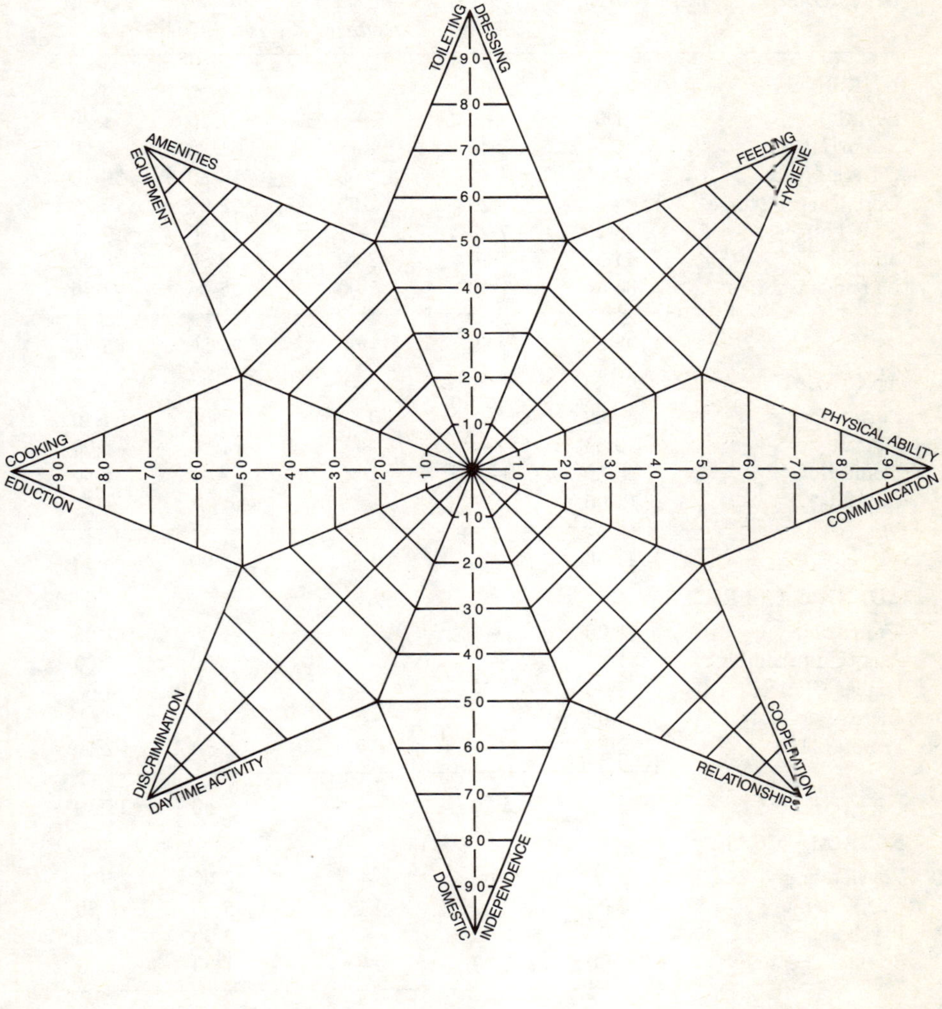

APPENDIX 2

Staffing Comparison of Mary Dendy and Community Care Arrangements

MACCLESFIELD HEALTH AUTHORITY: MARY DENDY HOSPITAL STAFFING COMPARISON

Group/Grade	*Current*	*Core & Cluster*	*Knutsford Cottage*	*Soss Moss Inc. I.C.U.*	*TOTAL*
NURSING					
D.N.S.	1·0	—	—	1·20	1·20
Senior Nurse	5·0	2·40	—	1·20	3·60
Charge Nurse	34·08	14·40	1·00	14·80	30·20
Dep. Charge Nurse	—	7·20	2·00	12·00	19·20
Staff Nurse	25·26	7·20	—	11·80	19·00
S.E.N.	44·31	7·20	2·00	8·80	18·00
Nursing Assistant	84·16	41·40	6·00	45·06	92·46
	193·81	79·80	11·00	94·86	185·66
ANCILLARY					
Porter/Driver	6·00	—	0·40	4·00	4·40
Hairdresser	0·63	—	—	1·00	1·00
Domestic*	28·85	—	1·50	—	1·50
Catering*	12·00	—	1·50	—	1·50
	47·48	—	3·40	5·00	8·40
ADMIN & CLERICAL					
Unit Admin.	1·00	—	—	1·00	1·00
Asst. Unit Admin	1·00	—	—	1·00	1·00
Higher Clerical	3·00	2·00	—	2·00	4·00
Clerical	2·00	—	—	3·00	3·00
Secretarial	2·54	—	—	2·50	2·50
	9·54	2·00	—	9·50	11·50
PARA-MEDICAL					
Physiotherapy	2·00	2·00	—	3·00	5·00
Occ. Therapy	7·00	2·00	1·00	5·50	8·50
Psychology	1·00	1·00	—	2·00	3·00
Speech Therapy	1·00	1·00	—	1·00	2.00
	11·00	6·00	1·00	11·50	18·50

*Subject to Competitive Tendering

CHAPTER 8

Case Study: Competitive Tendering—Greenbelt

Competitive Tendering and the National Health Service

The re-election of the Conservatives for a third term ensured that competitive tendering remained high on the political agenda. The Government quickly signalled its intentions by requesting Scottish Health Boards to tender for support services and in England extending mandatory competitive tendering to local authorities. Competitive tendering was given a further stimulus by the White Paper *Working for Patients* (Department of Health, 1989a). The establishment of a provider market linked by a patchwork of contracts will extend the competitive tendering process as it becomes the central mechanism to award contracts.

The White Paper represents a break with the traditional funding and organisational arrangements of the NHS, but details of how the provider market will operate have been sketchy and the numerous working papers have provided little reason to alter this judgement. Nonetheless the competitive tendering policy provides a legacy for management in terms of experience of drawing up contracts, agreeing standards, and monitoring performance.

The majority of clinical contracts will be placed with directly managed hospitals as the number of self-governing hospitals will initially be small and the private sector remains modest in size. In contrast to this the debate over the impact of competitive tendering has focused on when services have been contracted out. This tends to ignore the impact of competitive tendering on standards when services are provided in-house. The fragile relationship between standards and savings and the inherent difficulties of monitoring performance are seldom analysed. The implications of competitive tendering on other staff cannot be captured by an exclusive focus on financial savings. Consequently, this case study, which compares competitive tendering for domestic services in one Health Authority and examines in-house services and contracted-out services, has implications for the emergent provider market.

The Privatisation Initiative

Privatisation is an umbrella term for a range of initiatives which increase the role of the private sector in the economy. The injection of a commercial approach pervades the Government's restructuring of the public sector as the two recent White Papers on health care testify (Department of Health, 1989a,b). Similarly, for example, local financial management of schools introduced under the 1989 Education Reform Act has a commercial orientation, undermining the control of local Education Authorities by unleashing a market for school places with parents cast in the role of consumers.

Heald (1988) identifies four separate components which have been grouped under the term privatisation. First, charges can be levied on a service that continues to be provided by the public sector. Charges are an alternative to taxation and have been favoured by the Government as rises in dental, optical, and prescription charges demonstrate. Second, public enterprises have been transferred to the private sector through the sale of their assets. This has netted the Government billions of pounds. For example, British Gas sold in December 1986 raised £7·7b. Third, liberalisation refers to the removal of statutory barriers which prevent the private sector from competing in public sector markets. The liberalisation of the transport sector has ended the monopoly enjoyed by bus companies in urban and rural areas. Finally, services have been provided privately while remaining publicly funded. This has included contracting out work and proposals to issue educational and health vouchers which could be redeemed in the private sector.

The arguments in favour of privatisation stem from a belief that private sector provision is inherently more efficient and provides the consumer with greater choice than the public sector. This is due to the virtuous effects of competition and the stimulus to efficiency that the profit motive renders. The Adam Smith Institute has been a staunch proponent of privatisation and lobbied the Government to adopt privatisation. They argued that state provision of services is inefficient as there is no competition. Consequently, there are few incentives to be efficient and state bureaucrats attempt to maximise their own welfare which does not service public needs. Consumers are deprived of the opportunity to exercise choice in the market place. Consequently, the remedy suggested is the advent of competition which is a stimulus to efficiency.

The critics of privatisation have questioned the central tenet of the argument. Privatisation does not necessarily increase competition. The sale of state assets has created unaccountable private monopolies, British Telecom being a notable example. The embarrassment over their performance forced the Government to increase competition in its sales of the electricity industry. Similarly the concentration in ownership taking place in the contract cleaning industry has limited the competition occurring in competitive tendering exercises. In addition, the degree of competition in the nascent provider market has been questioned. The whole rationale of the planned development of hospital services with one District General Hospital per District serving a population of a quarter of a million people militates against the development of competition.

The efficiency of the private sector has been disputed. Privatisation of an industry may increase profits but this does not equate with increased efficiency. It may simply reflect a reduction in unprofitable but valued services, for example, the removal of rural telephone boxes. The trade unions argue that the ability of private firms to reduce costs when services are contracted out reflects inferior terms and conditions of employment, not greater efficiency. Market relationships have broader implications than simply cost considerations as Titmuss's (1970) study of blood donors in the USA illustrated. He examined blood donation arrangements in both countries and found that the level of serum hepatitis was higher in the USA than in Britain. He argued this was because in the USA, as donors were paid for blood donations there were incentives to lie about their attributes, while in Britain there was no financial incentive for donors to hide past illness. Consequently, changing incentives in an organisation by instigating financial rewards can have detrimental as well as positive effects.

In the competitive tendering debate there has often been a failure to differentiate between contracting out services, where a private firm takes over the supply of a service, and competitive tendering where local management have the opportunity to retain a service in-house if they compete effectively (Sheaff, 1988). The difference is important as competitive tendering enables management to exercise discretion in their approach which effects the consequences of competitive tendering.

Writers often focus on the origins of the policy in terms of government ideology which favours decreasing the size of the public sector and deregulating the labour market (Whitfield, 1983; Leedham, 1986). These approaches tend to ignore the manner in which managerial objectives have mediated the implementation of competitive tendering. Although some writers have rectified this situation, the emphasis is on the process of competitive tendering and the key actors involved.

Ascher (1987) suggests the results of the tendering exercise have been determined by political rather than economic considerations. Mailley (1987) emphasises the degree to which NHS managers have endeavoured to maintain service in-house. These approaches fail to specify the limits to managerial autonomy nor do they adequately address the material basis to competitive tendering and the links with the Government's strategy for the economy.

The Conservative Government's Approach to the Public Sector

The Government was elected on a platform committed to raising the competitiveness of the British economy. At the core of this strategy has been an attempt to restructure the economy by extending the scope of market relations through privatisation and deregulation. The means to restore the profitability of industry has been through opening up new markets to the private sector and the maintenance of low wages. Competitive tendering has been central to this policy and complements other initiatives. The partial abolition of the wages councils in 1986 was part of a package of measures to remove safeguards for the low paid. The legal restrictions on the trade unions and high levels of unemployment in the 1980s accentuated the difficulties of the low paid.

The Government portrays the British state as detrimental to the needs of capital. Its policies involve an explicit break with the Keynesian post-war consensus and the role of the welfare state has been criticised. Demand management policies are blamed for a neglect of the supply side of the economy, introducing rigidities into the economy. The public sector crowds out private industry as high taxes are levied to sustain public expenditure. This places an intolerable burden on the private sector which is exacerbated by the wasteful and bureaucratic nature of the public sector.

A second aim of government policy is to remove the rigidities in the economy to enable markets to work more efficiently. Trade unions affect the outcome of exchanges in the market. The Government's ideology of individualism views trade unions as coercive monopolies who use their market power to further the sectional interests of their members. Competitive tendering is complementary to the Government's aim of reducing trade union power.

Competitive tendering has created serious problems for the trade unions. It has opened up the spectre of large job losses and when services are contracted out conditions are less favourable to union membership as contractors are often hostile to unions. Union membership becomes fragmented and trade unions are traditionally strongest where trade union density is high. Finally, in an ideological climate hostile to trade unions their credability may be reduced if they are ineffective in combating government policy.

Cash limits have been the central policy the government has used to curb public expenditure. They were introduced in 1976 by a Labour Government to fulfil two functions. They needed to restore their credibility with the financial community and cash limits also helped to keep their income policy on course (Winchester, 1983). Since 1979 cash limits have had a more important role. The articulation of policy in cash terms was a natural outgrowth of the Government's early commitment to monetarism with the emphasis on reducing public expenditure and sustaining price stability. Cash limits have also introduced notions of ability to pay into the public sector. This eroded the traditional emphasis on comparability replacing it with market definitions of affordability and value for money.

The Government has encouraged the use of market forces and cooperation with the private sector as a way of increasing efficiency in the public sector. Consultants contracts were changed in 1980 to allow them to undertake more private sector work and still receive a full NHS salary. The 1988 Health and Medicines Act makes it easier for Health Authorities to raise their own income. *Working for Patients* by instigating a market for health services has provided scope for private sector expansion as the revised funding mechanism allows money to follow the patient regardless of where the patient is treated enabling Health Authorities to use private sector facilities. In the priority services *Caring for People* (Department of Health 1989c, 1989) also encourages local authorities to purchase services from the private sector. The Government has also encouraged a greater role for market forces in pay determination.

The Whitley System which has established pay in the NHS is a highly centralised system in which the trade unions are equal negotiating partners. The Government is antagonistic to the system as it rewards staff by length of service not primarily by performance. There is limited scope for variations in pay according to local market conditions and this inflexibility the Government deplores. The strengthening of management with the implementation of the Griffiths proposals and the shift of decision-making to unit level has increased managerial dissatisfaction with Whitleyism. Management want greater autonomy in determining pay so they are no longer bound by Whitley agreements.

The Government has eroded the Whitley system by establishing pay review bodies which cover more than 50 per cent of NHS staff. Increasingly pay targets are abandoned in favour of letting the market decide with increases in salaries for those with scarce skills. The importance of management has been reflected by steep rises in their salaries but they are subject to performance related pay. Furthermore, the pay of general managers has been removed from the Whitley system. The system is set for further devolution as self-governing hospitals will be allowed to set their own terms and conditions of employment and decide pay locally, creating a possible fatal haemorrhage for Whitley and the pay review bodies. Pay supplements decided by local management are being extended to difficult to recruit staff.

Competitive tendering has been part of the process of eroding Whitley. Health circular (83)18 on tendering procedures allowed bonus payments to be reduced below Whitley rates with staff side agreement in order to make an in-house tender competitive. This is one way in which competitive tendering has presented opportunities to management to re-assert managerial control and simultaneously generate financial savings.

This has been its attraction to the general managers in the NHS who in a climate of financial stringency, have seen the savings competitive tendering could bring, regardless of who won the tender. The process also enabled managers to negotiate changes in working practices due to the concern of staff not to jeopardise the chances of the in-house tender winning. Consequently, emphasis on the 'politics' of competitive tendering needs to move beyond individual's behaviour in the 'process' and acknowledge the economic interests that competitive tendering helped to serve.

The Evolution of Domestic Services in the NHS

Cleaning is the largest ancillary service in the NHS. In 1985/86 expenditure on domestic services in the NHS totalled £483m (National Audit Officer, 1987). The number of staff measured in Whole Time Equivalents (WTE) in 1985 totalled 54,220 (DHSS, 1987) a reduction from its peak of 68,579. This is due to the effects of technical change and the rationalisation of staff and frequencies that accompanied the introduction of bonus schemes in the late 1970s.

The majority of the expenditure (over 90 per cent) on domestic services is on labour costs and this naturally has been the target for reductions in the competitive tendering process. Domestic workers in the NHS are also characterised by their low pay.

The domestic function in hospitals has traditionally extended beyond cleaning to encompass other housekeeping duties. These include the distribution of linen, the labelling and distribution of staff uniforms, and serving meals and drinks. It is this patient contact that has established domestics as integral to the ward team. This reflects the evolution of hospital cleaning which has only established itself as a separate function since the 1960s.

The idea of employing specialist domestic managers was first suggested in a King's Fund report concerned with cleaning hospitals in the post-war era. The domestic supervisors who formed the nascent domestic departments in the 1950s were never intended to evolve into distinct departments. The domestic supervisors assisted the Matron and were under her control. The unplanned growth of domestic services in the 1950s led to appeals to formalise the process in the 1960s.

The catalyst for the establishment of separate domestic departments came from the implementation of the *Salmon Report* (MoH, 1966). This injected a new managerialism into the senior nursing structure. A corollary development was the absorbption by domestic staff of work previously performed by nursing staff.

The 1974 NHS reorganisation helped domestic management to gain the recognition and autonomy to which they aspired. The Hospital Management Committees were abolished and District functional managers were created. Domestic managers responsibility and authority were increased and crucially they held their own budgets. The 1974 reorganisation was subject to widespread criticism for creating a complex structure in which decision-making was too slow and distant from the hospital level.

The election of a conservative administration in 1979 brought further proposals for reorganisation of the NHS. *Patients First* (DHSS, 1979) sought to simplify the NHS by removing the area tier and devolving decision-making to local level while simultaneously strengthening accountability to Parliament. The 1982 reorganisation followed *Patients First* and required Health Authorities to arrange services into units of management. The emphasis on unit decision-making weakened the role of functional managers who frequently had to adopt an advisory role. Domestic managers became accountable to the Unit Administrator rather than the District Domestic Advisor. This pattern prevails currently although there is considerable diversity in sub-unit structures and attempts to restructure catering, cleaning, and laundry services into one hotel services department are common.

In February 1983 Norman Fowler announced the establishment of an inquiry into NHS management practices, led by Roy Griffiths. The central recommendation of the report was that general managers should be appointed at Authority and Unit level. The implementation of general management has led to greater emphasis on individual decisions rather than committee decisions and has attempted to increase the power and status of management in the NHS and confer on it greater legitimacy in order to weaken the professional ethos that pervades the NHS.

The implementation of Griffiths coincided with the competitive tendering exercise. The two measures shared the same pedigree. Consensus management symbolised the paternalistic management philosophy of the 1950s and 1960s. Industrial action in the 1970s and 1982 demonstrated that conflicts of interest existed as in any other organisation. General management was a culmination of the demise of this paternalistic ideology. The Government's quest for efficiency constantly reinforced to NHS managers the need to achieve their objectives in the least costly manner. This meant dispensing with some of the previous working practices. As early as 1984 the Tory Reform Group recognised the connection between General Management and competitive tendering:

> Private contractors will be natural allies of a Griffiths hospital general manager wishing to bypass pockets of resistance to new methods of working. (Tory Reform Group, 1984)

The weakening of functional management after the 1982 reorganisation and the implementation of Griffiths was to have a significant influence on the way in which competitive tendering was implemented. Performance related pay and fixed, short-term contracts have given general managers a powerful incentive to achieve their central objective of balancing their budget. Competitive tendering assisted this process.

The Development of Competitive Tendering in the NHS

Industrial action in the public sector in the winter of 1978/79 strengthened the Government's resolve to reduce trade union power and this coupled with its view of the inefficiency of the public sector, placed competitive tendering on the policy agenda. The deep recession stimulated the cleaning and catering trade associations to look for new markets in the public sector and they lobbied vigorously to encourage the introduction of comptitive tendering.

In 1980 and 1981, the Health Minister, Dr Vaughan, wrote to Health Authorities encouraging them to consider contracting out services in the ancillary services. The response from the NHS was unenthusiastic so the Government prepared a circular. This was never released in 1982 as planned. It was probably judged an inappropriate time to release the circular in the midst of a major pay dispute and in the aftermath of the 1982 reorganisation. The postponement was short-lived. In February 1983 DA (83)14 was published which confirmed the Government's intention to refund VAT paid by Authorities on private sector contracts. The measure evoked strong feelings among Authorities which were particularly angered at the short consultation period.

This reponse merely served to strengthen the Government's resolve. In September 1983 HC (83)18 was published which gave more specific instructions to Health Authorities. They were asked to test the cost effectiveness of their domestic, catering, and laundry services. Acceptance of the lowest tender was required unless 'compelling reasons' dictated otherwise. The intention to refund VAT on private contracts was maintained. Health Authorities had to submit a time-table for competitive tendering by February 1984.

In September 1983 the Government abolished the Fair Wages Resolution which although not universally welcomed by the contracting industries gave a further impetus to the use of private contractors in the NHS. The Fair Wages Resolution had prevented private contractors working on Government contracts from paying excessively low wages. Nonetheless, the widespread breach by Health Authorities who continued to specify rates of pay forced Kenneth Clarke to reiterate to the NHS that wage rates should not be stipulated.

Initially private contractors won the majority of domestic contracts, but increasingly the private contractors became agitated at their lack of success and a series of complaints against the NHS accused Health Authorities of deliberately trying to keep services in-house (Tory Reform Group, 1984; Sherman, J. 1986). This led to the chairman of the NHS Management Board intervening in January 1986 to curb the actions of Health Authorities who were requesting details of staffing levels and wages levels from contractors.

The competitive tendering exercise is estimated to have saved £105m (Table 22 below) of which half has come from savings made by in-house domestic contracts.

TABLE 22. *Estimated Savings from Competitive Tendering up to April 1988*

		Savings up to April 1988		
Service	*Expnd 1985/86* *£m*	*In-house* *£m*	*Contractor* *£m*	*Total* *£m*
Domestic	483	53·615	25·406	79·021
Catering	445	17·248	0·941	18·189
Laundry	231	7·072	1·579	8·654
TOTAL		77·935	27·926	105·861

SOURCE: NAO (1987) DHSS (1988)

The figures are only estimates and the National Audit Office (NAO) noted some inconsistency in the way savings were reported (NAO, 1987). For example, some Authorities included the cost of early retirement and redundancies while others did not. The timing of the tendering exercise affected the level of savings as many Authorities chose to tender after they had increased efficiency by investing in new equipment. The figures also ignore hidden costs which includes the management cost of implementing the policy.

The number of contracts won by private contractors and the number retained in-house are shown in Table 23.

These figures show that overall nearly 80 per cent of contracts are being won in-house. The particularly low level of penetration by private firms in catering is partly due to the larger capital outlays required than in domestics and the private firms dislike of fixed fee contracts which has discouraged tendering (Kelliher, 1987).

TABLE 23. *Contracts Awarded to April 1988*

Service	In-house	Contractor	Total
Domestic	775 (73%)	283 (27%)	1058
Catering	413 (95%)	21 (5%)	434
Laundry	151 (74%)	54 (26%)	205
TOTAL	1139 (79%)	358 (21%)	1697

SOURCE: Joint NHS Privatisation Research Unit (1988).

The figures also mask very great geographical variation in the penetration by private companies. In the Northern, North Western, and Trent Regional Health Authority, contractors were awarded less than 10 per cent of contracts up to September 1986. Conversely in North-West Thames Regional Health Authority the figure was 50–60 per cent (NAO, 1987). These variations reflect the poorer coverage of private firms in the North, and greater willingness to contract out services in the South of England.

Management Responses to Competitive Tendering

The accepted orthodoxy is that management is a reluctant partner in the competitive tendering exercise. This is attributed by Ascher (1987) to the process being imposed by government. Other writers (IPM/IDS, 1986; Mailley, 1987) emphasise the potential loss of control and flexibility to NHS managers if services are contracted out as well as uncertainty over their own future. Amongst personnel managers there is a desire not to jeopardise good industrial relations and concern to be a good employer (Cowan, 1984; IPM/IDS, 1986).

These responses give only a partial picture of NHS management views (Sheaff, 1988). The previous discussion on Griffiths indicated that general managers have the power and incentive to generate financial savings. Financial pressures have become more acute in the NHS since the early 1980s due to the demographic changes in the population, the rising cost and scope for technological intervention in health care, increased efficiency as manifested by higher throughput of patients with a stable budget and government strictures to Health Authorities to find efficiency savings, amounting to 0·5 per cent of their existing budgets in 1983/84. Consequently, general managers were likely to be well disposed towards competitive tendering as it offered the opportunity to reduce expenditure. It is also likely that attitudes to competitive tendering have changed as managers are encouraged to act commercially and have become more accustomed to cooperating with the private sector through income generation schemes. Finally, management cannot be treated homogenously but the differing perspectives within management needs to be unravelled.

Functional managers who are directly threatened if services are contracted out have been hostile to competitive tendering. The Association of Domestic Management opposed competitive tendering, concerned at the unfair advantage private contractors had obtained since the Government rescinded the Fair Wages Resolution (ADM, 1983). Personnel managers were concerned that competitive tendering would detract from the good employer philosophy that had prevailed in the NHS and this could sour industrial relations. They also expressed anxiety about the effects of having employees on different terms and conditions working alongside NHS staff if services were contracted out (IPM/IDS, 1986). To summarise, despite the reservations of particular groups of managers increasingly the wishes of general managers who have an interest in obtaining savings from the competitive tendering process have prevailed.

Trade Union Policy and Practice

A covert objective of the Government's tendering policy has been to reduce the power of public sector trade unions. The trade unions which organise ancillary staff in the NHS are NUPE and COHSE and to a lesser extent the GMB and T&GWU. These trade unions adopted an oppositional stance to competitive tendering. They initially tried to prevent Health Authorities complying with HC (83)18 and when this failed tried to influence the compilation of the specification. National union policy has discouraged involvement in preparing in-house tenders, due to the risk of the union being tarnished by acquiescence with worsening terms and conditions of employment. This position has not always been adhered to as the consequences of non-cooperation have often been greater deterioration of terms and conditions due to the loss of the contract to a private firm (Ascher 1987; Mailley 1987).

The unions have faced considerable difficulties in combating competitive tendering. The implementation of competitive tendering at local level over a lengthy period of time militated against effective national action. The emphasis on efficiency placed the unions in a position where they were susceptible to the criticism that they were defending outmoded working practices (Hastings *et al.*, 1982). Finally industrial action as a strategy is problematic due to the rivalry between trade unions in the NHS and because it does not immediately affect the employer but the user of the service. Yet users are an important constituency to be harnessed in action against privatisation. It is for these reasons that trade union policy at national level has frequently been to revert to the dissemination of information about contractors failures to discourage health authorities from using them.

The Impact of Competitive Tendering in the NHS: A Preliminary Evaluation

A central argument in favour of competitive tendering and the one which has most appeal to NHS managers is the money that competitive tendering saves. The source of these savings is disputed. For Forsyth (1982) it is the inherent innovation of the private sector and the lack of tolerance for trade union restrictive practices which accounts for the reduction in costs. Milne (1987) and Domberger (1987) both suggest that the introduction of competition is the catalyst which increases efficiency. Milne acknowledges that the reduction in costs was largely due to reductions in the specification yet this conflicts with his assertion that it is increased competition that increases productivity. Cowan (1984) cites the superior calibre of management which enables private contractors to generate savings. This argument ignores the savings which have been made under in-house managements.

The influence of competition has been questioned. The lack of interest amongst catering companies has been mentioned previously. Private sector interest has been sapped by their diminishing ability to win tenders and the damaging publicity that has plagued private contractors. The cost of preparing tenders is a further discouragement and has been estimated at £1,000–3,000 per tender (Hartley and Huby, 1985). Since 1983 there has been a trend towards concentration in the contract cleaning industry to the extent that two companies, BET and Hawley, held 53 per cent of NHS domestic contracts (LRD, 1987). Nonetheless there has been vigorous competition between the private sector and in-house tenders.

Other explanations are less comforting. The labour movement's analysis (LRD, 1987; ALA, 1988) suggests that financial savings are only achieved at the expense of a reduction in staffing levels, worse terms and conditions of employment, and lower standards of service. Job losses caused by competitive tendering up to mid-1986 were estimated at 9,500 ancillary staff in the NHS (LRD, 1987). A report from the Association of London Authorities highlights forty cases of reduced hours and staffing levels in cases where services were retained in-house (ALA, 1988).

Contractors have maintained a practice of paying Whitley rates. It is the reduction of the hours in the contract which has led to the biggest cuts in pay. Paradoxically the most protracted disputes have occurred in situations where existing contractors faced with increased competition have had to make radical reductions in hours. At Barking, for Crothalls to retain the contract, hours had to be reduced by 41 per cent. This led to domestics pay being reduced from £87 to £47 (Huws, 1985). Contractors also tend to employ staff for less than sixteen hours a week so they are not covered by employment legislation and are below the national insurance threshold.

Scientific evidence indicates the importance of cleanliness in providing good health care. A survey carried out in 1980 of 18,000 patients in forty-three hospitals discovered that one in ten patients developed infection after admission. This represents not only a 'cost' to the patient but a waste of resources for the NHS. Critics suggest that the use of private contractors leads to a lowering of standards.

The private contractors raison d'etre is to make a profit. The contract manager is accountable to the company and their shareholders. Any additional costs incurred in meeting the contract will impinge on the needs to maximise profit. Conversely, in-house services are under the direct control of the Health Authority and are geared to providing a service.

Although critics of competitive tendering usually reserve most criticism for private contractors, the competitive tendering process itself may reduce standards. This is a consequence of the Government's insistence on a system of competitive tendering which emphasises acceptance of the lowest cost tender rather than providing a cost effective service. This has detrimental effects, as the quality of training and equipment used is not given sufficient weight to sustain standards. Successful tendering becomes subject to the vagaries of the market forces—the ability to obtain cheap labour and the degree to which firms can cross subsidise activities to win tenders, by submitting loss leaders.

The NHS Joint Privatisation Research Unit documents sixty-four recorded failures by private companies between 1983–May 1987. Failures are interpreted broadly and include not only cases where contractors have been sacked but also cases where contractors have withdrawn or faced substantial complaints. Typical complaints include inadequate cleaning of toilets and ward areas, the discovery of food particles under beds and the use of inexperienced staff who are ignorant of cross infection hazards.

It is frequently nursing staff who have to cope with the reduction in domestic hours and standards. Domestics are widely regarded as part of the patient care team. The Government argued that a reduction in costs of hotel services would liberate money for patient care. Health Authorities rejected this division between patient care and ancillary services arguing domestics contributed to the patient care team (NHS Unlimited, 1984). Research (Hart, 1988) confirms that domestic work is more than just cleaning. Domestics performed an important informal role in patient care through their involvement with patients and they were a source of stability in a ward characterised by frenetic activity and changing personnel.

Efficiency measures which commenced in the 1970s with the introduction of Measured Day Work schemes affected the role of the domestic. By specifying an agreed level of pay for an agreed level of performance, managerial control was enhanced. This followed the dictum of scientific management which separated mental and manual work through a fine division of labour, with management allocating and planning work potentially increasing their control. Competitive tendering with its need to work to a measured contract specification has further reduced the autonomy of domestic staff. The reduction in hours and frequency of cleaning has restricted domestics' jobs to cleaning tasks.

These changes affect the boundary between nursing and non-nursing duties. Persistent shortages of nursing staff and changing theories of patient care with the adoption of the nursing process in the 1970s have also contributed to this shifting boundary. Competitive tendering has frequently increased the workload of nurses, because the tightness of contracts prevented domestics carrying out tasks other than cleaning. At Papworth Hospital competitive tendering led to a reduction in the night domestic service. This caused nurses to have to make patients' tea and collect the cups, tasks previously performed by domestics. Disagreements arose over which staff should unpack linen and clear up spillages at night (Hicks, 1985).

A related issue is flexibility. The ambiguity in the nursing and domestic role used to be resolved informally where standards and tasks would be established on the ward. This created flexibility for ward sisters who could rely on domestic staff to perform tasks beyond their work specification. Competitive tendering has reduced the scope for discretion by specifying the exact contract and by limiting hours preventing duties being performed outside of the contract.

Competitive tendering has made the monitoring of performance a salient issue. The DHSS does not differentiate between the monitoring of in-house and private contracts but it is probable that private firms will need closer surveillance. The profit margins and their need to make profit will tempt private firms to cut corners. This is lent credence by Williamson's work (Williamson, 1986). Williamson's theory is based on transactions costs and he argues that market relations are susceptible to 'opportunistic behaviour'. This is a situation where individuals pursue goals at variance with those employing their services creating inefficiencies. This particularly occurs where there is 'bounded rationality' which would be the situation in cleaning where uncertainty exists over the measurement of standards of cleanliness.

Consequently, the change from in-house provision to private provision has implications beyond financial considerations. It may be difficult for Health Authorities to monitor the performance of private contractors due to the uncertainty mentioned above. Health Authorities have few sanctions they can apply as contract staff are not directly under their control. Imposing financial penalties can make it harder for the contractor to rectify matters as terminating a contract requires DHSS permission and there is a significant cost involved in re-tendering.

Summary

Competitive tendering in the NHS was not entirely unknown in that certain Authorities had contracted out services prior to 1983, mainly due to labour shortages. Mandatory competitive tendering with the central goal of reducing expenditure was a different phenomenon which has generated a burgeoning literature. One problem associated with this literature is its treatment of management. It is usually assumed that management are hostile to competitive tendering and are portrayed as weak, with little discretion to influence policy implementation. Yet this seems implausible.

In a climate of financial stringency and attempts to strengthen NHS management, certain managers might welcome competitive tendering as offering opportunities to create financial savings. It may simultaneously enable managers to increase their managerial control by allowing them to negotiate local employment packages which deviate from Whitley agreements. However, the diversity of managerial goals in the NHS needs to be recognised. This situation is exacerbated by the lack of one clearly defined goal for the NHS which equates with the profit objective in the private sector, nor is there unanimity on how to achieve objectives in the NHS. Consequently, competitive tendering may be favoured by certain managers committed to financial objectives but rejected by others whose central concern is the maintenance of professional standards.

The issues of financial savings and the connections with service standards has only recently begun to be explored. It is frequently argued that competition creates financial savings yet this is asserted, not explained. Terminology including 'efficiency', 'savings' and 'competition' is used uncritically but the effects on staff and patients, difficulties for management and implications for service standards remained invisible.

As experience of competitive tendering has been gained a fuller appraisal of its impact has become possible. The cost savings have been valued and this has led to an extension of the competitive tendering process to additional services notably portering and pathology services. It has also provided the catalyst to change work organisation with hotel services departments emerging deploying staff more flexibly.

Nonetheless, management also recognise that savings frequently only resulted from the reduction of standards and the transfer of duties to nursing staff. Ironically as anxieties about nursing recruitment and retention have surfaced due to demographic pressure and the impact of Project 2,000 there have been attempts to reinstate the informal care role of the support worker (Ball, 1989) so that nurses can be divested of 'non-nursing duties' in order to use scarce nursing skills more productively. In addition the contracting arrangements in the provider market have provided a stimulus to increased managerial interest in setting standards for services. Recognition of the trade off's between costs and standards has led to a concern for increased standards in the second round of tendering with costs rising accordingly. This is the lead that needs to be followed as the NHS enters a new market-orientated era and is in contrast to the first round of tendering as illustrated by the case study that follows.

Greenbelt District

Greenbelt Health Authority covers a predominantly rural area punctuated by several major centres of population. The resident population of the District is approximately 290,000. The Authority employs over 6,000 staff and its total expenditure exceeded £62m in 1986/87. The management structure of the Authority will only be sketched as it has changed on a number of occasions since 1982. The salient points concern the increasing importance of decision-making at unit level after the 1982 reorganisation, the reduction in influence of functional managers and the implementation of general management.

Greenbelt had four management units for acute services, community services, mental handicap services and for mental health services. The units were headed by general managers who represented their units on the District Management Board (DMB), which was presided over by the District General Manager. The Acute unit accounted for £25m of expenditure (1986/87) and consisted of six hospitals which were situated in the main town of the Authority. The opening of the new District General Hospital (DGH) in 1984 led to a rationalisation of acute services.

The case study focuses on the provision of domestic services at the new DGH. The Hospital, situated on a greenfield site a couple of miles from the centre of the town, has 280 beds and provides the main Accident and Emergency Service for the Authority. As the Hospital was new, domestic staff were to be recruited after the contract was awarded, so there was no threat to existing jobs. Industrial relations in Greenbelt were cooperative and there is no militant legacy. The management style had the reputation for being more innovative than other Authorities in the Region. Its approach to competitive tendering was characteristic in terms of the rapidity and enthusiasm with which government policy was implemented.

Domestic Services in Greenbelt Health Authority

The attempt to reduce costs and increase productivity in ancillary services was a process initiated in the late 1960s. Trade unions who represented low paid workers viewed bonus schemes as an opportunity to increase ancillary workers' pay (Winchester, 1983). In Greenbelt bonus schemes began to be introduced for domestic staff in 1974. A senior manager stated that from 1977 bonus schemes led to an annual saving of £$\frac{1}{4}$m. This resulted from reducing staff levels, particularly by the removal of elder staff, who could not perform at the higher rates of work demanded of them.

Despite these changes management believed that there was still scope for further savings. There was opposition from nursing and medical staff to reductions in standards and frequencies. In an era of consensus management and before financial pressures were as acute as in the 1980s the nursing view prevailed. The opportunity to push through further savings came under the auspices of the Cleaning and Maintenance Research Services Organisation (CAMRASO) who had developed a method of measuring the cleanliness of hard surfaces. In 1983 trials we carried out which varied the cleaning routine (Appendix 1). The implementation of reduced cleaning frequencies led to further savings of £180,000 per annum on a District Domestic budget of over £2m.

Consequently prior to competitive tendering steps had been taken to achieve savings and improve productivity. There were limits to this process due to the resistance of medical and nursing staff to reduced standards, who prior to the advent of general management and the financial pressures of the 1980s were better able to resist reductions in standards. Nonetheless, these changes made senior domestic managers confident that they could meet the challenge of competitive tendering. This confidence proved to be unfounded.

The Competitive Tendering Process

Greenbelt management acted rapidly to implement Government policy on competitive tendering. They began to prepare for competitive tendering after draft circular DA(83)14 was issued in February 1983, prior to the compulsory imposition of competitive tendering in September. This reflected senior management's commitment towards competitive tendering which was symptomatic of an innovative management style. The decision to carry out a competitive tendering exercise was stimulated by the building of the new District General Hospital, which provided an opportunity to carry out a tendering exercise in a new environment which would be untainted by existing labour relations practices in the District.

In February 1983 a draft circular was issued for consultation purposes on the contracting out of domestic, catering, and laundry services in the NHS. The circular was discussed at the District Management Team (DMT) meeting of 3 March 1983. This was a forum for the most senior officers in the Authority, presided over by the District Nursing Officer, District functional heads including Finance, Personnel and Supplies. The DMT met a few days before the Health Authority and made recommendations which became policy if endorsed by the Authority meeting.

At the DMT meeting competitive tendering was discussed. Senior management welcomed the draft circular and viewed it as a constructive attempt to improve the performance of the Authority's in-house services by providing targets for managers; and acting as a spur to improve working practices. The District Adminstrator emphasised that the Authority had no particular desire to contract out services but was determined to ensure cost effectiveness.

He noted some specific points for consideration. The need for an accurate and clear specification was noted and that while briefing meetings should be arranged the danger of collusion by private firms had to be safeguarded against. The possible industrial relations consequences of the exercise were raised and the need to fully consult with staff to avoid jeopardising good relations was suggested. Finally the District Administrator was wary of the prescriptive nature of the circular and specifically wanted to retain the option of not accepting the lowest tender with the understanding that the costs of the service would be reduced to the lowest tender level over time. Simiarly he was concerned at contracting out a capital intensive service (e.g. laundry) which would be difficult to return in-house if the service became uncompetitive. Despite these reservations over the process the overall initiative was welcomed by the DMT.

The District Health Authority met a few days later on 8 March and considered the recommendations. The Health Authority was supportive of managements initiative. The limited influence of members is well documented (Haywood and Renade, 1985; Ham, 1986). Chris Ham's (1986) study in Bath and Croydon specifically investigates members influence in bringing competitive tendering on to the Authority's agenda and their involvement in the resolution of the tendering issue. He concludes that their role was limited, they merely responded to a central government initiative and then allowed officers to deal with the minutiae of the tendering exercise.

In Greenbelt members confined themselves to a general statement of intent, while emphasising the first consideration was to safeguard patient care:

> The market could be tested and tenders invited provided that comparisons of the bids by the commercial firms and by in-house services were fair and equitable. DHA minutes 8 March 1983

Members also drew specific attention to the need to closely monitor services if they were contracted out to prevent a deterioration in standards.

Having endorsed the DMT's decision to proceed with competitive tendering the Membership left the implementation of the policy to the District Administrator. He delegated a large part of the work to the District Domestic Manager who unlike other functional managers was not hostile to competitive tendering partly due to his private sector orientation where he had worked before entering the NHS. The District Supplies Manager and the Unit Administrator of the Acute unit were also heavily involved.

Preparing the Specification

The order in which services were tendered for was considered important. Domestic and Catering Services at the new DGH wre tendered for first. The new Hospital was a flagship contract and would attract considerable private sector interest. It was a natural choice to start with as there were no existing staff in post, reducing potential industrial relations difficulties and it could be carried out during the commissioning of the hospital minimising the disruption caused by the process.

Competitive tendering proved to be an extremely time consuming task for management. Three committees were established, the most influential being the Steering Committee which made policies and compiled the invitation to tender documents. The Steering committee consisted of the Unit Administrator, Hospital Manager, District Supplies Manager, Nurse Manager, Finance Representative, Management Services Representative and the District Domestic Manager. They compiled the specification although the bulk of the work was carried out by the Domestic department.

The invitation to tender document was a bulky document split into a number of sections. It included the conditions of contract which were divided into the special conditions of contract and the standard conditions of contract. The special conditions applied to the specific hospital as opposed to the standard conditions which were the conditions laid down by the Health Authority to cover all tendering exercises in the District. The special conditions stated the purposes of domestic services and drew attention to the relevant law that staff needed to be aware of. Finally it covered the financial requirements expected of the successful contractor, for example, the necessary insurance cover.

The operational policy stated the policies required to run an effective service for the needs of the hospital in conjunction with the contract specification. It included all areas to be cleaned and other services required, e.g. window cleaning or curtain changing, and made clear where for security reasons, cleaning would not be allowed when the department was closed. It also placed an obligation on the contractor to allow the Health Authority's Control of Infection Team to monitor the service and required a quality control system to be established by the contractor.

The specification detailed the exact frequency and type of clean required in all areas of the hospital. Each area was coded according to the differing cleanliness required in different parts of the hospital. Cleaning and nurse support duties were listed and a frequency was attached to the procedure. The specification represented the core of the tendering exercise and the level of services and consequently standards of cleanliness should have matched the requirements of the specification.

The other two committees had less gargantuan tasks than the Steering committee. The coordinating group, whose membership comprised hospital level domestic, administrative, and personnel representatives as well as staff side representatives, discussed the policies decided by the Steering Group. It acted as a purely consultative forum and consequently the ablity of the staff side to influence the specification was very limited.

During the summer of 1983 the documentation was prepared. Greenbelt was one of the first Health Authorities to tender for services with mandatory tendering only being announced in September, when Greenbelt was well advanced on its tendering exercise. Consequently officers in the authority had little guidance available to them on how they should carry out the policy.

Assessing the Tenders

The District Domestic Manager and the District Supplies Manager worked closely together and approached the National Trade Association of the contract cleaning industry for a list of private firms which might wish to tender. A regional list of approved firms did not exist at this point. Twenty companies were approached in August 1983 with a detailed questionnaire which included questions on the terms and conditions of employment, the financial position of the company and their experience of health service cleaning. Contractors were responsive to the questionnaires confident that they were likely to win and not yet wary of the health service as they were to become in the face of bad publicity and low success rates.

On the basis of the questionnaire responses, ten firms were invited to join the Health Authority's approved list of companies at the beginning of September. The companies were then invited for interview. In most instances the companies sent their Marketing Director and their Contracts Manager, who were interviewed by senior management.

The interviews were comprehensive and included questions on terms and conditions of employment, staff training and equipment to be used but focused particularly on the financial viability of the firm (which required bank references) and the nature of the staff to be employed, particularly the experience of the Contract Manager. Finally the firms were asked to give details of contracts in the NHS so that these managers could be approached and site visits carried out. This process led to a further elimination of five companies and the remaining five firms were invited to tender at the beginning of October 1983.

At the meeting of the District Management Team of 6 October 1983 a paper from the Unit Administrator was considered which set out the protocol for competitive tendering at the District General Hospital. The DMT agreed that tenderers should be required to quote for both three and five year periods. Minimum wages were not to be stipulated but the tender had to identify the proposed wages structure. The successful firm was also expected to satisfy existing occupational health requirements for staff.

The Health Authority held a briefing meeting on the site three weeks after tenders had been invited on 27 October 1983. It was believed this would be the fairest way to ensure that any additional information supplied was given to all contractors. The only reservation being that it might offer the contractors an opportunity to collude over the tender price. The trade unions asked to be involved in the briefing sessions but this was rejected by management.

The in-house tender was drawn up by the Steering Committee, the bulk of the work being carried out by the District Domestic Manager assisted by Management Services. This process created considerable tensions between Management Services and the District Domestic Manager. He felt that the number of hours proposed for the tender, which were based on work study hours as covered by Whitley agreements, was a reflection of negotiating strength between unions and management at national level rather than the actual hours needed to clean a hospital of that size.

The District Domestic Manager wished to reduce the number of hours in the contract to a more competitive level. Similarly he wanted to depress bonus scheme levels to below Whitley rates and used the provisions in circular HC(83)18 concerning in-house tenders as a justification for this:

> This would not rule out an undertaking in the tender to achieve specific savings under a revision of the bonus scheme if this had been agreed with staff interests.

Management services locally refused to adjust the standard hours or to change the performance level below Whitley agreements. The District Domestic Manager appealed to Regional Management Services who also rejected the argument leaving a tender which the domestic manager believed had too many hours included to make it competitive.

The closing date for the receipt of tenders was 25 November 1983 and tenders were opened on 28 November. The assessment team consisted of the Hospital Manager, the District Supplies Manager, a Finance Representative and two Health Authority Members. The appraisal team met on two occasions and each tender was scrutinised with the financial viability of each company being carefully considered. In accordance with DHSS guidelines the in-house tender was considered against the lowest tender from a commercial firm. This involved adjustments to the initial tender price to enable a fair comparison to be made. The in-house tender was removed at this stage because its price was over £60,000 more per annum than any of the private sector bids.

Two companies whose tender prices were competitive were allowed to reconsider their planned distribution of staff in the hospital because the Health Authority considered the distribution to be unbalanced. They were not allowed to change the price of the contract. Between 6 December when the Appraisal Team first considered the tenders, and 14 December when final recommendations were made detailed analysis of the tenders were made and the short-listed companies interviewed. The

TABLE 24. *Cost Comparisons of Tenders*

Contractor	*Total Cost Year 1 & 2* £	*WTE*	*Year 1*	*Year 2*	*Total Cost Labour Year 1 & 2* £	*Total Cost Materials Year 1 & 2* £	*Total Cost Equipment Year 1 & 2* £
A (In House)	596,074	57·89	296,881	299,193	567,050	20,709	8,315
B (Bonus Clean)	423,923	45·68	207,735	216,188	396,497	16,226	11,200
C	414,705	29·37	207,880	206,825	384,983	17,410	12,312
D	468,380	40·03	234,940	233,440	457,578	6,200	4,602
E	452,962	40·51	220,992	231,970	427,034	17,333	8,595

SOURCE: Greenbelt DHA Tender Document

TABLE 25. *Comparison of In-House and Bonus Clean Staffing and Cost Levels*

IN-HOUSE *Grade*	*WTE*	*Basic Rate £*	*Enhancements £*	*NI & Sup. £*	*Total £*	
Manager	1·00	—	—	—	64	(Cost of re-grading existing manager
Supervisors	3·63	75·92	9·41	12·70	355	
Other Staff	3·38	66·88	11·87	10·51	346	
Other Staff	49·88	65·84	6·01	8·93	4,029	
Other Staff	—	—	—	—	—	
TOTAL	57·89			Cost per week	4,794	
	Annual cost (× 52·143) 250,000 + 4% Pay Award + Contract Window Cleaning etc. =				284,590	
CONTRACTOR B						
Manager	1·00	150·00	—	17·10	175	
Supervisors	2·38	74·00	—	5·32	185	
Dom & Cl	34·00	65·84	9·38	5·38	2,740	
Dom & Cl	8·30	65·84	—	5·38	592	
TOTAL	45·68			Cost per week	3,692	
			Annual cost (× 52·143) =		192,514	

SOURCE: Greenbelt DHA Tender Documents.

details of the tenders are shown in Table 24. The difference in staffing levels and costs between the successful tender and the in-house service is shown in Table 25.

Bonus Clean who were awarded the contract were questioned closely about the low price of their tender. It was clear to Health Authority management that the contract was a loss leader because Bonus Clean's price was £25,000 per annum lower than other private firms' tenders which had similar staffing costs. The Marketing Manager acknowledged that it was a 'no profit' contract. He explained that Bonus Clean wished to establish themselves in the NHS market and winning the prestigious contract in a new hospital would assist in this process. It would also place them in an advantageous position to win other contracts in the Authority.

Greenbelt management's stance was that they had to provide a cost effective service and were unconcerned at Bonus Clean's loss leader behaviour provided assurances were given that the specification would be fulfilled. In retrospect some managers felt that the Marketing Managers approach, which was to win new contracts (but not to manage them profitably), was at odds with the Managing Director's need to make each contract operate at a profit. Consequently the assurances given by the Marketing Manager proved to be hollow.

Senior management accepted Bonus Clean's assurances and recommended to the District Health Authority that the tender be accepted. The decision was ratified by the Authority.

Bonus Clean won the contract on a price of £207,735 for the first year (Table 24). The labour intensive nature of domestic services is apparent from the tender documentation as £194,045 of the £207,735 contract price was attributable to labour costs. This represented 93 per cent of the total cost for a year. Consequently, the major factor in the discrepancy in price between the in-house tender and the contractor's price was in the cost of labour. This cost had two dimensions. First, the quantity of labour used and second, the terms and conditions under which that labour was employed. In terms of the quantity of labour used Bonus Clean planned to use nearly 500 hours per week less than the in-house team to clean the hospital (Table 26). Bonus Clean's employment terms were also inferior to the NHS in respect of bonus payments, holiday pay and sickness pay (Table 27).

Variations in Management Attitudes

The attitudes of managers were more diverse than the cautious welcome members gave to competitive tendering. The most enthusiastic supporters of competitive tendering came from within the senior ranks of administration. The District Administrator believed competitive tendering presented an opportunity to rigorously examine the standards of service required and bring about changes in working practices which would have been difficult to remove without the threat of competitive tendering. He suggested that it was an indictment of NHS management that the policy had to be imposed as this demonstrated lax managerial commitment. He viewed his role as ensuring that management commit-

ORDER NUMBER

PO NYAATP08

BOOK NUMBER

9433887

BAY NUMBER

2343-8

AUTHOR	Paton, C and Bach, S
TITLE	Case Studies in Health Policy and Management

ment existed for the exercise and fulfilling the Government's timetable for competitive tendering.

Foremost in senior managers support for competitive tendering were the financial benefits that accrued from the exercise. The Acute unit in Greenbelt had been struggling to remain financially viable since the new Hospital opened with the workload exceeding expectations. In 1986/87 the Acute unit overspent by £475,000 and a similar overspend was projected for 1987/88. The situation had been exacerbated by Government policy, consequently in 1987/88 the District had to find £527,000 in efficiency savings, these developments made competitive tendering a more alluring prospect to senior management.

Senior management also saw benefits in contracting out services and this appears to have been the initial preference of certain senior managers. Memories of the so-called 'Winter of Discontent' in 1979 and

TABLE 26. *Comparison of Proposed Staffing Levels between Bonus Clean and the In-House Service.*

	Whole Time Equivalents (WTE)	*Standard Hours (Per week)*
1 Bonus Clean	45·68	1,827
2 In-house	57·89	2,315
Difference (2–1)	12.21	488

SOURCE: Greenbelt DHA: Tender Documents.

TABLE 27. *Comparison of Terms of Employment between Bonus Clean and the NHS.*

	Bonus Clean	*NHS (current in-house service)*
Basic Pay	Whitley rates but 6–12 months in arrears.	Whitley rates, increases backdated to April plus 17·3% fixed bonus.
Enhancements	Double time for working Sundays.	Double time for working Sundays, evenings and Saturdays.
Bank Holidays	Double time *or* a day off in lieu.	Double time *and* a day off in lieu.
Holiday entitlement	10 days unpaid, after a year's employment.	20 days paid, after a year's employment.
Sick Pay	None.	Sick pay after 4 months employment.
Statutory Sick Pay	Ineligible below National Insurance threshold.	Eligible.
Employment rights	Ineligible as work less than 16 hours per week.	Mostly eligible as work over 16 hours per week.

SOURCE: Greenbelt DHA: Tender Documents.

the nurses' strike in 1982 were fresh in mind. This legacy of industrial action in which ancillary staff featured prominently made it attractive to divest themselves of this group of staff. The simplicity of only having to deal with one contract manager also proved attractive.

Functional managers were less sanguine about competitive tendering. The District Catering Manager submitted a paper to the Authority outlining his concerns:

> I am not in favour of contracting out catering services partly becaue of the involvement with other disciplines such as portering, domestic, and nursing. It would be difficult to achieve harmony of the service but more important I believe there would be a lowering of standards if the contractor could cater for a lower figure than we do already and still make a profit.

Domestic managers felt bitter about the imposition of competitive tendering, viewing it as a criticism of the way in which they managed the service. They felt singled out for treatment when other groups of staff appeared less efficient, yet these practices were condoned by management. They resented the quantity of work involved in the process and felt work preparing specifications would assist private contractors to take their jobs. Senior management were not viewed as supportive, a Domestic Manager commented:

> It was a 'save money at any cost' approach. They didn't understand the consequences on morale. I felt I was fighting our own management.

Nursing staff were also anxious about competitive tendering. Ward Sisters feared that if cleaning was contracted out they would have less control over domestics' work on their ward and the standards of cleanliness on the ward. However they acknowledged that the growth of domestic departments in the 1970s had already eroded the influence they could exert over how domestics carried out their work. Ward Sisters also were anxious that if domestic staff had to accept poorer terms and conditions of employment this would be demoralising and coupled with less hours in the contract could undermine standards.

Personnel managers expressed reservations about competitive tendering. Initial anxieties concerned the novelty of the process and possible inadequate knowledge to implement the policy smoothly. Industrial relations difficulties were largely discounted due to the acquiescent nature of ancillary staff in the District. Greater concern was expressed about the difficulties of recruiting staff if competitive tendering pushed down wage levels, and jeopardising the good employer image which Greenbelt tried to cultivate. Scepticism was expressed about if competitive tendering would reduce trade union influence because trade union power rested with nursing not ancillary staff in Greenbelt.

Personnel Managers acknowledged that competitive tendering had been finance orientated. The prime responsibility of District level officers for professional standards had been subservient to the Unit and District General Managers overriding need to balance the books. This had implications for personnel managers, one unit had decided the most efficient system involved employing some cleaners for five hours per week. This created difficulties for personnel managers who had the task of recruiting staff for those hours.

Personnel management had a limited role in competitive tendering and were not involved in either drawing up the specification or on the assessment team. They were important in persuading the trade unions to submit an in-house tender but mainly administered decisions taken rather than initiated those decisions. Nonetheless personnel officers saw the importance of competitive tendering as offering opportunities in the future to adopt a strategic view and be more active in the establishment of policy. This could be helped by the establishment of unit personnel officers who could work more closely as part of the unit management team.

The Trade Union Response

The trade unions did not appear to have a major role in competitive tendering for domestic services. This is partly attributable to the industrial relations in Greenbelt which did not have a history of strong trade union activity. Trade union organisation and strength was most developed amongst nursing staff in Greenbelt's large number of long-stay institutions.

Competitive tendering was a novel experience when the tender was prepared for the new Hospital. Consequently the trade unions at national level were still formulating their response. At local level, as there were no existing staff, it was a less contentious issue. The threat posed by competitive tendering was to future not current jobs. Trade union involvement was purely on a consultation basis. Management viewed competitive tendering as their function and did not involve the unions in the preparation of the specification. The unions were represented on one consultative committee but not on the key Steering committee which made policies and compiled the invitation to tender documents. They were also not involved in the assessment process.

When the contract was awarded the T&GWU started to recruit domestic staff. They were aware of their inferior terms and conditions of employment but there had been no industrial relations difficulties. The T&GWU requested a meeting with the Managing Director. At the meeting Bonus Clean agreed to some improvements and decided to recognise the local branch of the T&GWU. The T&GWU Branch Secretary felt that by pushing up the labour costs of Bonus Clean the union had helped to prevent them winning other contracts in Greenbelt. The T&GWU Branch Secretary cooperated with management when the contract was put out to tender for the second time, which meant colluding with management on reducing the bonus paid. However he felt this was serving his members better than by refusing to cooperate and risking the service being contracted out.

The Experience of Private Provision of Domestic Services

When Bonus Clean were awarded the contract the Hospital had planned to open in May 1984. However a series of delays prevented the opening until October 1984. Patients were not admitted until December 1984. Nonetheless Bonus Clean began to prepare for the start of the contract by recruiting staff from July. The critical appointment being the contract manager. Bonus Clean had to be very flexible during this period and despite the delays in the opening no extra costs were incurred by the Authority.

Throughout the Commissioning period a satisfactory level of cleanliness was maintained. This was during a period of considerable upheaval with large flows of traffic in equipment and furniture through the hospital. Bonus Clean were cooperative in making the adjustments required of them often at short notice. However at this stage there were no patients in the Hospital so the cleaning task was considerably easier.

The Health Authority felt that the contracting out of the service did not diminish their responsbility for ensuring that a satisfactory service was provided. A monitoring system was instigated which started in February 1985. The monitoring system consisted of a monitoring officer taking approximately 1,500 observations per month. This consisted of physically checking for signs of dust and dirt. Each observation was categorised as acceptable or a failure depending on the cleanliness expected as specified in the tender. A performance figure was calculated using the following formula:

$$\text{Performance (\%)} = \frac{\text{number of satisfactory inspections}}{\text{number of observations}} \times 100$$

The results were prepared monthly and discussed by the Hospital Managers with Bonus Clean. Bonus Clean were meant to have their own quality control system, but the proformas used by Bonus Clean supervisors were treated with suspicion by hospital management who, as the contract proceeded, questioned the thoroughness of the process.

The first full month of monitoring by the Health Authority in February 1985 showed a deterioration in the fabric of the carpets on certain wards. This was drawn to the attention of Bonus Clean who rectified the situation quickly. Hospital management suspected the deterioration occurred due to the lack of training of newly appointed staff and the company not having recruited the actual number of staff as detailed in their tender document.

Hospital management were tolerant of the lapses in standards assuming that the situation would improve as staff became better trained and staffing levels improved. The District Domestic Manager who was responsible for maintaining standards of cleanliness took a less lenient attitude. After informal approaches to the Contract Manager had limited effect, he formally met with her on 11 March 1985 and catalogued a series of complaints. The marked deterioration in the standards of cleanliness of the carpets on a number of wards and the growing number of stains indicated that the frequency of cleaning in the contract was not being adhered to. Other concerns included inadequate dusting and poorly cleaned windows. In a letter to the contracts manager on 15 March confirming their conversation at the meeting of 11 March, the District Domestic Manager gave the contractor fourteen days to correct these faults.

On 18 March the situation had deteriorated to the extent that the District Domestic Manager was forced to write to Bonus Clean's Area Manager and mentioned nineteen areas of the hospital, including two operating theatres, which were not cleaned to an adequate standard. The District Domestic Manager forcefully expressed his concern:

> It does appear that failure by staff employed to adhere to the frequencies laid down in the schedules for this department is a result of insufficient hours being employed within this area and inadequacies of training. As an example, this morning your staff had left a solution of Hycoline in the tank of the scrubbing machine which was left in a dirty condition in the theatre cleaner's cupboard, which was stored in an upright position. The member of staff on duty this morning when asked why she had not emptied the machine, replied that she had not been taught how to empty it. It appears that when the monitoring officer discussed the shortcomings of the service with your supervisor, the impression was given that she did not consider it her duty to carry out a quality control check of work carried out by your operatives.

An additional concern was lapses of security that were occurring when Domestics omitted to lock rooms after evening cleaning. This led the Unit Management Team to have their first detailed discussion about low standards of cleaning in the hospital on 23 May 1985. As a result of these criticisms and complaints Bonus Clean corrected these faults on the wards but at the expense of other departments where standards began to fall.

These poor standards of cleanliness can be gauged from the Domestic Monitoring reports (Appendix 2). During the whole contract period Bonus Clean averaged a 69 per cent performance but this dropped to 42 per cent in the closing month of their contract. Complaints continued to focus on the appearance of the hospital and included the presence of stains on carpets, scuffed floors, dirty toilets, and the absence of domestic staff who dusted wards correctly. Appendix 3 documents these complaints in detail.

Management Action to Improve the Service

Although standards improved marginally in the Autumn of 1985 the situation was sufficiently serious that management adopted a number of measures to try and improve standards. The approach adopted consisted of using the monitoring system to impress upon Bonus Clean the magnitude of the problem. The Health Authority instigated a monitoring system in February 1985 but this was very much an *ad hoc* development as management increasingly recognised that they needed to ensure that they were obtaining the service they were paying for and that the service was of the required quality.

Contracting out services posed new problems for management. Previous management control procedures relied on Greenbelt's disciplinary and grievance procedures. These were not applicable to Bonus Clean's staff as Greenbelt had no managerial authority over them. However monitoring was not initially assigned great importance as evidence by the lack of a full-time monitoring officer until October 1985, a year after Bonus Clean started their contract.

Consequently as the situation deteriorated the monitoring officer's reports were used to cajole Bonus Clean to improve standards. In addition the District Domestic Manager suspected that staffing levels were below that specified in the contract. He authorised the Monitoring Officer to carry out a survey of Bonus Clean's staffing levels in January 1986 which revealed staffing levels below that agreed in the contract. A further contentious issue concerned the discrepancy between the quality control sheets completed by the contractors supervisors and the Health Authorities own monitoring procedure. To try and overcome these differences in February 1986 it was agreed that there should be closer liaison in monitoring, with Bonus Clean adopting the monitoring system used by the Health Authority in order that the standard of service could be monitored on a comparable basis.

The difficulty for Greenbelt Management was trying to keep Bonus Clean's management role separate from the Authority's monitoring role.

This arose because of the inadequate nature of Bonus Clean's quality control system. Departmental managers were also unclear about their monitoring role which was a source of frustration to hospital management and senior Domestic Managers:

> It was felt necessary to reiterate to Heads of Departments the established procedures for registering complaints . . . Mr X stresses that without feedback from Heads of Departments relating to discrepancies and complaints, the District Officer and Hospital Manager would not be able to monitor the contractor satisfactorily.
>
> Heads of Departments Meeting Minutes, 28 November 1986

The District Domestic Manager recirculated the appropriate specification to each Head of Department to enable them to exercise closer monitoring. The results of this close monitoring effort was to establish greater dialogue between both sides but Bonus Clean did not accept all the criticisms made by Greenbelt management. First, they argued that the Authority's Monitoring Officer was monitoring the contract to a higher specification than that agreed in the contract and that despite the veneer of objectivity the monitoring process was subjective and harshly applied. Second, they argued that domestics were experiencing a high level of hostility from nursing staff on the wards and this hindered their work. They cited the problems of spillages at night not being reported, domestics being asked not to vacuum due to the noise it created and domestics being asked to distribute meals and feed patients unassisted by nursing staff. Finally the Managing Director of Bonus Clean claimed that they were in danger of losing money on the contract due to rises in labour costs since the contract was awarded.

Despite numerous meetings with Bonus Clean it was becoming clear to senior management that stronger action needed to be taken to try and rectify the situation. The contract contained penalty clauses which allowed the Health Authority to:

> deduct from any monthly sum payable to the contracts such proportion thereof as is fair and reasonable having regard to the period of the relevant failure and to the terms of the agreement.

The District Supplies Manager advised caution in deducting money from Bonus Clean as he favoured cooperation as the way to improve standards rather than confrontation. The Unit General Manager, Hospital Manager and District Domestic Manager, however, believed a tougher approach was needed as standards continued to decline. Nonetheless they recognised that penalising Bonus Clean financially made it harder for local management to rectify matters as they were already severely constrained financially by more senior management in Bonus

Clean. It became a finely balanced judgement the extent to which penalty clauses were invoked as they feared that Bonus Clean might terminate the contract immediately, leaving the Hospital without a service.

Terminating the Contract

The catalyst for invoking penalty clauses was a letter from the Managing Director of Bonus Clean at the end of February 1986 which claimed that throughout the contract period they had sustained losses but had accepted them in the belief that other contracts would become available in Greenbelt. However it was clear to Bonus Clean that business expansion in Greenbelt was now unlikely. Consequently to ensure an adequate level of service Bonus Clean requested an additional £66,805 per annum. An increase of 32 per cent on the initial contract price of £207,735.

Greenbelt management were furious at this attempt to exert pressure on them but for legal reasons wanted Bonus Clean to terminate the contract. Furthermore management wanted to invoke penalty clauses but realised if they did Bonus Clean would simply terminate the contract immediately leaving the Hospital without a service. Consequently the penalty clauses were set at a level that would make Bonus Clean terminate the contract but not immediately. As a result the Unit General Manager wrote to the Managing Director on 5 March 1986:

> We recognise that the profit margin on your contract price was low, if not non-existent, and this was pointed out to your Marketing Manager when he was interviewed by our Assessment Team before the contract was let. His response was that he agreed that the price was low, but that a Board decision had been taken to provide the service in the Hospital at virtually no profit to Bonus Clean in order to gain a foothold in the NHS Domestic Services Market.
>
> We accepted this explanation in good faith, and are now somewhat dismayed that your Company has changed its mind midway through the Contract. This will, no doubt, reflect in references for Bonus Clean which we will be asked to provide in future. We, therefore, do not agree to any increase in the Contract price over what was agreed initially, and, I understand that you will now wish to terminate the Contract in accordance with the conditions laid down in the current documents.
>
> We will expect you to continue to provide the level of service laid down in the Contract, at the present price, and, if you fail to meet this requirement we shall have no alternative but to with-hold an appropriate proportion of the contract price until such times as the contract is terminated.

Bonus Clean duly terminated the contract and gave six months notice leaving hospital management until September to re-tender and replace Bonus Clean.

Explanations for Low Standards under Bonus Clean

The low standards of cleanliness under Bonus Clean were reflected in the Domestic Monitoring Reports and resulted from low staffing levels and poorly trained staff. They were unable to keep staffing up to the planned level that was specified in the contract. They experienced a high turnover rate, one senior Domestic Manager claimed staff turnover exceeded 60 per cent during the contract period. They were meant to provide Hospital Management with their staff attendance records but only complied with this request once in January 1986 when input hours were 1,677 hours, an equivalent of 41·92 WTE. This is below the figure their contract specified (Table 26). The Monitoring Officer queried these figures contending that standards did not reflect these hours.

Bonus Clean engaged in deliberate understaffing to make profit on an explicitly 'no profit' contract. Bonus Clean admitted the contract was a loss leader which was apparent to Greenbelt Management at the assessment stage as Bonus Clean's price was £25,000 per annum lower that other private firms' tenders which had similar staffing costs. However during the period Bonus Clean were at the Hospital other contracts were awarded in-house. They realised they would win no further contracts in Greenbelt and attempted to make the contract profitable.

Training

Bonus Clean in their tender document emphasised the importance they attached to properly trained staff:

> Bonus Clean believe that thorough training of all staff is of vital importance to the efficient running of hospital cleaning services. The company is therefore committed to ensuring that all grades of staff have adequate initial training as well as planned on-going training programmes during their employment.

The reality proved to be very different with the Training Officer only visiting the Hospital once during the contract period. Domestic staff received no training when they started employment. A domestic stated that she had been interviewed on a Tuesday and started work in the Operating Theatre that evening without either training or medical check.

The lack of training manifested itself in three ways. First, staff did not understand the coding system used to prevent cross infection.

Domestic staff would not clean cubicles which contained infectious patients through ignorance of correct procedures. Second, staff were not made sensitive to the environment in which they worked. Complaints occurred over staff wearing open footwear which was a health and safety hazard and about staff forgetting to lock doors which had clear security implications. Finally staff were not taught correct cleaning procedures leading to gaps being left on floors and a lack of appreciation of the need to use different materials in different colour coded areas.

Low staffing levels and inadequate training contributed to poor standards. This situation was exacerbated by the inadequate equipment used which was frequently commented on by Health Authority staff. Bonus Clean used a twelve inch machine to clean the corridors yet, when the in-house team took over they used a thirty-six inch wide machine, a three fold increase. This situation was made worse by not having on site facilities to maintain and repair equipment. The Contract Manager had limited autonomy to rectify this situation. She did not have her own budget and could not make decisions about the purchase of new equipment or the employment of extra staff.

The cleanliness of a Hospital affects the spread of infection. Methicillin-resistant Staphylococcus Aureus (MRSA) is a micro organism that can cause infection which contributes to death (*Journal of Hospital Infection*, 1983; Sanderson, 1986). MRSA is spread directly between people or indirectly via infected dust. Consequently, the incidence of MRSA is a good indicator of the standards of cleanliness in a hospital.

During 1985 there were outbreaks of MRSA and in October nine patients were MRSA positive. In 1986 sixty patients were MRSA positive, infection was most virulent during August 1986 when the Domestic Performance Figures plummeted to 41 per cent (Appendix 2). In 1987 the situation improved with twenty-one cases recorded up to September but it must be noted improving standards after Bonus Clean departed was a gradual process. From August 1987 to June 1988 the number of MRSA cases were negligible.

The difficulties with MRSA cannot be solely attributed to standards of cleaning, as screening processes and nursing practices have an impact on the spread of MRSA. Nonetheless these practices remained constant during the whole period and the correlation between the performance of Bonus Clean and the incident of MRSA is suggestive of a strong link.

The poor standards of cleanliness and subsequent cross-infection outbreaks stemmed from low staffing levels, minimal training and inadequate equipment. The standards of supervision and quality control procedures were also deficient. Staff shortages led to frequencies not being adhered to and a lack of continuity on wards as staff were shifted to cover other wards. The poor terms and conditions of employment encouraged staff to take on a second job and the absence of sick pay discouraged staff from notifying the Hospital of their absence. This created further fluctuations in staffing levels at short notice. The Contract Manager struggling to deal with this welter of problems had little discretion to manage the service. In this environment standards deteriorated until the contract was terminated.

The Service Returns In-house

Following the March 1986 termination of the Domestic Contract the Health Authority re-tendered for domestic services, senior management had dual concerns. First, they needed to maintain a service until September when the new service was due to begin, conscious that Bonus Clean had little incentive to maintain the service. Second, a new service had to be ready to commence in September.

It was decided to maintain a hard line with Bonus Clean and that deductions should continue subject to the agreement of the Authority's solicitors. The Authority were facing legal action from Bonus Clean in connection with the deductions they had made from the January and February invoices. It was also agreed to obtain an independent check of the quality of clean from CAMRASO, the independent research organisation for the cleaning industry and to recruit staff temporarily to maintain standards if necessary.

The procedure for competitive tendering followed the earlier arrangements. The termination of the contract coupled with the inability of private firms to cope with the surge in competitive tendering discouraged private sector interest, and no external tenders were received. The specification was adjusted to take into account changes in frequencies suggested by ward staff. The in-house tender was the subject of vigorous debate particularly concerning the inclusion of a bonus scheme which was absent from the first in-house tender.

The District Domestic Manager argued for the inclusion of a 17·3 per cent bonus payment, which was calculated as adding £31,852 to the overall labour costs, he argued that it would reduce the problems of recruitment which Bonus Clean had experienced. Second, it would forestall action by the staff side to improve conditions of service bringing them into line with other hospital staff. Finally by paying adequate salaries it would place control firmly back in management's hands by enabling them to demand high standards.

The Acute Unit General Manager was suspicious of this logic and wanted to prevent costs rising too sharply. The Unit General Manager suspected that the District Domestic Manager was trying to take advantage of the absence of competition to increase the tender price.

TABLE 28. *Comparison of Costs and Staff Levels between Bonus Clean and the In-House Service.*

	WTE	*Cost (£)*
(A) Bonus Clean (1983/84 Tender Price)	45·68	216,188*
(B) In-house Service (1983/84 Tender Price)	57·89	299,193
(C) In-house Service (1986/87 Tender Price)	53·23	313,164

Difference C–A £85,000:
£40,000—increase in staffing
£32,000—Bonus Payments
£10,000—improvements to specification
£3,000—residences supervision

*The budget allocated in 1986/87 was £230,000
The figures have not been adjusted for inflation

SOURCE: Tender Documents, Greenbelt DHA.

Clearly a sharp rise in price would have reflected badly on the Unit General Manager. However there was a need to raise standards.

A compromise was reached and the in-house service was awarded the contract at a price of £313,164 per annum. This was £85,000 per annum higher than Bonus Clean's price. The increase related mainly to the higher staffing levels and the addition of a bonus scheme (Table 28). Signficantly the staffing levels and contract price in real terms were lower than the previous in-house tender in 1983/84 even though a bonus scheme was excluded from that tender. By September after a difficult few months when the service had declined to the lowest levels of the whole contract the in-house service was ready to resume.

Service Standards and Work Organisation

The new in-house Domestic Manager took up her post in the Autumn and faced a formidable task. First, the Hospital was very dirty and neglected at the end of Bonus Clean's tenure. Second, the new in-house staff were predominantly the same staff who had worked under Bonus Clean and were demoralised by the criticism they were subject to indirectly as employees of Bonus Clean. They were also anxious that supervision would be tightened and the pressure of work increased, Third, the Hospital was experiencing a serious outbreak of MRSA which spread from a single ward to two other wards by October 1986.

The Domestic Managers approach placed firm emphasis on the value of good training. The contract contained seven days training for each domestic and when domestics started work they were placed beside an experienced worker for up to a fortnight. An induction checklist was completed (Appendix 4) which ensured staff were aware of correct cleaning procedures and the importance of health and safety.

Greenbelt management spent nearly £12,000 on new machinery for domestic work in the Hospital. This ended the shortages of equipment and the use of modern equipment with wide cleaning heads increased the effectiveness of the service. The Domestic Manager also altered the shift pattern reducing the number from three to two. She believed that Bonus Clean had domestics in the wrong place where they were not needed and cleaned the wards in the afternoons when the wards were busy with visitors. Domestics were assigned to particular wards which eliminated the variations of personnel on a ward and allowed the domestic to become fully integrated into the ward team. Consequently tighter managerial control was exercised both informally through the Ward Sister and formally through tighter supervision with the existence of a bonus scheme acting as an added incentive.

This led to rapid improvements in cleaning standards at the Hospital. By December the domestic monitoring performance had improved to 69·76 per cent from 41·77 per cent in August/September 1986. This led the Hospital Manager to comment in a letter to the Domestic Manager on the:

> Noticeable improvement in the cleaning standards within the CGH since the change to the contract. I am very pleased that we have been able to demonstrate that the same staff with an alternative management approach can produce the results.

The Hospital Manager was relieved that standards had risen because previously low cleaning standards had undermined the quality of care the hospital was providing by appearing to condone low standards in one highly visible respect. This had contributed to perceptions of low morale in the Hospital.

Furthermore the Hospital Manager had to justify the increase in expenditure on domestic services and a rise in standards was the most tangible justification. He was also able in conjunction with the domestic department to use the re-tendering exercise to review the provision of domestic services and to implement changes in working practices. However the Hospital Manager believed the blame for making unpopular changes could be placed on the Government as competitive tendering was imposed by them.

Part-time working dated from the introduction of bonus schemes and was confined to weekends and evenings. Bonus Clean's employees had predominantly worked for less than sixteen hours a week enabling Bonus Clean to avoid coming under the regulations of employment legislation. Greenbelt domestic management followed suit and having [illegible]amined the critical periods of domestic activity employed domestics [illegible]art-time to cover the busy early afternoon period. Functional flexibility was increased, with domestic contracts no longer specifying the work location but requiring domestics to be prepared to work at any hospital across the Acute Unit.

The Impact on Nursing Services

Nurses are often the recipients of duties shed by domestic staff in their attempts to remain competitive and win tenders (Hicks, 1985; Hart, 1988). This proved to be the case in Greenbelt where nursing staff were particularly critical of Bonus Clean. The Control of Infection Nursing Officer's views were typical. She argued that appropriate standards were not set as it was difficult to [illegible] correct frequencies in a new hospital. The contract[illegible]d didn't understand abo[illegible]r use which allowed bac[illegible]

> There is a differenc[illegible]ls of the patient were [illegible]

Nursing staff were con[illegible]w standards provided by[illegible]e context to which Bonu[illegible]e provision of linen. A n[illegible]d Sisters on 29 Novemb[illegible]

> Should the contract[illegible]

The use of domestics' [illegible]d that domestics should *assist* (emphasis added) nursing staff in the distribution of meals. Yet when domestics distributed meals this left them insufficient time for cleaning. However, it was clearly a matter of interpretation to determine the extent to which assistance with meals meant the distribution of meals.

The shortcomings of Bonus Clean revealed the full extent of domestic support duties in the pre-competitive tendering era. This encouraged the re-adoption of non-nursing duties by domestic staff after the termination of the contract and removed the ambiguity noted above. Instead of 'assist with meals', the new specification read:

> 'Distribute meals under the direction of nurse in charge and collect trays, crockery, cutlery after meals'.

The enlargement of domestic duties undermined the demarcation of duties which had created the tensions under Bonus Clean. This helped to develop the domestics' informal patient care role aided by the increased continuity of staff on the ward, enabling domestic staff to be reincorporated into the ward team increasing their job satisfaction. Domestic staff commented that being on the same ward enabled them to exert informal job control over their work. They knew the standards expected of them by the Ward Sister and worked to these standards rather than rigidly following the frequencies required of them in the Blue Book.

CONCLUSION

Management in Greenbelt moved quickly to implement competitive tendering which built on earlier efficiency measures, notably the introduction of bonus schemes. Competitive tendering was qualitatively different in that it directly threatened domestic managers' jobs in a way bonus schemes never had, focusing as they did on staff working practices. Competitive tendering also created great uncertainty for those managers as the extent of competition and likely tender prices were unknown. Not surprisingly, these managers were opposed to competitive tendering.

For senior managers the incentives were different. Competitive tendering offered managers the opportunity to generate financial saving, evaluate services and change working practices. They welcomed competitive tendering and used their discretion in the process to fulfil their objectives. Senior management influenced the process at a number of stages and most significantly at the assessment stage. The lowest tender was rejected yet another tender which was a loss-leader and which proved not to be viable was accepted.

Management had hoped that contracting out would relieve them of managing ancillary staff and allow them to devote time to more pressing problems. Instead they realised the need to establish a monitoring process to ensure contract standards were fulfilled. The monitoring and cajoling of Bonus Clean proved to be a time consuming and frustrating process and the subjectivity of assessing cleaning standards led to disagreements with Bonus Clean over the standards require.

The experience of Bonus Clean had contradictory effects on the in-house provision. It acted as an impediment to the reduction of frequencies and costs which frequently characterise in-house tenders. Yet Bonus Clean had established a baseline cost and Greenbelt management viewed Bonus Clean's contract hours as adequate if proper training and supervision existed and staffing levels in the contract were fulfilled. Consequently the in-house service worked to a similar contract to Bonus Clean but standards were raised significantly.

Domestic management also learnt lessons from Bonus Clean and experimented with a greater use of part-timers and increased functional flexibility. Competitive tendering enabled domestic management to increase their control over staff by a tight specification of what constituted 'domestic work'. The process of competitive tendering acted to push down wages with management negotiating a 17·3 per cent fixed bonus on a 95 performance which according to Whitley agreements attracted a 26·7 per cent bonus. The ability of management to negotiate locally and undercut Whitley rates was legitimated by the tendering process and the need to remain competitive. Therefore competitive tendering in Greenbelt enabled management to reinforce managerial prerogatives as well as generating financial savings.

APPENDIX 1

The Camraso Trials

The Cleaning and Maintenance Research Organisation (CAMRASO) measure the cleanliness of hard surfaces by weighing moistened filter papers before and after cleaning.

Two hospitals were chosen in Greenbelt for three, fifteen day trials. The cleaning routine was varied and the level of soiling tested until frequencies were obtained which gave an acceptable standard and there was no increased risk of cross infection. The findings are summarised below:

Frequency of Cleaning Pre-Camraso and Post-Camraso.

Technique	*Trial 1 (fx)*	*Trial 2 (fy)*
Vacuum	7 times per week	3 times per week
Damp mop only	3 times per week	—
Scrub	1 per 3 weeks	—
Wet mop and dry off	3 times per week	—
Spot mop	—	3 times per week
Spray clean	—	1 per week

fx=pre-CAMRASO frequencies
fy=post-CAMRASO frequencies

SOURCE: The CAMRASO Project: An evaluation of cleaning methods within Greenbelt. RHA, October 1983.

APPENDIX 2

Domestic Monitoring Performance Figures 1985–1988

Year	*Month*	*Performance*	*Year*	*Month*	*Performance*
BONUS CLEAN PERFORMANCE					
1985	February	80·72%	1986	January	57·73%
	March	64·76%		February	51·29%
	April	67·03%		March	67·83%
	May	71·57%		April	66·32%
	June	78·07%		May	53·38%
	July	79·20%		June	72·21%
	August	84·40%		July	66·04%
	September	87·25%		August } September }	41·77%
	October	93·00%		Contract terminated	
	November	82·73%		October } November }	No formal monitoring
	December	69·62%			
			Mean	$\frac{1376 \cdot 69}{20} \times 100 = 68 \cdot 83\%$	
IN-HOUSE PERFORMANCE					
1986	December	69·76%	1987	September	82·08%
1987	January	77·31%		October	80·72%
	February	74·77%		November	85·48%
	March	74·91%		December	88·84%
	April	82·99%	1988	January	82·50%
	May	75·72%		February	82·59%
	June	82·21%		March	87·79%
	July	82·70%		April	87·87%
	August	79·18%		May	91·93%
			Mean	$\frac{1469 \cdot 35}{18} \times 100 = 81 \cdot 60\%$	

SOURCE: Greenbelt DHA Domestic Monitoring Officer Reports

Performance is calculated by: $\frac{\text{Number of Satisfactory Inspections}}{\text{Number of Observations}} \times 100$

APPENDIX 3

Complaints against Bonus Clean 1985/86

Complaint	*Month*	*Source*
Stains on carpet not removed on four wards, damp dusting not being carried out.	March	District Domestic Adviser (DDA) letter to Contract Manager, 15.3.1985.
Scrubbing machine in dirty condition and left full of toxic Hycolin in the operating theatres. Staff not trained to empty machine.	March	DDA letter to Area Manager, 18.3.1985.
Floor scrubbed and dirty in all departments. Lapses in security in X-ray department.	April	DDA letter to Contract Manager, 3.4.1985.
Toilet Cleaning inadequate 1985.	July	Monitoring Report July.
Ward fridges not cleaned.	November	Letter from senior nurse to Contract Manager, 25.11.1985.
Cleanliness in operating theatres poor, staff not moving X-ray equipment but cleaning around it, lack of training of domestic staff.	November	Notes of a meeting with ward sisters, 29.11.1985.
Window cleaning services inadequate, removal of spillages from wards poor.	December	Notes of a meeting between Greenbelt management and Bonus Clean, 11.12.1985.
Food particles on carpets, balls of fluff on stairways, cobwebs at corners of windows in outpatients; build up of lime in taps in bathrooms on wards, rubbish not emptied from bins in the General Office.	May	Complaints forms dated 2.5.1986, 4.5.1986, 16.5.1986.

APPENDIX 4

Domestic Services Department

INDUCTION CHECKLIST

Initial here when completed

1 TIME SHEETS
- a Method of completion
- b To whom given/when
- c Procedure/method of payment
- d Pay queries

2 ANNUAL LEAVE
- a Entitlement
- b Method of applying
- c Public holidays, Statutory days, lieu days

3 SICKNESS
- a Certification: Self Certificate
  Doctors Certificate
- b Notifying Domestic Office when sick—time

4 ROSTER
- a Hours worked, days off
- b Working areas—flexibility

5 REST BREAKS
- a Coffee break—where taken/time taken
- b Meal break—entitlement/where taken/time taken
- c Eating on wards

6 HEALTH AND SAFETY
- a Staff responsibilities under HASAW Act 1974
- b Accident reporting
- c Fire procedure
- d First Aid procedure
- e Smoking policy
- f Colour coding

7 PERSONAL HYGIENE
- a Hair
- b Personal hygiene
- c Issue/wearing/laundering of overalls
- d Issue/wearing of protective clothing
- e Footwear

Initial here when completed

8 SECURITY
- a Issue of locker/security of personal belongings
- b Security of cleaning cupboards/materials
- c Reporting untoward occurrences
- d Confidentiality
- e Theft of hospital property
- f Security of keys

9 DISCIPLINARY PROCEDURE

10 GRIEVANCE PROCEDURE

11 TRADE UNION MEMBERSHIP

12 SOCIAL CLUB MEMBERSHIP

INDUCTION CHECKLIST TRAINING

1 CLEANING MATERIALS
- a General purpose liquid
- b Glitto scouring powder
- c Cream cleanser
- d Nigel/7142 floor cleaner
- e Carpet Cleaning solution
- f Oven cleaner
- g Aerosol furniture polish
- h Soda crystals
- i Plastic sacks—colour coding

2 CLEANING PROCEDURES
- a Floor mopping
- b Vacuuming
- c Damp dusting
- d High/low level dusting
- e Sanitary Areas: Baths
  Toilets
  Showers
  Wash hand basins
  Sluice areas
- f Carpet shampooing
- g Cooker
- h Refrigerator
- i General kitchen cleaning
- j Washing of crockery
- k Refuse disposal

3 NURSING SUPPORT DUTIES

Initial here when completed

I confirm I have been informed, shown and fully understand the above conditions.

Signed ....Date ....

Signed ....Date ....

References

ALLEN, I., WICKS, FINCH, J., LEAT, D. (1987) *Informal Care Tomorrow*, Policy Studies Institute, London.

ALLISON, G. (1971) *Essence of Decision*, Little Brown, Boston.

ANONYMOUS EDITORIAL (1983) Methicillin-Resistant Staphylococcus. Aureus, *Journal of Hospital Infection*, No. 4, pp. 327–9.

ASCHER, K. (1987) *The Politics of Privatisation*, Macmillan, Basingstoke and London.

ASSOCIATION OF DOMESTIC MANAGEMENT (1983) *Competitive Tendering for Domestic Services.*

ASSOCIATION OF LONDON AUTHORITIES (1988) *Privatising Health Care.*

AUDIT COMMISSION (1986) *Making a Reality of Community Care*, HMSO, London.

BALL, J., HURST, K., BOOTH, M., FRANKLIN, R. (1989) *'... But who will make the beds?'—A Research-based strategy for Ward Nursing Skills and Resources for the 1990s*, Mersey RHA, The Nuffield Institute, University of Leeds.

BATES, T., HAMM, J. (1989) 'Data unto the Day Patient', *Health Service Journal*, 2 March.

BEECH, R., CRAIG, M. AND BEVAN, G. (1987) 'Estimating Catchment Populations: Implications for Target Allocation', *Hospital and Health Service Review*, Vol. 83, No. 2, pp. 77–90.

BEST, G., PARSTON, G., ROSENHEAD, J. (1986) 'Robustness in Practice—The Regional Planning of Health Services', *Journal of Operational Research*, Vol. 37, No. 5.

BRUNT, J., PEEL, V. (1989) 'Reducing Waiting Lists: An Initiative in Bolton', *Health Services Management*, February.

BURN, J. M. B. (1983) 'Responsible use of Resources: Day Surgery', *British Medical Journal*, 5 February.

COLLEGE OF HEALTH (1989) *Guide to Hospital Waiting Lists 1989*, College of Health, London.

CONSTABLE, J. AND MCCORMICK, R. (1987) *The Making of British Managers*, BIM.

COTTRELL, K. M. (1980) 'Waiting Lists: Some Problems of Definition and a Relative Measure of Waiting Times', *Hospital and Health Services Review*, August.

COWAN, N. (1984) 'Privatisation in the NHS: Minor Surgery or Amputation?', *Personnel Management*, October.

COYLE, A. (1985) 'Going Private: The Implications of Privatisation for Women's Work', *Feminist Review*, No. 21.

CULLIS, J. G., JONES, P. R. (1983) 'Inpatient Waiting: A Discussion and Policy Proposal', *British Medical Journal*, 12 November.

CULYER, A. J., CULLIS, J. G. (1976) 'Some Economics of Hospital Waiting Lists in the NHS', *Journal of Social Policy*, July.

DEPARTMENT OF HEALTH (1989a) *Working for Patients*, Cmnd 555, HMSO, London.

DEPARTMENT OF HEALTH (1989b and 1990) *Working Papers 1-10*, HMSO, London.

DEPARTMENT OF HEALTH (1989c) *Caring for People*, Cmnd 849, HMOS, London.

DHSS (1971) *Better Services for the Mentally Handicapped*, Cmnd 4683, HMSO, London.

DHSS (1975) *Reduction of Waiting Times for Inpatients Admissions Management Arrangements*, August.

DHSS (1976) *Priorities for Health and Personal Social Services in England: A Consultative Document*, HMSO, London.

DHSS (1979) *Patients First*, HMSO, London.

DHSS (1981) *Growing Older*, HMSO, London.

DHSS (1987) *Health and Personal Social Services Statistics for England*, HMSO, London.

DOMBERGER, S., MEADOWCROFT, S., AND THOMPSON, D. (1987) 'The Impact of Competitive Tendering on the Costs of Hospital Domestic Services', *Fiscal Studies*, November.

DON, B., LEE, A., GOLDACRE, M. J. (1987) 'Waiting Lists Statistics III. Comparison of Two Measures of Waiting Times'. *British Medical Journal*, 14 November.

DONALDSON, L., MARATOS, J. I., RICHARDSON, R. A. (1984) 'Review of an Orthopaedic Inpatients Waiting List', *Health Trends*, No. 16, pp. 14–15.

DUTHIE, H. B. (Chairman) (1981) *Orthopaedic Services: Waiting Time for Outpatient Appointments and Inpatient Treatment: Report of a Working Party*, DHSS, HMSO, London.

ETZIONI, A. 'Mixed Scanning: a 'Third' Approach to Decision Making', *Public Administration Review*, December.

ENTHOVEN, A. C. (1985) *Reflections on the Management of the National Health Service*, Nuffield Provincial Hospitals Trust, London.

FABRIZIO, C., BUCKENHAM, M. (1988) 'Care for People with Mental Handicap', *Nursing Times*, 19 October.

FEINMANN, J. (1987) 'Oh, Why Are They Waiting?' *Health Service Journal*, 19 March.

FORSYTH, M. (1982) *Reservicing Health*, Adam Smith Institute, London.

GLENNERSTER, H. (1984) *Progress for Partnership*, Martin Robertson, Oxford.

GLENNERSTER, H., KORMAN, N., AND MARSDEN-WILSON, F. (1983) *Planning for Priority Groups*, Martin Robertson, Oxford.

GOFFMAN, E. (1961) *Asylums*, Penguin, London.

GOLDACRE, M. J., LEE, A., DON, B. (1987) 'Waiting List Statistics, I: Relations Between Admissions from Waiting List and Length of Waiting List', *British Medical Journal*, 31 October.

GRIFFITHS, M., PEACOCK, M., SLACK, R. (1988) 'Working at the Weekend', *Health Service Journal*, 6 October.

GRIFFITHS, R. (1988) *Community Care: Agenda for Action*, HMSO, London.

HALPERN, S. (1986) 'Waiting for the Blitz', *Health Service Journal*, 7 August.

HALPERN, S. (1987) 'Playing the NHS Waiting List Game', *Health Service Journal*, 26 February.

HAM, C. J. (1981) *Policy Making in the National Health Service*, Macmillan, London.

HAM, C. (1986) *Managing Health Services; Health Authority Members in Search of a Role*, School for Advanced Urban Studies, Study No. 3, Bristol.

HAMBLETON, R. (1986) 'Rethinking Policy Planning' School for Advanced Urban Studies, Bristol

HARRISON, S., MARNOCK, G., HUNTER, D., POLLITT, C. (1989) *The Impact of General Management in the NHS*, The Nuffield Institute, Open University.

HART, E. (1988) *'I Love my Work, I Hate My Job'. A Study of Hospital Domestics*, Economic and Social Research Council. Information Bulletin, No. 9/88.

HARTLEY, K. AND HUBY, M. (1985) 'Contracting Out in Health and Local Authorities: Prospects, Progress and Pitfalls', *Public Money*, September.

HASTINGS, S. AND LEVINE, H. (1982) *Privatisation*, Spokesman.

HAYWOOD, S., RANADE, W. (1985) 'Health Authorities: Tribunes or Prefects?' *Public Administration Bulletin*, April.

HEALD, D. (1983) *Public Expenditure*, Basil Blackwell, Oxford.

HEGINBOTHAM, C. (1988) 'Just Consumerism and Social Care', *THS*, Vol V, Nos VI.

HEPPENSTALL, I. (1985) 'Entering the Twilight Zone', *Health Service Journal*, 8 August.

HICKS, C. (1985) 'Who Cleans Up After?', *Nursing Times*, 9 January.

HM TREASURY (1986) *Using Private Enterprise in Government*, Report of a multi-Department Review of Competitive Tendering and Contracting for Services in Government Departments, HMSO, London.

HUDSON, B. (1987) 'Steering a Course through the Myths of Community Care', *Health Service Journal*, 28 May.

HUDSON, B. (1988) 'Tried and Tested in Wales', *Health Service Journal*, 26 May.

HUNTER, D., JUDGE, J., PRICE, S. (1988) 'Time to act on Griffiths', *Health Service Journal*, 10 November.

HUNTER, D., JUDGE, K. (1988) 'Griffiths and Community Care—Meeting The Challenge', *King's Fund Institute*, London.

HUNTER, D., WISTOW, G. (1987) *Community Care in Britain—Variations on a Theme*, King Edward's Hospital Fund for London, London.

HUWS, U. (1985) 'A Very Ordinary Picket', *New Socialist*, January.

INCOME DATA SERVICES (1988) Pay in the Public Sector, *IDS Report No. 526.*

INSTITUTE OF PERSONNEL MANAGEMENT/INCOME DATA SERVICES (1986) *Competitive Tendering in the Public Sector*, IPM.

JAMES, E. (1989) 'Eyes Open to Bright Ideas', *Health Service Journal*, 5 January.

JAY COMMITTEE (1979) *Report of the Committee of Enquiry into Mental Handicap Nursing and Care*, Vol. 1, Cmnd 7468, HMSO, London.

JOINT NHS PRIVATISATION RESEARCH UNIT (1987) *Contractors' Failures the Whole Story 1983-1987.*

JONES, C., BASSETT, S. (1988) 'Happier in the Community', *Health Service Journal*, 5 May.

JONES, K. (1976) *Issues in Social Policy*, Routledge and Kegan Paul, London.

KELLIHER, C. AND MCKENNA, S. (1987) 'Contract Caterers and Public Sector Catering', *Employee Relations*, 9:1.

KELLIHER, C. AND MCKENNA, S. (1988) 'The Employment Implications of Government Policy: A Case Study of Public Sector Catering', *Employee Relations*, 10, 2.

KING'S FUND CENTRE (1980) *An ordinary Life*, Project Paper 23, King's Fund Centre, London.

KING'S FUND (1987) *Planned Health Services for Inner London, Back to Back Planning*, King Edward's Hospital Fund for London, London.

KIRKMAN-LIFF, B. L., LAPRÉ, R., KIRKMAN-LIFF, T. L. (1988) 'The Metamorphosis of Health Planning in the Netherlands and the USA', *International Journal of Health Planning and Management*, Vol. 3, No. 2, pp. 89–108.

LABOUR RESEARCH DEPARTMENT (1987) *Privatisation, Paying the Price*, LRD Publications Ltd.

LEE, A., DON, B., GOLDACRE, M. J. (1987) 'Waiting List Statistics, II: An Estimate of Inflation of Waiting List Length', *British Medical Journal*, 7 November.

LEE, K., MILLS, A. (1982) *Policy Making and Planning in the Health Sector*, Croom Helm, London.

LEEDHAM, W. (1986) *The Privatisation of NHS Ancillary Services*, WEA.

LINDBLOM, C. E. (1959) 'The Science of 'Muddling' Through', *Public Administration Review*, Spring.

LINDBLOM, C. E. (1979) 'Still Muddling Not Yet Through', *Public Administration Review*, November/December.

LONDON HEALTH EMERGENCY (1988) *Community Care: Agenda for Disaster*, London Health Emergency, London.

LOURIE, J. A., (1978) 'Notes of an Orthopaedic Waiting List', *British Journal of Clinical Practice*, No. 32, pp. 224–5.

MAILLEY, R. (1987) 'Competitive Tendering Approaches Adopted in the NHS', *Health Care Management*, 1, 1.

MALIN, N. (Ed.) (1987) *Reassessing Community Care*, Croom Helm, London.

MANSELL, J. (1986) *The Natural History of the Community Mental Handicap Team.* Paper given at University of Loughborough, 22 September.

MANSELL, J., FELCE, D., JENKINS, DE KOCK U., AND TOOGOOD, S. (1987) *Developing Staffed Housing for People with Mental Handicaps*, Costello, London.

MARTIN, F. (1984) *Between the Acts: Community Mental Health Services 1959-83*, Nuffield Provincial Hospitals Trust, London.

MAYNARD, A., SMITH, J. C. C. (1983) 'The Elderly. Who Cares? Who Pays? *Nuffield/York Portfolio,* No 1, Nuffield Provincial Hospitals Trust, London.

MAYS, N. AND BEVAN, G. (1989) *Resource Allocation in the National Health Service*, Bedford Square Press, London.

MILNE, R. (1987) 'Competitive Tendering in the NHS: An Economic Analysis of the Early Implementation of HC(83)18, *Public Administration*, Summer.

NATIONAL AUDIT OFFICE (1986/87) *Competitive Tendering for Support Services in the NHS*, No. 318.

NATIONAL DEVELOPMENT TEAM FOR MENTALLY HANDICAPPED PEOPLE (1984) *Fourth Report.*

NHS MANAGEMENT BOARD (1988) *Review of Resource Allocation Working Party—Final Report*, Department of Health, London.

NHS UNLIMITED (1984) *Contracting Out 'Ancillary' Services: The Health Authority View.*

PALMER, J., JENKINS, J. (1982) 'The Wessex Behaviour Rating System for Mentally Handicapped People: A Realibility Study' *British Journal of Mental Subnormality*, December.

PATON, C. (1985) *The Policy of Resource Allocation and its Ramifications*, Nuffield Provincial Hospitals Trust, London.

PATON, C. (1990) *US Health Politics*, Gower, Aldershot.

PAUL, J. (1984) 'Contracting Out in the NHS: Can we afford to take the risk?', *Critical Social Policy*, 10.

PETERS, T. J. AND WATERMAN, R. H. (1982) *In Search of Excellence: Lessons from America's Best-run Companies*, Harper and Row, London.

PETERS, T. J. (1987) *Thriving on Chaos: Handbook for a Management Revolution*, Macmillan, London.

PHILLIPSON, C. (1988) *Planning for Community Care: Facts and Fallacies in the Griffiths Report,* Working Paper No. 1, Centre for Social Gerontology, University of Keele.

PORTER, K. M. (1985) 'Orthopaedic Audit—Review of Inpatient Waiting Lists', *British Medical Journal*, No. 291, pp. 1216–7.

PUBLIC ACCOUNTS COMMITTEE (1988) *Fiftieth Report: Use of Operating Theatres in the NHS*, HMSO, London.

RADICAL STATISTICS HEALTH GROUP (1987) *Facing the Figures What Really is Happening to the National Health Service?*, Radical Statistics, London.

RATHWELL, T. (1987)*Strategic Planning in the Health Sector*, Croom Helm, London.

RAYNES, N. (1987) 'Managing before Training: A Cautionary Tale in Care in the Community', *Hospital and Health Services Review*, May.

ROBB, B. (Ed.) (1967) *Sans Everything: A Case to Answer*, Nelson, London.

ROSENHEAD, J. (1980) 'Planning under Certainty: A Methodolgy for Robustness Analysis', *Journal of the Operational Research Society*, Vol. 31, No. 4, pp. 331–41.

ROYAL COLLEGE OF SURGEONS OF ENGLAND (1985) *Commission on the Provision of Surgical Services. Guidelines for Day Case Surgery*, July.

RYAN, J., THOMAS, F. (1987) *The Politics of Mental Handicap*, Free Association Books, London.

SANDERSON, H. F. (1982) 'What's in a Waiting List', *British Medical Journal*, 6 November.

SANDERSON, P. J. (1986) 'Staying One Jump Ahead of Resistant Staphylococcus Aureus', *British Medical Journal*, Vol. 293, No. 6547.

SECOND REPORT FROM SOCIAL SERVICES COMMITTEE SESSION 1984/85 *Volume 1 Community Care with special reference to Adult Mentally Ill and Mentally Handicapped People*, HMSO, London.

SHEAFF, M. (1988) 'NHS Ancillary Services and Competitive Tendering', *Industrial Relations Journal*, Summer.

SHEARER, A. (1986) *Building Community with People with Mental Handicaps, their Families and Friends*, King's Fund Centre, London.

SHERMAN, J. (1985) 'Waiting for the Big Bite', *Health and Social Service Journal*, 27 June.

SHERMAN, J. (1986) 'Curbing the Tender Benders' *Health and Social Service Journal*, 16 January.

STEINBRUNER, J. (1974) *The Cybernetic Theory of Decision*, Princeton University Press, New Jersey.

STOCKING, B. (1985) *Initiative and Inertia*, Nuffield Provincial Hospitals Trust, London.

TITMUSS, R. (1970) *The Gift Relationship: From Human Blood to Social Policy*, George Allen and Unwin, London.

TOMLINSON, D. (1988) 'Let the Mental Hospitals Close', *Policy and Politics*, July.

TORY REFORM GROUP (1984) *High Noon in the NHS*, Tory Reform Group, London.

TOWNSEND, P., DAVIDSON, N. (1982) *Inequalities in Health, The Black Report*, Penguin, London.

WERTHEIMER, A. (1988) 'Speaking Up to Win Independence' *The Guardian*, 31 August.

WHITE, G. AND PALMER, J. (1987) 'Contracting Out and the Cleaning Up Question', *Personnel Management*, May.

WHITFIELD, D. (1983) *Making it Public. Evidence and Action Against Privatisation*, Pluto Press, London.

WILLIAMSON, O. (1986) *Economic Organisation, Firms Markets and Policy Control*, Wheatsheaf.

WINCHESTER, D. (1983) 'Industrial Relations in the Public Sector', in BAIN, G. (Ed.) *Industrial Relations in Britain*, Basil Blackwell, Oxford.

WISTOW, G. (1988) 'Joint Working', *Community Care*, 30 June.

WOLFESNBERGER, W. (1972) *The Principle of Normalisation in Human Services*, NIMR, Toronto.

YATES, J. (1987) *Why are we Waiting? An analysis of Hospital Waiting Lists*, Oxford University press, Oxford.

YATES, J., DAVIDGE, M., HORLEY, M., VICKERSTAFF, L. (1987) 'The Anatomy of Large Inpatient Waiting Lists', *The Lancet*, 4 April.

Case Studies in Health Policy and Management